Case Studies in Geriatric Medicine

This case-based approach to geriatric medicine is suitable for all health professionals and trainees who provide care for the elderly, including interns, residents, geriatric fellows, physicians in practice, and nurse practitioners. Illustrated with more than 40 cases based on the authors' experience in clinical practice, the examples range from the healthy elderly to those with advanced cognitive or physical impairments. Discussions are evidence based with extensive references, emphasizing differential diagnosis, atypical presentations in late life, age-appropriate medical management, interdisciplinary methods, and care in the context of different health care settings. The authors have distilled a wealth of practical and clinical experience in this area to produce a user-friendly guide to geriatric medicine. This is the ideal study guide for certifying examinations and highly suitable as a textbook for courses in geriatric medicine and gerontology.

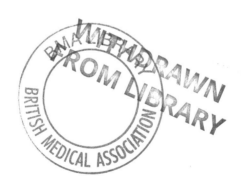
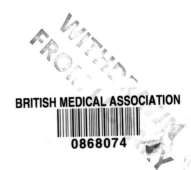

Case Studies in Geriatrics

Judith C. Ahronheim, M.D.

State University of New York – Downstate Medical Center,
Brooklyn, New York, USA

Zheng-Bo Huang, M.D.

Weill Medical College of Cornell University, New York, USA

Vincent Yen, M.D.

New York Medical College, Valhalla, New York, USA

Christina M. Davitt, M.S., G.N.P

Seton Hall University Law School, Newark, New Jersey, USA

David Barile, M.D.

Drexel University College of Medicine, Philadelphia,
Pennsylvania, USA

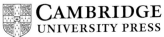

CAMBRIDGE
UNIVERSITY PRESS

CAMBRIDGE UNIVERSITY PRESS

Cambridge, New York, Melbourne, Madrid, Cape Town, Singapore, São Paulo

Cambridge University Press
The Edinburgh Building, Cambridge CB2 2RU, UK

Published in the United States of America by Cambridge University Press, New York

www.cambridge.org
Information on this title: www.cambridge.org/9780521531756

First published 2005

Printed in the United Kingdom at the University Press, Cambridge

A catalog record for this book is available from the British Library

Library of Congress Cataloging in Publication data

ISBN-13 978-0-521-53175-7
ISBN-10 0 521 53175 6 paperback

Contents

Preface

Case Studies in Geriatric Medicine condenses a rapidly growing body of knowledge about aging and geriatric care. The intent of this volume is to reach clinicians at all levels of experience – to intercept the student before nonage-adjusted principles become too firmly imbedded, and to enhance the well-honed skills of the experienced health care provider. The case-based learning approach will propel the reader to think about the total patient, to consider the medical as well as the psychosocial, ethical, and complex interdisciplinary aspects of caring for elderly patients.

Cases are identified by the patient's symptom or syndrome, so the reader can arrive at "the right answer" through a process of question and answer. Cases are grouped by syndrome category (for example, early, moderate, and late dementia; hypothermia and hyperthermia), and categories or individual cases may be studied in or out of sequence as desired. The question and answer format will serve as a skill enhancer and a supplemental guide for geriatric certifying examinations, and hopefully will make the learning process enjoyable. Current and some "classic" references are provided throughout for additional reading.

As the body of knowledge has expanded, basic geriatrics principles have endured. Awareness of these principles is essential to the mastery of geriatric medicine.

Chronologic and biologic age are not well matched

While some people are "old at 18," many 90-year-olds appear or act in ways that are surprisingly youthful. Behavior that is merely youthful should not be regarded as inappropriate; depression and social crises should not be considered to be "expected at that age." New physical complaints should not be ignored or ascribed to "old age."

When considering treatment options, clinician as well as patient should resist age biases, but must also realistically consider projected life span, benefits, and burdens.

Evidence-based geriatric practice is encumbered by pitfalls of aging research

Cross-sectional studies by age group differ in their definition of the age groups under study; for example, one must question the validity of comparing subjects "under 65" with "65 and older" if the average age of the two cohorts varies only by a few years. Longitudinal studies are plagued by dwindling numbers in the oldest age groups, and the findings may be confounded by extrinsic factors that have changed over time. Many studies exclude subjects over 75 years of age, and most studies of older adults include few patients in the oldest age groups. Biologic heterogeneity increases with age, making it practically impossible to draw conclusions about an aged cohort when one can be studied. A carefully selected "healthy" cohort of people over 85 may represent a biologic elite and their study results cannot be extrapolated to the majority.

All of these factors must be carefully considered when applying research findings to elderly patients.

Disease more often presents "atypically" in the elderly

This important observation is related to physiologic changes of aging and the existence of overt and occult disease of late life. Atypical presentations are given little emphasis in most general medical textbooks but are to be expected in geriatric practice. Among frail elderly, "atypical" presentations are in fact "typical."

Silent pathology is often present

A quiescent process, such as atherosclerosis, may remain silent until an additional insult is superimposed. Diminished reserve, such as impaired baroreceptor function, may not be apparent until the organism is stressed. Disorders not yet symptomatic, such as preclinical Alzheimer's disease, may remain asymptomatic unless acute illness occurs, or an iatrogenic factor, such as a medication, is added.

Drugs are potential poisons

Compared with younger adults, older patients take more drugs, develop more adverse effects, and tend to exhibit a certain spectrum of effects, such as altered mental status, urinary symptoms, weakness, or changes in behavior. If a symptom occurs, the first question should be "what medications has the patient taken?" More often than not, it is prudent to discontinue a medication rather than add one.

Older patients often have multiple diseases and functional impairments

Although the astute clinician seeks to "unify" multiple symptoms and explain them on the basis of one pathologic process, diverse symptoms in an elderly patient are more often due to several problems occurring at one time in more than one organ system. These problems may be etiologically unrelated but physiologically intimately interrelated. Thus, a health care provider must not only sharpen his or her "subspecialty" skills, but must become a skillful generalist who treats the complex patient as a unified whole.

Geriatrics is a multidisciplinary field

The primary care provider for the complex geriatric patient requires the assistance of professionals from the fields of social work, rehabilitation, nursing, nutrition, podiatry, dentistry, and other disciplines, such as the medical subspecialties. Family, friends, or neighbors are often an integral part of this multidisciplinary team.

Geriatrics is an interdisciplinary field

The primary care provider is the gatekeeper and needs to organize all of the people in the item above for the benefit of the patient.

Case 1

▸▸ Annual physical

An 84-year-old widow lives alone in her apartment in a "continuing care retirement community" where payment includes full medical care. She is summoned to the medical clinic for her "annual physical."

The patient says she can't understand why she is there, because she feels "just fine." You explain the need for periodic health screening, doing so in a loud voice, since she has obvious hearing loss. "You don't have to shout," she says, a little annoyed. "I'm not hard of hearing."

You review the past year with her, asking about any falls, incontinence, and recent losses. You ask her how she is managing in her apartment, focusing on activities of daily living (like bathing, dressing, and grooming) and instrumental activities of daily living (like paying bills, taking medication, and driving). She says that she gave up driving when she moved into the retirement community because "everything is so convenient here."

The patient mentions that she enjoys a cocktail with the ladies once in a while, but doesn't think she drinks too much. She has been taking calcium supplements and a daily multivitamin but has declined hormone replacement therapy in the past. She says that she walks for 30 minutes every day on the paved oval in the complex and she has convinced some of her friends to join her. She takes no other medications.

In the chart, there is an advance directive that designates the patient's daughter, who lives nearby, as her health care agent (medical power of attorney).

On physical examination, she appears robust and has a normal gait. Her blood pressure is 126/80, her pulse 72 and regular. The examination is completely normal, including breast, rectal, neurologic, and mental status examination. Tympanic membranes are normal and well visualized. Stool is guaiac negative. She refuses pelvic examination, stating that she is "too old for that."

Case Studies in Geriatric Medicine, Judith C. Ahronheim *et al.* Published by Cambridge University Press.
© J. C. Ahronheim, Z.-B. Huang, V. Yen, C. M. Davitt, and D. Barile

Questions

1. Is the patient "hard of hearing" or not? What is going on?
2. What is the rationale for offering a pelvic exam and Pap smear to an 84-year-old widow?
3. What other health screening should she undergo?
4. What immunizations are recommended?
5. Why has this patient chosen to live in a "continuing care retirement community?" What other options are available?

Answers

1. She is hard of hearing, as is obvious to the speaker but less so to the listener, a common inconsistency in the setting of progressive sensorineural hearing loss (presbyacusis), which occurs commonly in late life. Most people with presbyacusis will hear better when spoken to loudly, but if loud speaking is perceived as shouting, the patient might be experiencing the "recruitment phenomenon." People with normal hearing can hear and understand an increasing number of speech stimuli as the loudness is increased above a whisper (see Figure 1). With presbyacusis, there is a leveling off of the amount that can be heard as loudness increases. Thirty percent of people with presbyacusis experience the recruitment phenomenon, in which the amount that can be heard actually decreases as a particular state of loudness is reached. Such people have a great deal of difficulty being fitted with hearing aids, which amplify extraneous noise as well as sounds that the patient wants to hear. The best approach is to speak distinctly, in an ordinary or slightly loud voice, looking directly at the patient, ensuring good eye contact.

   The patient can undergo audiologic evaluation consisting of audiometry (pure-tone testing) and speech testing. Audiometry is performed by presentation of tones through the use of earphones, applying sounds of varying loudness in decibels and different frequencies (Hertz). In presbyacusis, high-frequency sounds are generally lost first. Speech testing consists of the delivery of monosyllabic words at a comfortable level of loudness, a level at which normal young people will understand 100% of what is heard. Certain patients may perform fairly well in audiometry but poorly on speech testing. Such patients are said to have problems with "discrimination" and often fail to distinguish between rhyming words with high-frequency, voiceless consonants, such as "thin" and "shin," or "cap" and "tap."

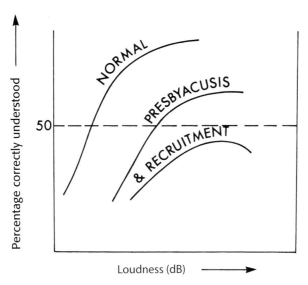

Figure 1   The recruitment phenomenon. People with normal hearing can comprehend more spoken words as loudness in decibels (dB) increases above a whisper. In presbyacusis, the curve shifts to the right. In the recruitment phenomenon, hearing and comprehension begin to decrease as a particular state of loudness is reached.

2. Most elderly women have not been adequately screened for cancer of the cervix, and many have never had a Papanicolaou (Pap) smear or have not seen a gynecologist since menopause. The incidence of carcinoma *in situ* (cervical intraepithelial neoplasia), detected by Pap smear, decreases dramatically with age over 30 years, and in older women newly diagnosed noninvasive and invasive cervical cancers are virtually all in patients who have been inadequately screened. A general consensus exists that screening can be discontinued after age 65 or 70 if prior screening has been adequate and normal, because the risk of interventions from false positive examinations outweighs the benefits, and because a speculum examination can be very uncomfortable in late life, especially among women with untreated atrophic vaginitis. Also, with advancing age, there is an increase in the rate of false positive smears – i.e. smears interpreted as "squamous atypia;" in most cases, though not all, these findings represent benign enlargement of cell nuclei seen in atrophic epithelium, which reverts to normal after a course of topical estrogen, and which differs in appearance from nuclear changes in precancerous cells.

   Despite consensus to liberalize cervical cancer screening requirements in late life, gynecologic examination provides the opportunity to screen for other important pathology, including gynecologic malignancies that occur most often in the elderly. Despite the high incidence of false negatives, many cases of endometrial cancer can often be detected on speculum examination or Pap smear. Vulvar cancer is frequently missed but curable if detected early. Vaginal cancer is rare, but is almost exclusively a disease of late life.

Recommendations to discontinue screening or reduce frequency from annual to every 2–3 years at most do not apply for women in certain high-risk groups, such as those with prior treatment of cervical cancer or those with high risk of papilloma virus exposure. One should be sure to inquire about sexual activity and screen any woman who has begun a new sexual relationship in late life as the thinning and dryness of the vaginal mucosa increases susceptibility to sexually transmitted diseases. Likewise, the incidence patterns of cervical cancer differ among groups; for example, the incidence of invasive cervical cancer continues to rise with age among African American women and does not plateau among the oldest old.

3. In an elderly person, a screening test should be able to detect disease for which corrective action can be taken, including cure, amelioration, or improvement in quality of life.

Intraocular pressure should be measured annually by an ophthalmologist since open angle glaucoma can remain asymptomatic for years and is a preventable cause of blindness.

All patients should have an annual full body skin examination to detect cancerous and precancerous lesions. The incidence of basal and squamous cell carcinoma, as well as malignant melanoma, increases with age, and most are curable if detected at an early stage.

Recommendations for other forms of periodic health screening are generally based on studies performed in people under the age of 75 years, so special considerations may modify official recommendations made by professional groups.

Cholesterol screening is controversial in people over the age of 75 (see Case 13). However, many people are curious about their cholesterol level and highly motivated to improve their health. Furthermore, elevated cholesterol may be an added incentive for people to exercise and improve their diet. No action should be taken on elevated cholesterol done without measurement of high and low density subfractions, since the predictive value of total cholesterol declines with age.

The incidence of breast cancer rises with age in women until, approximately, age 80. However, the impact of screening (including mammography) on mortality is controversial, and there is a paucity of data in women over the age of 75. Several factors complicate this issue in the older age group. Studies in which outcomes focus on all-cause mortality may obscure any reductions in cancer-related mortality, as elderly women will have higher death rates overall. Statistically, healthy women aged 70 and older may have lower breast cancer-specific mortality than the average middle-aged woman (Walter *et al.*, 2001).

Mammography itself may have enhanced positive predictive value in older women. The ratio of fatty to glandular tissue increases with age, improving the ability to visualize abnormalities radiographically. Conversely, the use of hormone replacement therapy can increase radiographic density, making tumors harder to detect. Decision to perform mammography should take into account the patient's overall quality of life and estimated life expectancy, and ability to tolerate the physical or emotional stress of a positive exam and the consequent workup.

The incidence of colon cancer rises dramatically with age and there is little controversy regarding the outcome of minimally invasive treatment. Colonoscopy is well tolerated when patients are sedated, but, because not all older patients are able to prepare adequately for the procedure, it may be difficult from a practical standpoint for many patients to complete an outpatient colonoscopy (or the alternative, an air contrast barium enema). Sigmoidoscopy is less sensitive, detecting about 80% of cancers, and is actually less well tolerated because patients may not receive sedation.

Currently, the American Cancer Society (ACS) recommends that screening colonoscopy be performed every 10 years in people over 50 (more often if they have a family history of colon cancer or adenomatous polyps). The limited sensitivity of solitary annual fecal-occult blood testing can be enhanced by multiple and more frequent testing.

Not ordinarily included in official health screening recommendations, blood tests are virtually routine in office practice. Those that are particularly useful for the elderly include complete blood count (CBC), blood glucose, and thyroid function tests. CBC may be a useful adjunct in screening for colon cancer or for other conditions very common in late life, including vitamin B12 and iron deficiency. Although more expensive, serum levels of B12 and ferritin are more sensitive measurements of these conditions. Plasma glucose should be checked on a regular basis because the incidence of type II diabetes rises dramatically with age; the sensitivity of that test is enhanced if the sample is taken after a meal rather than in the fasting state, although use of nonfasting glucose for screening is controversial. Although controversial (see U.S. Preventive Services Task Force, 2004) most geriatricians recommend that thyroid function tests should be performed in all elderly persons because thyroid disease is difficult to diagnose on clinical grounds, as discussed in Case 41.

Screening for alcoholism, depression, and dementia should be considered because these problems are often missed by primary care physicians. These aspects of screening and their limitations are discussed in Cases 4, 11, and 27.

4. Influenza vaccine should be given annually in late autumn to all people over the age of 50. Although viruses other than influenza virus often cause deaths that occur

during influenza epidemics, influenza is the only respiratory virus for which an effective vaccine exists. A large proportion of older adults have at least one risk chronic medical condition that increases the risk of influenza-associated complications, and people aged 65 and over are five times more likely than younger adults to die from these complications. Community-wide immunization is particularly important in closed communities such as skilled nursing facilities, where epidemics can be curtailed only when the vaccination rate approaches 75%.

Pneumococcal vaccine is generally recommended for all elderly persons because it is the most common form of community-acquired pneumonia in that age group and because the risk of mortality increases with age. However, the efficacy in older individuals has been questioned, especially for the oldest old and those with serious chronic illnesses. Limited efficacy might be related to rapid decline in the levels of protective antibody in these groups. Efficacy of revaccination as well as its timing are uncertain. For example, increase in antibody level following revaccination is lower and shorter in duration than following initial vaccination. Since the vaccine is generally safe, and since it does seem to protect against the development of pneumococcal bacteremia ("invasive disease"), it is generally recommended. More controversy exists regarding revaccination of older adults, which is currently recommended after 5 years only for people who received primary vaccination prior to the age of 65 (Centers for Disease Control, 1997). However, revaccination recommendations are not based on actual efficacy data. Status of the evidence regarding pneumoccal vaccine in the elderly is discussed in the references (see Artz *et al.*, 2003).

Tetanus and diphtheria are rare, but mortality and the most severe morbidity among adults occur primarily in the underimmunized, older population. Although many elderly men received primary immunization during military service, elderly men and women attended school prior to school immunization programs. If immunization history is not known, or if a booster has not been given in the past 10 years, primary series should be given. Tetanus and diphtheria toxoid may be given alone or together as the usual adult preparation (Td).

5. Most people aged 65 and over are able to live independently with little assistance. It is not widely recognized that fewer than 5% of Americans aged 65 and older live in nursing homes, although, among those aged 85 and older, over 18% reside in nursing homes.

Increasing frailty and dependence on assistance can lead to a change in living situation. Some seniors choose to live in an "age exclusive" community where everyone is over a certain age, usually 55; others prefer to live nearer to their children, or where the cost of living is lower, or where health care is more readily available. A "continuing care retirement community," also known as a "life care community," is one option in a broad spectrum for the elderly. A life care community offers several levels of care in one location. One entrance option is that the senior pays an "entrance fee" and monthly charges that vary with the level of care required. Housing is in a private apartment, and varying levels of assistance are provided, depending on need. There is usually a wide range of activities offered, transportation for shopping and recreation, full meals, maintenance services, and housekeeping on site. Medical care may be provided on site as well. People generally move in when they are relatively healthy, but, when they become more frail, they move to an area with more assistance in the complex or to an on-site nursing home. Contractual arrangements made at the time of entrance will specify the levels of care provided and the accompanying charges.

Other housing options include government-funded senior housing, which are rental apartments designed to meet the needs of people who no longer wish to care for a single family home but who do not need daily assistance. These apartments may have alarm pull cords in the bathroom and be designed to accommodate persons in wheelchairs. One may also find "congregate" housing in an apartment building setting. Seniors who need a bit more assistance may live on one floor of the building and receive one or more meals a day, medication reminders, and some assistance with daily activities. "Assisted living residences" are facilities where seniors live in their own room or apartment, have on-site help with daily activities including taking medications, receive full meals, and have activities and transportation provided. The cost of assisted living residences vary depending on the services, amenities, and location, but generally cost less than a skilled nursing facility (nursing home), which provides the highest level of assistance. Residents of a nursing home receive the highest level of assistance, up to 24-hour assistance with activities, medication administration, meal service or feeding, daily monitoring by nursing staff, and can receive physical therapy or other skilled services. Increasingly, nursing homes in the United States are delivering various types of acute and subacute care previously available only in the hospital setting.

Various forms of available housing in the United States are reviewed in the references (see Administration on Aging and American Association of Homes and Services for the Aging).

Caveats

Hearing aids are very expensive and are not reimbursed by Medicare. Many states now require that patients be able to purchase a hearing aid trial for a modest amount, so that, if they are not satisfied with the results, the apparatus can be returned. Unfortunately, not all elderly are aware of this option and it is not uncommon for an unscrupulous merchant to take advantage of this fact.

With age, the glands that produce cerumen tend to produce a harder wax than previously, and impacted cerumen can compromise hearing. Complete occlusion may cause rapid onset of hearing loss, often unilaterally, but can be remedied with irrigation of the external auditory canal or by extracting the wax.

REFERENCES

Administration on Aging (2004). http://www.aoa.gov/eldfam/Housing/Housing.asp; accessed February 10, 2005.

American Association of Homes and Services for the Aging (2004). www2.aahsa.org; accessed February 10, 2005.

Artz, A. S., Ershler, W. B., and Longo, D. L. (2003). Pneumococcal vaccination and revaccination of older adults. *Clinical Microbiology Reviews*, **16**, 308–18.

Centers for Disease Control (1997). Prevention of pnuemococcal disease. Recommendations of the Advisory Committee on Immunization Practices. *Morbidity and Mortality Weekly Report*, **46**, 1–24.

U.S. Preventive Services Task Force (2004). Clinical guidelines: screening for thyroid disease. Recommendation statement. *Annals of Internal Medicine*, **140**, 125–7.

Walter, L. C., Eng, C., and Covinsky, K. E. (2001). Screening mammography for frail older women: what are the burdens? *Journal of General Internal Medicine*, **11**, 779–84.

BIBLIOGRAPHY

Abati, A., Jaffurs, W., and Wilder, A. M. (1998). Squamous atypia in the atrophic cervical vaginal smear: a new look at an old problem. *Cancer*, **84**, 200–1.

Burke, G. L., Arnold, A. M., Bild, D. E. *et. al.* (2001). Factors associated with healthy aging: the cardiovascular health study. *Journal of the American Geriatrics Society*, **49**, 254–62.

The Expert Committee on the Diagnosis and Classification of Diabetes Mellitus (2003). Follow-up report on the diagnosis of diabetes mellitus. *Diabetes Care*, **26**, 3160–7.

Feig, S. A. (2000) Age-related accuracy of screening mammography: how should it be measured. *Radiology*, **214**, 633–40.

Fletcher, S. W. and Elmore, J. G. (2003). Mammographic screening for breast cancer. *New England Journal of Medicine*, **348**, 1672–80.

Jackson, L. A., Neuzil, K. M., Yu, O. *et al.* (2003). Effectiveness of pneumococcal polysaccharide vaccine in older adults. *New England Journal of Medicine*, **348**, 1747–55.

Lackner, T. E., Hamilton, R. G., and Hill, J. J. (2003). Pneumococcal polysaccharide revaccination: immunoglobulin G seroconversion, persistence, and safety in frail, chronically ill older subjects. *Journal of the American Geriatrics Society*, **51**, 240–5.

Modlin, J. (2001). Recommendations of the Advisory Committee on Immunization Practices. *Morbidity and Mortality Weekly Report*, **50**, 1–46.

Moore, A. A. and Siu, A. (1996). Screening for common problems in ambulatory elderly: clinical confirmation of a screening instrument. *American Journal of Medicine*, **100**, 430–43.

National Cancer Institute (2003). Seer incidence and U.S. death rates, age-adjusted and age-specific rates, by race. Cervix Uteri Cancer (invasive). http://www.seer.cancer.gov/csr/1975–2000/results_single/sect_05_table.02.pdf; accessed July 28, 2003.

National Cancer Institute (2003). Seer incidence and U.S. death rates, age-adjusted and age-specific rates, by race and sex. Breast cancer (invasive). http://www.seer.cancer.gov/csr/1975–2000/results_single/sect_04_table.03.pdf; accessed July 28, 2003.

Sarkisian, C. A., Liu, H., Guttierez, P. R. *et al.* (2000). Modifiable risk factors predict functional decline among older women: a prospectively validated clinical prediction tool. *Journal of the American Geriatrics Society*, **48**, 170–8.

Saslow, D., Runowicz, C. D., Solomon, D. *et al.* (2002). American Cancer Society guidelines for the early detection of cervical neoplasia and cancer. *Cancer Journal for Clinicians*, **52**, 342–62.

Sawaya, G. F., Grady, D., Kerlikowske, K. *et al.* (2000). The positive predictive value of cervical smears in previously screened postmenopausal women: the Heart and Estrogen/Progestin Replacement Study (HERS). *Annals of Internal Medicine*, **133**, 942–50.

Sawaya, G. F., Brown, A. D., Washington, A. E. *et al.* (2001). Current approaches to cervical-cancer screening. *New England Journal of Medicine*, **344**, 1603–7.

Van Wessen, G. A., Kuyenhoven, M. M., and De Melker, R. A. (1997). Why do healthy people fail to comply with influenza vaccination? *Age and Ageing*, **26**, 275–9.

Walter, L. C. and Covinsky, K. E. (2001). Cancer screening in elderly patients: a framework for individualized decision making. *Journal of the American Medical Association*, **285**, 750–6.

Case 2

▸▸ Office visit

An 84-year-old woman lives in the same continuing care community as the patient in Case 1, and is summoned for her annual physical. She has been living there for just a year and greets you happily, stating that she has been looking forward to this visit because there are a number of things she has been wanting to talk to you about.

She explains that she used to be "tall and slim, with a nice, flat tummy," but now her abdomen sticks out and she has trouble finding clothing to fit her, because of "that hump," indicating her upper back. She is annoyed that she is "covered with wrinkles," but knows she can't do anything about that. She is more concerned about her memory, which is not as good as it used to be, and would like to discuss this with you. She is socially and physically active, plays bridge every Wednesday evening, and goes for long walks, wearing her "Nikes." She refuses to play shuffleboard because "that's for old people," and she thinks it's the "most boring game on earth." She reads the newspaper every day and is distressed about the recent downturn in the stock market. She says, "I hope . . . what's his name? He's in charge of the . . . what's it called? You know. Anyway, I hope he can straighten things out. Why can't I remember his name?"

The patient has never smoked. A retired kindergarten teacher, she shares her apartment with her husband of 50 years. He is a retired engineer who is in apparently good health. They have no children. She drives by herself to the local grocery store and to the beauty parlor weekly, but says her husband worries about her driving because she has had two "fender benders" in the last year.

The patient is robust, friendly, and cooperative. She leaps onto the examining table with great agility, still wearing her Nikes. She appears to be a little hard of hearing, and she explains that she isn't wearing her hearing aid, which she refers to as "that awful thing." She has moderate kyphosis and a protuberant abdomen, her "bête-noir." Her blood pressure is 130/70, and

Case Studies in Geriatric Medicine, Judith C. Ahronheim *et al.* Published by Cambridge University Press.
© J. C. Ahronheim, Z.-B. Huang, V. Yen, C. M. Davitt, and D. Barile

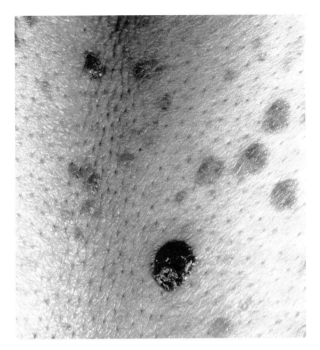

Figure 2   Seborrheic keratoses.

her pulse is 64 and regular. Barefoot, she is 5 feet 3 inches tall and weighs 140 pounds. Her upper arms, she points out, are "flabby." She has "horrid brown things" (dark brown keratotic lesions that have a stuck-on appearance; see Figure 2) covering her back and a few on her anterior thorax and under her breast. She has a bruit over her right carotid artery. There is a grade I/VI systolic ejection murmur heard best over the apex. The rest of the physical examination is normal.

Blood count and screening blood chemistries are normal. Her EKG shows normal sinus rhythm with a left axis deviation.

Questions

1. How should you approach the problem of her:
   a. skin lesions?
   b. hearing problem?
   c. sagging skin?
   d. carotid bruit?
   e. heart murmur?

2. What should the patient be told about her:
   a. figure problem?
   b. memory problem?
   c. electrocardiogram?
3. Why has she lost height?
4. At the age of 50 years, she was considered a slim 130 pounds. Should she now go on a diet?
5. Is this patient too old to drive?

Answers

1a. Her skin lesions are seborrheic keratoses (see Figure 2). These are benign lesions, which increase in incidence with age. The etiology is not known. Since they are benign, they do not need to be removed unless the patient finds them cosmetically disagreeable. Individual lesions, strategically located, may become irritated when clothing or underwear rubs on them, and can be removed surgically or with electrodesiccation. Reassurance as to the benign nature of seborrheic keratoses is called for. Seborrheic keratoses sometimes resemble the nodular form of malignant melanoma, except that the latter tend to be more darkly pigmented and grow rather rapidly. If there is any doubt as to the diagnosis, a biopsy must be done.

1b. The patient should be questioned as to why she is not using her hearing aid (amplification). Hearing aids of all varieties amplify not only what a person wishes to hear, but unwanted ambient noise as well – a situation that is often intolerable. Those who experience the recruitment phenomenon (see Case 1) may find this particularly annoying. Many individuals dislike wearing a behind-the-ear hearing aid for cosmetic reasons. In-the-ear amplification may be a suitable alternative, although impaired manual dexterity may hinder the ability to change the tiny battery and adjust the volume control.

1c. The patient's skin sags because of age changes in collagen and elastin. This process is irreversible and, to date, not preventable. Skin wrinkling is due largely to sunlight, wind, smoke, and other environmental ravages. This is termed "photoaging" or "extrinsic aging," and is to be distinguished from intrinsic aging of the skin. Daily life-long use of sun-blocking creams with a skin protection factor (SPF) of at least 15, avoidance of excessive sunlight exposure, and abstaining from smoking reduce the degree of skin wrinkling. Topical tretinoin (Retin-A) shows some promise in the treatment of fine wrinkling (rhytids) and other signs of photoaging. The major side effects are dry skin and erythema. Although the literature reports successful cosmetic results with topical tretinoin, facialplasty, botulinum toxin, glycolic peels, and laser resurfacing in "elderly" or "aging" patients, no specific data exist in the over-80 age group. The patient's comorbid medical conditions must be taken into account when individualizing a treatment plan, especially if plastic surgery is being considered.

Skin dryness can be minimized with the use of emollient creams and by reducing bathing time and water temperature.

1d. This patient has an asymptomatic carotid bruit, an incidental finding in more than 10% of people over the age of 65. Although asymptomatic carotid bruit is associated with an increased risk of stroke, this association declines with age, so, by age 70 years, it may be no greater than for patients without bruits. The Asymptomatic Carotid Atherosclerosis Study (see Executive Committee, 1995) demonstrated a statistically significant benefit of carotid endarterectomy for the prevention of stroke for patients with asymptomatic high grade (>60%) stenosis found on ultrasound. However, subjects were aged 40–79, with low surgical risk, limiting generalizability of the study to the geriatric population at large.

Age alone is the greatest independent risk factor for stroke. Stroke prevention in this patient should focus on attention to known modifiable risk factors, should they arise (see Case 17).

1e. Depending on the population studied, 30–60% of people over 65, and as many as 80% of people 80 years of age and older, have heart murmurs. Systolic murmurs can be due to the same pathology seen in any age group, but are commonly due to sclerosis of a nonstenotic aortic valve, and may be heard in the "wrong location" because of the flow dynamics and because of anatomic alterations in thoracic cage – e.g. this patient's kyphosis. Once considered a benign lesion, aortic sclerosis is associated with an increased risk of cardiovascular morbidity and mortality. There is currently no evidence that a sclerotic but nonstenotic aortic valve is the cause; rather, it may serve as a marker for coexisting coronary artery disease, as risk factors for coronary artery disease and aortic sclerosis are similar.

Additional causes of heart murmurs would need to be investigated, including anemia or hyperthyroidism, which can cause a "flow murmur." Because potentially progressive lesions, such as aortic stenosis, may be present, follow-up is desirable.

2a. The patient's abdomen may be protruding because of age-related redistribution of fat from the extremities to the trunk, and the protruberant appearance may be exaggerated because of her kyphosis, which is most likely due to osteoporosis. Abdominal tone can be improved with isometric exercises but spinal flexion exercises (such as "sit ups") should be avoided because of the risk of compression fractures. Erect posture and exercises that emphasize gentle thoracic extension are recommended because they help to increase flexibility and muscle tone. Management of osteoporosis is discussed in Case 25.

2b. Patients who complain that they have memory problems usually do not have dementia, but their concerns need to be addressed. Significant pathology is generally brought to a physician's attention by family members and not by patients themselves. This woman's obvious clarity of mind on the interview and her discussion of current events make significant pathology unlikely.

Self-reported memory loss is part of a complex of symptoms sometimes called "mild cognitive impairment" (MCI). Patients with MCI have objective memory impairment but normal general cognitive function and no impairment in activities of daily living. Other terms applied to this general concept have included "benign senescent forgetfulness," "age-associated memory impairment," and others. These concepts, as well as MCI, have been determined by a variety of diagnostic or definitional criteria, so the notion of an intermediate state between normal aging and dementia is imprecise. There is substantial evidence that patients with MCI are at greater risk than their same-age cohorts for developing dementia with time, but criteria do not exist to determine the level of risk and what form the dementia might take. If she is very concerned, a close friend or family member could be asked to confirm or refute the patient's observations. MCI is discussed in detail in the references (see Petersen *et al.*, 2001).

Likewise, it is common for cognitively normal people to experience difficulty with name retrieval, even in midlife. Whether this frequent complaint – in the absence of measurable memory problems – is a very early predictor of dementia is an intriguing question that requires further study.

2c. She should be told that her EKG is normal for her age. Left axis deviation is the most commonly found abnormality in the elderly, but, when seen alone, has no prognostic significance (see Case 11).

3. She has lost height because of progressive kyphosis from wedging and compression of individual vertebrae. Other factors that contribute to age-related loss of height include decrease in the intervertebral disc spaces from desiccation of the nucleus pulposus and degeneration of the disc. There is also slight flexion at the knee and hip with age. All of these factors can lead to considerable loss of height over time.

4. Ideal body weight is generally expressed as body mass index (BMI), which is calculated by dividing weight in kilograms over height in meters squared. When asked what her height was at her "tallest," she reported that she was "always 5 feet 6 inches tall." Based on that, and her weight at age 50, her BMI was once a "slim" 21. However, although she has gained 10 pounds over the years, she has apparently lost three inches in height. It is illogical to now calculate her BMI based on crown to floor height. One approach would be to use her maximum height of 5 feet 6 inches to calculate her current BMI, which would yield a BMI of 22.6, which is much lower than her BMI calculated on her current height of 5 feet 3 inches, which would be

24.8. This approach has not been validated, however, and does not take into account other age-related anthropomorphic changes, such as loss of bone and muscle mass.

Another approach is to measure tibial length, which does not change, and which can be used to derive height, using a validated equation (see Chumlea and Guo, 1992), but this measurement may have substantial intra- and interrater variability, and calculations have not been validated in all races. Skinfold thickness can also be expected to be less accurate in the elderly because of increased skin laxity (the patient herself has made this observation). For clinical purposes, obesity is often judged by inspection.

A modest increase in weight with age is common, because of changes in metabolism and decreased exercise. Epidemiological studies have shown a "J"-shaped association between weight and longevity, with greatest longevity being among the slightly overweight. Although these studies failed to exclude groups who are thin but have high mortality, such as smokers and individuals with serious illness, a more recent prospective study of BMI in subjects 50–74 years old suggested the impact of obesity on mortality declines with age (see Bender *et al.*, 1999). Since BMI could be misleadingly high in subgroups of older cohorts (and since no separate data exist in people over 75), it is difficult to draw conclusions about the impact of excess body weight in late life.

5. Among older drivers, function rather than age per se determine a person's ability to drive. The vast majority of motor vehicle accidents occur in young men, but, among all age groups, those 85 and older have the highest accident rate per mile driven. Still, compared with motor vehicle accidents caused by young males, those caused by elderly men and women occur at slower speeds and result in fewer fatalities. Fortunately, most older drivers recognize their deficits and take precautions, such as driving at slower speeds, and avoiding night driving and poor road conditions.

Although specific medical and functional impairments can increase crash risk, physiologic changes may account for this. Visual changes that occur with age have the greatest impact, and these are not tested in vision exams given for licensure. In addition to decreased visual acuity, aging is associated with decreased dynamic visual acuity, poor adaptation to change in light, heightened sensitivity to glare, and deterioration in depth perception. Poor adaptation to light changes and sensitivity to glare make night time driving more challenging. Although aging is associated with decreased reaction time, it does not appear to play a significant role in crash risk, possibly because the older driver compensates for physical limitations by, for example, driving at slower speeds and avoiding dense traffic. In addition, road signs are distanced far enough to take into account slow reaction time, assuming the driver observes the speed limit.

This patient's history does not suggest any of the most common disorders that affect driving in the elderly, including diseases that impair alertness, mobility, control, or the limb strength needed to maneuver the automobile safely. Diabetics on insulin have a high crash risk, but diabetics that are well controlled without hypoglycemic episodes do not appear to have driving difficulties. Coronary artery disease in and of itself also does not carry any increased incidence in crashes but acute cardiac or cerebrovascular disorders can cause sudden loss of control. Medications are well known to affect driving ability, and those that cause sedation or otherwise impair cognition are particularly important (see Case 20).

Although this patient appeared "too bright" to the physician to have dementia, or even MCI, her complaint of memory problems should be explored and followed, because subtle changes in executive function may exist before frank symptoms of dementia occur. Likewise, the comprehensive evaluation should look for factors that might be impairing her driving, and correct them if possible. If no apparent problems exist, the physician should suggest the patient take a driving test or a course for older drivers.

The approach to the elderly driver is discussed further in Case 3 and in the references (see American Medical Association, 2003).

Caveats

1. Another common form of skin lesion that occurs in the elderly is the actinic ("senile," "solar") keratosis. Actinic keratoses are tan-colored, relatively flat, rough lesions that occur predominantly in sun-exposed areas, such as the forehead, dorsum of the hands, and shoulders, and are most common in fair-skinned people. These lesions should be removed because they occasionally progress to squamous carcinoma, although metastatic disease is unusual.

   Actinic keratoses occur in most Caucasian elderly. In contrast, actinic keratoses and skin cancers are rare in deeply pigmented people. Seborrheic keratoses, however, are common.

2. Basal cell carcinoma, which this patient does not have, is the most common tumor affecting light-skinned elderly. It also is related to sunlight exposure and is increasing in frequency. Although this tumor rarely metastasizes, it should be removed because it has a tendency to enlarge and erode adjoining structures. Basal cell carcinoma is unusual in dark-skinned people.

3. Although sunlight exposure may produce skin lesions and extrinsic aging, avoidance of the sun can lead to vitamin D deficiency. It is estimated that 15 minutes two to three times a week is all that is required for a light-skinned individual to achieve adequate vitamin D status. More exposure is required in dark-skinned people, who also are less likely to develop extrinsic aging and skin cancer.

REFERENCES

American Medical Association (2004). Physician's Guide to assessing and counseling older drivers. www.ama-assn.org/ama/pub/category/10791.html; accessed February 10, 2005.

Bender, R., Jockel, K., Trautner, C. *et al.* (1999). Effect of age on excess mortality in obesity. *Journal of the American Medical Association*, **281**, 1498–504.

Chumlea, W. C. and Guo, S. (1992). Equations for predicting stature in white and black elderly individuals. *Journals of Gerontology*, **47**, M197–203.

Executive Committee for the Asymptomatic Carotid Atherosclerosis Study (1995). Endarterectomy for asymptomatic carotid artery stenosis. *Journal of the American Medical Association*, **273**, 1421–8.

Petersen, R. C., Stevens, J. C., Ganguli, M. *et al.* (2001). Practice parameter. Early detection of dementia: mild cognitive impairment (an evidence-based review). Report of the Quality Standards Subcommittee of the American Academy of Neurology. *Neurology*, **56**, 1133–42.

BIBLIOGRAPHY

Attenhofer Jost, C. H., Turina, J., and Mayer, K. (2000). Echocardiography in the evaluation of systolic murmurs of unknown cause. *American Journal of Medicine*, **108**, 614–20.

Benavente, O., Moher, D., and Pham, B. (1998). Carotid endarterectomy for asymptomatic carotid stenosis: a meta analysis. *British Medical Journal*, **317**, 1477–80.

Gilchrest, B. A. (1997). Treatment of photo damage with topical tretinoin: an overview. *Journal of the American Academy of Dermatology*, **36**, S27–36.

Ingall, T. J., Dodick, D. W., and Zimmerman, R. S. (2000). Carotid endarterectomy – which patients benefit? *Postgraduate Medicine*, **107**, 97–100, 104–6, 109.

Kakaiya, R., Tisovec, R., and Fulkerson, P. (2000). Evaluation of fitness to drive: the physician's role in assessing elderly or demented patients. *Postgraduate Medicine*, **107**, 229–34.

Kuczmarski, M. F., Kuczmarski, R. J., and Najjar, M. (2000). Descriptive anthropometric reference data for older Americans. *Journal of the American Dietetic Association*, **100**, 59–66.

Lawrence, N. (2000). Treatment and emerging treatments for photoaging. *Dermatologic Clinics*, **18**, 99–112.

Matarasso, A. (1997). Facialplasty. *Dermatology Clinics*, **15**, 649–58.

Otto, C. M., Lind, B. K., and Kitzman, D. W. *et al.* (1999). Association of aortic valve sclerosis with cardiovascular morbidity and mortality in the elderly. *New England Journal of Medicine*, **341**, 142–7.

Owsley, C., Ball, K., and McGwin, G. *et al.* (1998). Visual processing impairment and risk of motor vehicle crash among older adults. *Journal of the American Medical Association*, **279**, 1083–8.

Sherris, D. A., Otley, C. C., and Bartley, G. B. (1998). Comprehensive treatment of the aging face – cutaneous and structural rejuvenation. *Mayo Clinic Proceedings*, **73**, 139–46.

Shorr, R. I., Johnson, K. C., Wan, J. Y. *et al.* (1998). The prognostic significance of asymptomatic carotid bruits in the elderly. *Journal of General Internal Medicine*, **13**, 86–90.

Sims, R. V. (1998). A preliminary assessment of the medical and functional factors associated with vehicle crashes in older adults. *Journal of the American Geriatrics Society*, **46**, 556–61.

Shua-Haim, J. R. and Gross, J. S. (1996). The co-pilot driver syndrome. *Journal of the American Geriatrics Society*, **44**, 815–7.

Weiler, J. M., Bloomfield, J. R., Woodworth, G. G. *et al.* (2000). Effects of fexofenadine, diphenhydramine and alcohol on driving performance. *Annals of Internal Medicine*, **132**, 354–63.

Willett, W. C., Dietz, W. H., and Colditz, G. A. (1999). Guidelines for healthy weight. *New England Journal of Medicine*, **341**, 427–34.

Wilson, P. W. and Kannel, W. B. (2002). Obesity, diabetes and risk of cardiovascular disease in the elderly. *American Journal of Geriatric Cardiology*, **11**, 119–23, 125.

Case 3

▶▶ A bad driver

A 78-year-old man is brought to your office by a friend who is concerned about his progressive decline in function. She reports that the patient's memory has deteriorated and that he has trouble walking, often complaining of pain in his hip. She knows that he takes medications for his pain and wonders if these medications are causing his memory problem.

The patient is aware of his memory disorder and is actually concerned that he is getting "Alzheimer's disease," which his mother had, although at an older age. He focuses, however, on his "leg problem," for which he was supposed to have surgery. He is looking forward to discussing this with you because he wanted to have a "second opinion."

The friend reports that the patient still goes to work every day, but the office functions poorly because of his inability to manage the work and his confusion about existing projects. Without the patient present, she confides to you that the business is in a "shambles" and that she has noticed problems in his self-care, noting that there is often a "smell of urine."

The friend is particularly concerned about his driving, but, when she mentions this, the patient becomes angry, stating, "Oh, there's nothing wrong with my driving!" She gently disagrees, stating that the patient has made serious errors on the street, on more than one occasion turning into incoming traffic. She says, "It is only a matter of time before there is a bad accident. I won't drive with him anymore!"

The patient is a widower who lives alone and has no known living relatives. He has a small publishing business and the friend has been a client for a number of years. He lives in a major urban area which has excellent public transportation, with access to persons with disabilities. When asked why he doesn't use the bus instead of driving, he says, "Oh, I still have a special pass and can have free parking – the parking lot attendants all know me, and my driving is just fine!" He mentions this rationale several times during the visit.

Case Studies in Geriatric Medicine, Judith C. Ahronheim *et al.* Published by Cambridge University Press.
© J. C. Ahronheim, Z.-B. Huang, V. Yen, C. M. Davitt, and D. Barile

On physical examination, the patient ambulates independently using a cane. An odor of urine is noticeable. He is alert and interactive, fully cooperating with the examination and his memory is grossly intact. He shows you a list of medications (tamsulosin, donepezil, oxycodone with acetaminophen, cyclobenzaprine, and tolterodine), but the doses on the list that he hands you are different from those on the bottles, and medication bottles contain the wrong medications or mixtures of pills. He knows the indications for his medications, but is unable to match the indication with the correct drug.

Mini-Mental Status Examination (MMSE) was performed. He was able to recall only one of three objects and couldn't recall the date, giving a score of 27 of 30 possible points. Except for a limited range of motion in his left hip, the remainder of the examination, including visual acuity, is normal.

Questions

1. What could be impairing the patient's driving?
2. What can the physician do about this situation?
3. What does the law require?

Answers

1. The patient has two important risk factors for driving: his painful hip and his cognitive dysfunction. Impaired gait alone can negatively impact driving performance. A call to the patient's orthopedic surgeon revealed the patient had severe osteoarthritis of his hip, and total hip replacement had been recommended. Further inquiry revealed the patient's pain medications were prescribed by at least two other physicians. Three of his medications – oxycodone, the centrally acting muscle relaxant cyclobenzaprine (Flexeril), and the antocholinergic tolterodine (Detrol) – have the ability to worsen cognitive function and impair driving ability.

This patient has had probable Alzheimer's disease. Dementia, even in the early stages, is a risk factor for accidents. In addition to memory loss and confusion, dementia-related deficits that impair driving ability include visual spatial problems and impairments in visual tracking and attention, processing of visual cues and other information, executive function, and judgment. This patient's prior intellectual abilities were well above average, so his modestly reduced score on the MMSE probably underestimated his significant functional deficits (see Case 9). Although he is aware of his memory problem, he is likely to be unaware of its severity and its impact on his function, and has either forgotten his driving errors or is unwilling to acknowledge them.

Not all studies demonstrate that patients with early dementia have a crash risk greater than age-matched controls. In general, it is important to assess the patient's function rather than rely on a specific diagnosis.

2. In general, health care providers need to recognize the importance of driving to a patient's independence and well being, as well as the risk to others from impaired drivers, and should be prepared to help patients to gain access to community transportation services where they exist and enlist friends and family to find alternatives. Unlike the suburban dwelling patient in Case 2, this patient lives in a major urban setting and has access to public transportation and other alternatives to driving his car. In this case, however, his dementia will impair his independence more rapidly than the absence of driving.

Repeatedly reminding the patient about his driving deficits may only make him angry. Since the patient does not admit to driving problems, he would feel any instructions by the physician to give up driving would be unjustified. The physician could, however, recommend a "refresher" course for older drivers, and if the patient were willing to attend one, or to take a driving test (or lived in a jurisdiction that required retesting), someone in authority could tell him he should no longer drive and this might reinforce the problem sufficiently for the patient. In the United States, only a few jurisdictions have developed mechanisms in which physicians may report an impaired driver to the motor vehicle bureau, and such reporting is, in any case, problematic (see below).

Friends or family sometimes manage the situation by disabling or removing the vehicle, but this would seem to be a drastic solution for someone with early dementia and fairly good insight into his situation. Moreover, families are often reluctant to stop their loved one from driving because of the loss of independence for the senior and the increased burden to the family who must now provide transportation.

Hip surgery might improve his physical function and would eliminate the need for analgesics, but will not improve or forestall his dementia. The primary care provider can, however, take a central role in ensuring that harmful medications are not prescribed and can work with friends and family to develop strategies for preventing this patient from driving.

Often, the approach to this problem is a process over time that involves the health care team and a committee of friends, family, or trusted professionals (such as an attorney or clergy). Sadly, it is often a "seminal event," such as an injury to the patient, that serves to put the forces in process to solve the problem, which often involves a guardianship proceeding or placement in a skilled nursing facility or some other higher level of care, as the dementia progresses. In this case, the patient's desire for hip surgery and the consensus that he would benefit from it (aside from driving) diverted attention from his driving and failing business. He underwent surgery and rehabilitation, and eventually moved to a nursing home. Sadly, he became very depressed in his new environment, and he underwent a rapid functional decline.

Approach to the elderly driver with medical impairments is discussed in detail in the references (see American Medical Association, 2004)

3. Laws in the United States regarding mandatory reporting, age-associated retesting for licensure, and reporting of potentially problematic elderly drivers vary from state to state. Most states do not require vision retesting for license renewal and only a few have separate requirements for older adults, such as periodic vision or driving tests. However, research has not shown a consistent decrease in crash rate where mandatory screening has been instituted. Furthermore, there appears to be a reluctance on the part of government to involve itself actively in this matter, perhaps because of cost or voter demographics. Many seniors feel threatened by any limitations made on their primary mode of transport, and one study has demonstrated an increased incidence of depression among seniors who have stopped driving for various reasons.

Physician reporting of most impairments has generally not been mandated because such reporting is seen as a violation of patient confidentiality, which in turn discourages a patient from seeking help. A physician is permitted to breach confidentiality under the "duty to warn," but this is limited to situations where an *identified* third party would be at risk of harm – for example, a patient who informs his psychotherapist he is going to kill someone. In contrast, while the impaired driver may put others at risk, it is not possible to identify any *specific* individual who would be helped by reporting someone to the motor vehicle bureau. In any case, taking away his driving privileges would be insufficient if he still had access to a car, just as the younger impaired driver may continue to cause accidents despite prior convictions for driving while impaired and despite loss of license.

Some professional organizations recommend that all patients with Alzheimer's disease be advised to stop driving completely. However, most states do not have specific policies concerning patients with dementia. In some states, physicians are protected from liability if they report a patient to the Department of Motor Vehicles; in other states, they are not. Although there seems to be a conflict between patient confidentiality and public safety, the ultimate solution lies in practical solutions provided through a collaborative effort between the health care team, the patient, and his friends and family.

REFERENCE

American Medical Association (2004). Physician's guide to assessing and counseling older drivers. www.ama-assn.org/ama/pub/category/10791.html; accessed February 10, 2005.

BIBLIOGRAPHY

Coley, M. J. and Coughlin, J. F. (2002). State older-driver relicensing: conflicts, chaos and the search for policy consensus. *Elder's Advisor: Journal of Elder Law and Post-Retirement Planning*, **3**, 43–56.

Davitt, C. M. and Timiras, M. L. (2002). The elderly driver. In *Clinical Geriatrics*, eds., R. A. Norman and T. S. Dharamarajan. New York: CRC-Parthenon Press, pp. 118–92.

Dubinsky, R. M., Stein, A. C., and Lyons, K. (2000). Practice parameter: risk of driving and Alzheimer's disease (an evidence-based review). Report on the Quality Standards Subcommittee of the American Academy of Neurology. *Neurology*, **54**, 2205–11.

Fozard, J. L., Vercryssen, M., Reynolds, S. L. *et al.* (1994). Age differences and changes in reaction time: the Baltimore Longitudinal Study of Aging. *Journals of Gerontology*, **49**, P179–89.

Kakaiya, R., Tisovec, R., and Fulkerson, P. (2000). Evaluation of fitness to drive: the physician's role in assessing elderly or demented patients. *Postgraduate Medicine*, **107**, 229–34.

Levy, D. T., Vernick, J. S., and Howard, K. A. (1995). Relationship between driver's license renewal policies and fatal crashes involving drivers 70 years or older. *Journal of the American Medical Association*, **274**, 1026–30.

Marottoli, R. A. (1997). Driving cessation and increased depressive symptoms: prospective evidence from the New Haven EPESE. *Journal of the American Geriatrics Society*, **45**, 202–6.

Sims, R. V. (1998). A preliminary assessment of the medical and functional factors associated with vehicle crashes in older adults. *Journal of the American Geriatrics Society*, **46**, 556–61.

Case 4

▸▸ Early dementia

Mrs. N, a 77-year-old woman, is brought to your office as a new patient. She says she "feels fine," but knows that her daughter is concerned about her. Mrs. N has been living alone in her own home since her husband died 3 years ago. Her daughter tells you that she has noticed a change in her mother over the last 18 months. Her memory is "failing" and has gradually worsened. Although her clothes are clean, her outfits sometimes don't quite match. The home, once spotless, has started to look cluttered. The daughter has noticed her mother's mail left unopened on the table and wonders if she is paying her bills. One troubling behavior is that the patient phones her daughter repeatedly, "asking the same questions over and over."

Her daughter feels that the patient has been anxious and a little depressed since her husband died. She has been feeling well, is eating well, and has maintained a normal weight. She is being treated for hypertension, urinary incontinence, and osteoarthritis of the knee. She has no history of diabetes, transient ischemic attack (TIA), stroke, or major depression. She had a wrist fracture at the age of 60 after slipping on a wet surface at home. She denies smoking or any alcohol use. Six months ago, her daughter took the patient to a neurologist to evaluate her for "memory problems." The workup included blood tests and neuroimaging, and a diagnosis of "vascular dementia" was made and aspirin (81 mg per day) was prescribed. The patient's other medications include enalapril, oxybutinin, and ibuprofen.

On physical examination, the patient appears healthy and well groomed. Her affect is not depressed, and she is pleasant and interactive. Blood pressure is 130/80, pulse is 70 and regular, and her weight is 128 pounds. Lungs are clear, and there are no heart murmurs. Left dorsalis pedis pulse is faintly palpable and right dorsalis pedis pulse is 1+; otherwise, peripheral pulses are full and equal and there are no neck bruits. Neurologic examination reveals normal gait, affect, and strength in all muscle groups, and bilaterally intact deep tendon reflexes. She has bilateral palmomental reflexes, but grasp

Case Studies in Geriatric Medicine, Judith C. Ahronheim *et al.* Published by Cambridge University Press.
© J. C. Ahronheim, Z.-B. Huang, V. Yen, C. M. Davitt, and D. Barile

and snout are negative. Speech is fluent, but she has some word-finding difficulty. Cranial nerves are intact and there is no tremor and no Babinski. On Folstein Mini-Mental State Examination (MMSE), she scores 25 out of 30; she recalls only one of three objects, is unable to draw a figure, and does not know the day of the week or the date. She is able to subtract serial 7s without difficulty. When asked questions about current events, she turns to her daughter and says, smiling, "Oh, she is the expert on those things."

Questions

1. What disease has caused Mrs. N's memory disorder?
2. What workup should be done?
3. What information does neuroimaging provide?
4. What information does the mental status testing provide?
5. What causes this disease?
6. What treatment can be offered?

Answers

1. The patient's memory impairment and disturbance in executive functioning (reduced ability to perform her accustomed activities of daily living on account of her cognitive deficits) indicate that she has dementia. Her ability to focus during mental status testing, and particularly her ability to subtract serial 7s, indicate that she does not have superimposed delirium (see Case 20). The insidious onset and slow progression suggests a neurodegenerative process rather than a structural lesion. The presence of a palmomental reflex is nonspecific, but patients with Alzheimer's disease often exhibit one or more "primitive reflexes," such as grasp, snout, and palmomental. These are thought to be due to deterioration in cortical inhibitory centers that ablate these reflexes after infancy. These signs are sometimes seen in clinically normal elderly or in those with other neurologic diseases.

   If the onset were acute or subacute, especially if there were a history of head trauma, subdural hematoma would have to be considered. Subdural hematoma generally (though not invariably) presents with altered mental status out of proportion to "hard" neurologic signs, and symptoms are manifest over a period of a few days or, less often, weeks. Delirium is often present but cognitive symptoms may resemble dementia.

Although the diagnosis of vascular dementia was previously made, the history of gradually declining memory, the clinical course to date, and findings on the physical examination are consistent with probable Alzheimer's disease. It is possible that Mrs.N's diagnosis of vascular dementia was based on her history of hypertension and diminished pedal pulses, coupled with abnormal neuroimaging. Vascular dementia (also called "multi-infarct" dementia), classically attributed to small, lacunar infarcts, is often assumed to be the primary cause if the patient has risk factors for stroke, such as diabetes or hypertension. Traditional diagnostic criteria for vascular dementia include abrupt onset or stepwise deterioration, a history of stroke, or focal neurologic signs and symptoms suggesting a vascular component (see Rosen *et al.*, 1980). However, at autopsy, most patients with the clinical diagnosis of vascular dementia have evidence of neurogenerative dementia, such as Alzheimer's disease. There is currently no reliable way to distinguish vascular dementia clinically from neurodegenerative dementias when they do coexist. The hippocampus, which is responsible for memory, is vulnerable to hypoxia and other ischemic insults, so it is possible that vascular stresses can produce memory loss, leading to what could logically be called vascular dementia. Overall, the precise contribution of stroke and cerebral atherosclerosis to the dementing process is not known. However, there is some evidence that vascular disease and associated risk factors play a partial role in the etiology of Alzheimer's disease. This issue is reviewed in detail in the references (see de la Torre, 2002).

Other important causes of progressive dementia include dementia with Lewy bodies (DLB) and Parkinson's disease (PD). Although patients with probable Alzheimer's disease may have some physical and cognitive features of these diseases, such as a flat affect, stereotypic gait, or delusions, these features are far more prominent and tend to occur much earlier in DLB and PD. Patients who satisfy clinical criteria for probable Alzheimer's disease often have neuropathologic evidence of one or more coexisting dementing processes, including vascular changes, DLB, or PD. These and other forms of progressive dementia are discussed in subsequent cases (see Cases 5–9).

Potentially reversible causes of dementia include medications, vitamin B12 deficiency, hypothyroidism, syphilis, Lyme disease, severe depression, and normal pressure hydrocephalus. These, and a variety of metabolic derangements (such as hypo- and hypernatremia, hypercalcemia, and others) can cause dementia-like illness or delirium. Drug side effects are the most common cause of reversible cognitive impairment. Virtually any centrally acting agent can impair cognition, with the most common offending agents including: anticholinergic agents, such as first-generation antihistamines, antispasmodics, tricyclic antidepressants, and others; benzodiazepines and other sedative–hypnotics; and phenothiazines, baclofen, muscle relaxants, opioid analgesics, and cimetidine. Antihypertensive agents that can cause memory loss include highly lipid-soluble beta blockers, such as propranolol, and older agents such as methyldopa, clonidine, and reserpine. This patient was taking an angiotensin-converting enzyme (ACE) inhibitor, a class that is well tolerated in dementia. The only possible offending agent in her regimen is oxybutinin. Although this short-acting anticholinergic agent would not cause progressive deficits, regular use could worsen or unmask an underlying dementing process and would be worth discontinuing long enough to observe for any improvement. As a rule of thumb, if a change in mental status occurs with the addition (or sometimes cessation) of a medication, drug-induced cognitive impairment should be considered.

Vitamin B12 deficiency can produce psychiatric disorders but these do not usually resemble a "typical" dementia such as Alzheimer's disease. Hypothyroidism can cause depression and severe hypothyroidism can impair cognitive function (see Case 41). Unfortunately, correction of these disorders, which are common in elderly patients and therefore often coexist with dementia, rarely improves the cognitive disorder. Rather, patients with reversible dementia have a higher risk of developing full blown dementia in the future, presumably because of subclinical brain changes that predisposed to the reversible process. Tertiary syphilis is a rare cause of dementia in older adults today and there are few descriptions of tertiary syphilis among the elderly; classically, the presentation does not resemble Alzheimer's disease.

Lyme disease should be considered in a patient who has spent time in an endemic area, especially if other symptoms of Lyme disease exist or if there is a history of tick bite or erythema migrans.

Depression is an important cause of memory loss in the elderly, and frequently coexists with dementia. When depression is so severe that it alone produces a dementia syndrome, it can usually be distinguished on clinical grounds by an experienced examiner, and there is frequently a past history of major depression. This patient does not appear clinically depressed, but more careful questioning should be undertaken. "Pseudodementia" of depression is discussed in detail in Case 7.

The classic triad of dementia, urinary incontinence, and gait apraxia of normal pressure hydrocephalus (NPH) occurs only in some patients with NPH, and patients with other forms of dementia often have urinary incontinence and gait disturbances, as do many elderly without dementia. Because of the difficulty in interpreting neuroimaging in this disease, NPH may be overdiagnosed. Misdiagnosis may be one reason for inadequate outcomes following ventriculoperitoneal shunting. NPH is discussed in further detail in the references (see Bech-Azeddine *et al.*, 2001).

2. The most important part of the workup in this patient has been done – a careful history to ascertain the nature and onset of symptoms and the pattern of

progression. In addition, this patient has had a thorough physical examination, including neurologic and mental status testing. More exhaustive neuropsychologic testing is generally appropriate only when there is a diagnostic difficulty, such as the need to distinguish deficits from severe depression or other psychiatric illness, if the presentation is atypical.

The remainder of the workup should include a complete drug review, including queries about nonprescription medications, and laboratory studies including comprehensive metabolic panel, serum B12 level, and TSH. Serologic tests for syphilis and Lyme titers should only be done if there is high pretest probability of infection, because they lack specificity and positive tests may lead to unnecessary treatment and concerns.

3. Neuroimaging techniques such as computed tomography (CT) and magnetic resonance imaging (MRI) are employed to rule out structural causes of cognitive impairment, such as subdural hematoma or a neoplasm. There is no typical presentation of a brain neoplasm, but it is unlikely to resemble the typical course of Alzheimer's disease, and such a finding on imaging in someone like the current patient might actually represent an incidental finding – e.g. a calcified meningioma. Although one study found one brain neoplasm in a series of 100 cases, no information was given about that one patient's presentation (Chui and Zhang, 1997). Neuroimaging is almost universally recommended as part of a routine dementia workup, but the yield is almost negligible if history and physical and neurologic examination do not suggest a structural lesion. Still, neuroimaging is justified if the physician is uncertain about the diagnosis and the patient could easily tolerate the procedure. Neuroimaging is necessary if a structural lesion is suspected – especially if the onset is acute or subacute – and if diagnosis would change management.

A reversible lesion would be extremely unlikely in Mrs. N, who has a typical Alzheimer-like history. Importantly, the findings on neuroimaging (such as a silent stroke, "diffuse/ periventricular white matter changes," or "leukoariosis") should not divert attention from the diagnosis of neurodegenerative dementia in a patient like this. CT and MRI are not sensitive enough to distinguish between atrophy of Alzheimer's disease and age-related cortical atrophy seen in elderly persons with normal cognition. Although statistically, "white matter changes" are associated with a higher risk of developing dementia, they are present in many cognitively normal elderly and, in any case, they do not differentiate one form of dementia from another. In particular, they do not distinguish vascular dementia from Alzheimer's disease or other neurodegenerative dementias. "Silent strokes" are common, and such a finding might reinforce the need for stroke prophylaxis, such as daily aspirin, but evidence does not exist that this would alter the course of her dementia.

4. The widely used 30-point MMSE (Folstein *et al.*, 1975) and other screening tests can help to validate reports by informants or can be used to screen for abnormalities, but alone cannot make a diagnosis of dementia. The MMSE measures a broad range of cognitive functions, including orientation, immediate and delayed recall, attention, and visual–spatial function. A score of 23 or less is considered to be consistent with dementia, but educational level, age, depression, and other conditions that affect cognitive function can alter performance on this test. A score as low as 19 might be normal for someone with less than 5 years of education, whereas a score as high as 28 might be abnormal for a college-educated person. The MMSE does not distinguish among various forms of dementia, and is therefore not diagnostic of Alzheimer's disease, but this patient's deficits (delayed word recall and orientation to time) are typical for a patient with early Alzheimer's disease.

   Communication difficulties between patient and examiner, such as hearing or visual impairment and language or cultural differences, are also likely to affect scores. The Clock Drawing Test may overcome some of these difficulties. In this test, the patient is asked to draw a circle, placing the numbers at the appropriate positions, and then to set the time to a particular time. The Clock Drawing Test is a measure of executive function, including planning and visuospatial construction, which may be abnormal before memory deficits are measurable. It is easy to administer but does not test memory and should be used in conjunction with a test like the MMSE, along with an informant interview, such as IQCODE (see Case 9), for maximum screening sensitivity and specificity. Less than a perfect clock, with all elements present in the correct location, should prompt further investigation.

   This patient's clock (see Figure 3) was incorrectly drawn, suggesting executive dysfunction.

5. The cause of Alzheimer's disease (AD) is not known but a combination of genetic and nongenetic factors are believed to exist. Familial (generally "early" onset) AD can be caused by a mutation in one of several genes, namely, the amyloid precursor protein (APP), presenilin 1, or presenilin 2 genes, which leads to increased production of a relatively insoluble form of beta amyloid (Abeta), and a cascade of events that ultimately leads to central nervous system dysfunction. Genetic polymorphisms have also been associated with early AD as well as the far more common late-onset form – notably, the epsilon 4 allele (Apo ε4) of the apolipoprotein E gene. This allele is associated with an elevated risk of developing AD, but is not invariably associated and perhaps acts with other cofactors to promote late-onset, "nonfamilial" AD. The mechanism is not known, and the association of this allele with Abeta production or deposition is less clear.

   Old age is the most important risk factor for AD, which may exist in as many as 50% of people aged 85 and older. Less is known about extrinsic factors such as

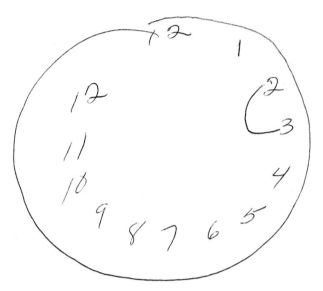

Figure 3   Clock drawing test. The patient was unable to draw a simple clock and place the clock's hands correctly.

toxins, history of head trauma, or infection with atypical agents such as prions or slow virus. Head trauma may increase the risk of AD, acting as a cofactor, perhaps in patients who lack intrinsic neuroprotective factors for genetic reasons. There is currently no evidence that this disease is infectious, as investigators have failed to transmit AD to laboratory animals.

6. Acetylcholinesterase (AChE) inhibitors are frequently employed in an effort to enhance cognitive function. AChE inhibitors act by inhibiting acetylcholinesterase, the enzyme responsible for the degradation of acetylcholine. AchE inhibitors interfere with the hydrolysis of acetylcholine at the synaptic cleft, enhancing cholinergic transmission in the brain. The cholinergic system appears to be the predominant neurotransmitter that is deranged in AD. Agents currently in use include donepezil (Aricept), rivastigmine (Exelon), and galantamine (Reminyl). These agents have greater affinity for acetylcholinesterase, which operates mostly in the brain, than for butyrylcholinesterase, which operates mostly in the periphery, including cardiac and smooth muscle, and are generally well tolerated when dosed properly. An earlier agent, tetrahydroaminoacridine (Tacrine), is rarely used today because of a high incidence of hepatotoxicity. Clinical trials of AChE inhibitors have demonstrated modest improvement in measures of cognitive function, activities of daily living, and psychiatric symptoms, and anecdotal experience suggests a few patients exhibit substantial, though temporary, improvement. On the whole, however, observable clinical benefit and improved quality of life have not been demonstrated in

substantial numbers of patients with AD (although other forms of dementia, such as DLB, may respond more overtly). Objective measurements show a delay in loss of function (i.e. higher level of function at any given level of deterioration), but there is no evidence that these agents retard neural degeneration. AchE inhibitors occasionally cause gastrointestinal symptoms and rarely cause cholinomimetic adverse effects, such as bradycardia.

A newer agent, memantine (Ebixa), is a N-methyl-D-aspartate (NMDA) receptor antagonist which blocks the effects of glutamate, an excitatory neurotransmitter that can cause neurotoxicity in excessive concentrations. Like older agents, positive effects are measurable in clinical trials of patients with moderate to severe dementia, whereas observable clinical benefit is minimal. Although promising, more study is needed to determine the role of this agent – specifically, to determine if it enhances neuroprotection and delays progression.

In patients with risk factors for stroke, or if neuroimaging showed an old infarct, there might be justification to prescribe aspirin for stroke prevention, but there is no evidence from clinical trials that aspirin alters the course of progressive dementia, which is generally due to factors other than stroke. However, there is evidence that anti-inflammatory agents may reduce the risk or delay the progression of AD; whether this suggests an inflammatory or vascular etiology for AD, or is further evidence of coexisting but undiagnosed vascular disease in AD patients, remains to be determined.

Important nonpharmacologic treatment approaches in early dementia include identifying and treating superimposed illness that can reversibly worsen cognition (e.g. infection or metabolic disease), and avoiding medications that can do this. Interpersonal methods are very important and include engaging the patient in the present, since the recent past is commonly forgotten, while tapping into the distant past, if pleasant reminiscences can be elicited. This issue is discussed in greater detail in Case 5.

Devices to promote the safety of frail elderly, such as systems to alert apartment management or alarm devices that the patient can wear, have limited value in the patient with dementia, who often cannot remember how to use these devices or that they possess them. Likewise, medication reminders, such as marked boxes or even phone calls, are not reliable and may give family and neighbors a false sense of security about safety concerns. Family and other caregivers are a critical part of the treatment team. The establishment of a long-term supportive relationship with the caregiver, in addition to the patient, can be immensely helpful, and their ability to cope should be periodically assessed, along with the patient's medical status, as the former can have a direct effect on the latter. An interdisciplinary approach with a nurse practitioner, social worker, or others can add substantially to the level of care and attention given.

Caveat

HIV infection should be considered in the differential diagnosis of dementia in any patient who has risk factors for HIV infection, even though it is much less common among the elderly than among younger adults. It can be mistaken for other forms of dementia in the elderly, especially if HIV/AIDS is not suspected, and dementia alone can be the presenting sign. HIV dementia is generally accompanied by ambulation dysfunction in younger adults, but this is not a helpful distinguishing sign among the elderly, when gait abnormalities are common, and which eventually accompany most forms of late-life dementia.

REFERENCES

Bech-Azeddine, R., Waldemar, G., Knudsen, G. M. *et al.* (2001). Idiopathic normal-pressure hydrocephalus: evaluation and findings in a multidisciplinary memory clinic. *European Journal of Neurology*, **8**, 601–11.

de la Torre, J. C. (2002). Alzheimer disease as a vascular disorder: nosological evidence. *Stroke*, **33**, 1152–62.

Folstein, M. F., Folstein, S. E., and McHugh, P. R. (1975). Mini-Mental State. A practical method for grading the cognitive state of patients for the clinician. *Journal of Psychiatric Research*, **12**, 189–98.

Rosen, W. G., Terry, R. D., Fuld, P. A. *et al.* (1980). Pathological verification of ischemic score in differentiation of dementias. *Annals of Neurology*, **7**, 486–8.

BIBLIOGRAPHY

Chui, H. and Zhang, Q. (1997). Evaluation of dementia: a systematic study of the usefulness of the American Academy of Neurology's practice parameters. *Neurology*, **49**, 925–35.

Crum R. M., Anthony, J. C., and Bassett, S. S. *et al.* (1993). Population-based norms for the Mini-Mental State Examination by age and educational level. *Journal of the American Medical Association*, **269**, 2386–91.

Goebels, N. and Soyka, M. (2000). Dementia associated with B-12 deficiency: presentation of two cases and review of the literature. *Journal of Neuropsychiatry and Clinical Neurosciences*, **12**, 389–94.

Karlawish, J. H., Casarett, D., Klocinski, J. *et al.* (2001). The relationship between caregiver's global ratings of Alzheimer's disease patients' quality of life, disease severity, and the caregiving experience. *Journal of the American Geriatrics Society*, **49**, 1066–70.

Kirby, M., Denihan, A., Bruce, I. *et al.* (2001). The clock drawing test in primary care: sensitivity in dementia detection and specificity against normal and depressed elderly. *International Journal of Geriatric Psychiatry*, **16**, 935–40.

Knopman, D. S., DeKosky, S. T., Cummings, J. L. *et al*. (2001). Practice parameter: diagnosis of dementia (an evidence-based review). Report of the Quality Standards Subcommittee of the American Academy of Neurology. *Neurology*, **56**, 1143–53.

Lambert, J. C., Mann, D., Goumidi, L. *et al*. (2001). Effect of the APOE promoter polymorphisms on cerebral amyloid peptide deposition in Alzheimer's disease. *Lancet*, **357**, 608–9.

Massoud, F., Devi, G., Moroney, J. T. *et al*. (2000). The role of routine laboratory studies and neuroimaging in the diagnosis of dementia: a clinicopathological study. *Journal of the American Geriatrics Society*, **48**, 1204–10.

Mehta, K. M., Ott, A., Kalmijn, S. *et al*. (1999). Head trauma and risk of dementia and Alzheimer's disease: the Rotterdam study. *Neurology*, **159**, 748–54.

Nolan, K. A., Lino, M. M., Seligmann, A. W. *et al*. (1998). Absence of vascular dementia in an autopsy series from a dementia clinic. *Journal of the American Geriatrics Society*, **46**, 597–604.

Nussbaum, R. L. and Ellis, C. E. (2003). Genomic medicine. Alzheimer's disease and Parkinson's disease. *New England Journal of Medicine*, **348**, 1356–64.

Reisberg, B., Doody, R., Stoffler, A. *et al*. for the Memantine Study Group. (2003). Memantine in moderate-to-severe Alzheimer's disease. *New England Journal of Medicine*, **348**, 1333–41.

Small, J. B., Viitanen, M., and Backman, L. (1997). Mini-Mental State Examination item scores as predictors of Alzheimer's disease: incidence data from the Kungsholmen Project, Stockholm. *Journal of Gerontology*, **52A**, M299–304.

Tariot, P. M., Farlow, M. R., Grossberg, G. T. *et al*. for the Memantine Study Group (2004). Memantine treatment in patients with moderate to severe Alzheimer disease already receiving donepezil. *Journal of the American Medical Association*, **291**, 317–24.

Tierney, M. C., Herrmann N, Geslani, D. M. *et al*. (2003). Contribution of informant and patient ratings to the accuracy of the mini-mental state examination in predicting probable Alzheimer's disease. *Journal of the American Geriatrics Society*, **51**, 813–18.

Trinh, N., Hoblyn, J., Mohanty, S. *et al*. (2003). Efficacy of cholinesterase inhibitors in the treatment of neuropsychiatric symptoms and functional impairment in Alzheimer disease. A meta-analysis. *Journal of the American Medical Association*, **289**, 210–16.

Case 5

▸▸ Moderate dementia

Mrs. N's cognitive function continued its gradual decline over the next 2 years. She refused to move out of her own home, despite the pleas of her daughter that she move in with her. Mrs. N's daughter, whom we met in Case 4, works full time and is a divorced mother of a teenaged daughter, but has been increasingly involved in her care. Unfortunately, she lives 30 miles away and has been able to visit only on weekends, but she calls her mother daily and reminds her to take her medications, which include donepezil (Aricept), enalapril (Vasotec), and baby aspirin.

Last week, Mrs. N fell while walking in the street at night by herself. She was unable to get up and was brought by ambulance to the local emergency room, where she was found to have a fracture of the right clavicle. She was given a supportive sling to wear and acetaminophen with codeine for the pain as needed. She was sent home to live with her daughter "temporarily" until she recovers. Mrs. N's son, who lives in another state, has told his sister, "Mom has got to go into a nursing home," but she protests that she promised her mother she "would never do that."

Mrs. N's daughter now reports that the police have found her mother wandering three times in the past 2 months. There has been no change in mental status since the fall but the daughter is afraid of what will happen if this behavior continues because no one is at home to watch her mother. In addition, the patient, who often naps during the day, is awake for part of the night and the family's sleep is interrupted by the disturbance and concern that the patient will fall or leave the house. Her hygiene has been deteriorating and her daughter says, "It's a real struggle to get her to take her bath at night! Can't you give her something to calm her down or get her to sleep?"

On physical examination, the patient is thin, her posture is stooped, and she has poor hygiene. She walks with a cane but does not use it consistently. The nurse, who has recorded her weight as 120 pounds, reports the patient had difficulty standing on the office scale. The patient is alert and interactive,

Case Studies in Geriatric Medicine, Judith C. Ahronheim *et al*. Published by Cambridge University Press.
© J. C. Ahronheim, Z.-B. Huang, V. Yen, C. M. Davitt, and D. Barile

but seems impatient and says several times, "I want to go home." She is wearing the sling but tugs at it repeatedly, saying it "annoys" her. She has a fading hematoma over her left eye, which is tender to touch. Her abdomen is soft and rectal examination reveals moderate amount of soft stool, which is negative for occult blood. The patient whispers to you that she is "being held prisoner against her will" and wishes you could "spring her out." The daughter tells you the patient has accused her of stealing her money as well.

Except for her Mini-Mental State Examination score, which is now 14/30, the neurologic examination is unchanged from her baseline.

Questions

1. How can you explain Mrs. N's decline in mental status?
2. What can be done about her wandering?
3. What can be done about her night time sleeplessness?
4. What accounts for Mrs. N's suspiciousness, and how can it be managed?
5. Is the patient's son correct that his mother must enter a nursing home?
6. How can the primary care provider support the patient's family caregivers?

Answers

1. A hematoma on the face following a fall raises concern and, if there had been any worsening of mental status following the fall, or new neurologic findings, a subdural hematoma would need to be ruled out. Mrs. N, who takes aspirin, should continue to be observed for new changes and brain imaging performed if necessary. If pain from her fracture is severe enough to require opioid analgesia, this should be given at the lowest effective dose with close observation of mental status, ambulation, and bowel function. Abrupt changes in mental status in patients with underlying dementia can also mean other serious problems, such as infection or stroke, or even seemingly trivial problems such as urinary tract infection or fecal impaction. However, there has been no recent change, and this patient's cognitive decline can be explained by the natural progression of Alzheimer's disease, which occurs relentlessly, though perhaps more slowly with the cholinesterase inhibitor that was prescribed 2 years ago. At that time, the patient had already demonstrated some difficulty with instrumental activities of daily living (IADLs), like housekeeping and managing money, but she is now having problems with basic activities of daily

living (ADLs), including dressing and grooming. If the patient survives for a few more years, her memory and intellectual function will continue to decline and more advanced functions such as speech and motor function may eventually be lost.

2. Although neuroleptic and other sedating medications are often prescribed for wandering, with the expectation that they will have a calming effect, wandering generally does not improve with medication, which can create problems of their own. Neuroleptics, which block dopamine, can cause extrapyramidal symptoms ("drug-induced parkinsonism;" EPS), increasing the risk of falls. To prevent wandering, doses must be sufficient to sedate or immobilize the patient and this can seriously endanger safety and health. In some cases, neuroleptics can cause restlessness (akathisia), which increases psychomotor activity, prompting the clinician to increase the dose mistakenly, which merely worsens the problem. Benzodiazepines, which are very sedating, are particularly likely to worsen confusion and can increase agitation, sometimes by producing disinhibition. Benzodiazepines should be entirely avoided if possible in patients with dementia.

Wandering is best treated with nonpharmacologic methods. Environmental modification can be very helpful, such as putting up a large STOP sign over the door, disguising the door by covering it with a sheet or curtain, or installing a set of bells or a door alarm to alert the caregiver if the door is being opened. Locks can be placed higher on the door frame out of reach or can be changed to a new system that the patient might not be able to figure out. Interpersonal methods, including distraction, are helpful, and a well-structured, daily routine that includes exercise and supervised walking may decrease the restlessness that leads to wandering. Community organizations, caregiver support groups, and consumer-oriented literature are important resources for patients, providing creative ways of handling difficult day-to-day situations. Resources are discussed in detail in the references (see Alzheimer's Association; Mace and Rabins, 2001).

Around-the-clock observation and close interaction with the patient would be ideal, but is usually impractical in most homes today, as traditional caregivers (typically, though not invariably, the oldest adult daughter or a daughter-in-law) are generally in the work force, often "sandwiched" between caring for an elderly relative and young children. If resources permit, home attendant services can take the place of, or augment, family support. A patient with dementia who wanders and is suspicious is the most challenging, and requires devoted, well-trained, or creative split-shift caregivers, who will also watch the patient if she is up at night.

3. Many patients with dementia have a reversed sleep–wake cycle, with exaggeration of physiologic age-related changes in sleep (see Case 22). If the patient sleeps all day, a hypnotic agent at night will either fail to work or, if adequate doses are given to have any effect, will increase the risk of falls and other problems linked to sedation. If there is a caregiver, he or she can keep the patient alert during the day with activities,

such as walking, conversation, or even board games, and this may increase night time sleeping. An ideal but costly solution would be a salaried, well-rested caregiver to ensure the patient's safety at night, while accommodating the patient's altered sleep pattern.

An additional problem that occurs in dementia is "sundowning," in which the patient becomes more confused in the late afternoon or evening. This can increase the risk of falling, agitation, wandering, and injury. Although the exact mechanism is not known, one small study linked sundowning to disturbances in circadian body rhythms including body temperature regulation caused by Alzheimer's disease itself. Small doses of neuroleptic agents (see below) may be helpful in patients with dementia-associated nocturnal agitation or sleeplessness, but should be used only if nonpharmacologic methods fail.

4. Mrs. N's suspiciousness and apparent paranoia are neither universal nor unusual in Alzheimer's disease, and could be secondary to memory loss – e.g. the patient may have misplaced her money and insist that it was stolen. However, marked suspiciousness and paranoid delusions, such as the idea that she is being held prisoner, may be due to neurologic or neurohormonal alterations of the disease itself.

Paranoia and delusions may produce harmful or disruptive behavior, and (in contrast to wandering) should be managed pharmacologically, usually with low doses of "atypical" neuroleptics like risperidone or olanzapine, which are less likely than older, nonspecific, dopamine-blocking agents to cause EPS. However, regular use even of these agents may impair gait in susceptible people and they would need to be used very cautiously in this patient who has experienced falls. Dementia itself can increase the risk of falling due to inattention to environmental hazards, lack of awareness of physical impairments, visual–spatial deficits, and progressive cerebrocortical deterioration. Pharmacologic treatment of delusions and paranoia should be limited to symptoms that are bothersome to the patient, that interfere with her care, or that endanger her or her caregivers. Arguing or attempting to reason with her may be counterproductive.

During a clinical encounter, it is important to speak slowly and distinctly, avoiding complex topics, being mindful of coexisting problems, such as low vision or hearing loss. In order to maximize the patient's attention, it is best to choose a "good time" for conversation, when agitation and distraction are minimized. The patient should be given adequate time to answer questions. Orienting her to time or location may be helpful but is not essential, since this information can be quickly forgotten and repeated correction will only increase anxiety and confusion. If the patient appears to be reaching his or her tolerance limit, a different activity should be selected, such as moving on to the physical examination, which can be performed in short segments if necessary.

5. This patient's wandering, falls, and need for assistance with ADLs and IADLs make her an unsuitable candidate for independent living. However, there is no "rule" or specific set of criteria that demands nursing home placement – whether the patient enters a nursing home or remains at home with caregivers is, rather, a function of the family's ability to care for the patient or harness available resources. Most communities have some services that can help maintain a person with dementia at home. Unfortunately, government entitlements for the elderly do not cover these services on a consistent basis. A home attendant can be employed to assist in caring for the patient in her own home, but 24-hour care would be needed in this patient's case and this would be very costly – often more than a nursing home. In the United States, entitlements are complex and may vary from state to state. In the home (and except for home hospice), Medicare only pays for "skilled care" – i.e. services that require the supervision of a registered nurse and are ordered by the attending physician. Most patients with dementia need "custodial" (unskilled) care – namely, assistance with ADLs – which must be paid out of pocket, unless the patient has Medicaid and lived in one of the very few states that paid for this type of care. Medicaid is health insurance for the poor and is a federal–state partnership, so states vary greatly in the amount of funds designated for various services. Private long-term care insurance covers many custodial services, but is expensive and would have had to have been purchased before the onset of a disabling illness. Some policies will not pay for care related to a "mental" illness and classify Alzheimer's disease as such, or have other restrictions as to their use.

An adult day care center can provide structured activities, meals, administration of medications, and physical therapy, and serves as a respite for family caregivers; however, only Medicaid and certain types of private long-term care insurance will pay for this usually costly service. An assisted living residence can provide a home health aide, meals, medication assistance, and some limited activities, but would only be appropriate for this patient if there were a dedicated dementia ("Alzheimer") unit on site. The Program of All-inclusive Care for the Elderly (PACE) is available in a few communities for frail older patients who are "dually eligible" for both Medicare and Medicaid. PACE programs encompass assisted living, adult day care, and home care. Local social service agencies or privately employed geriatric care managers can assist the family in accessing these services and can help determine eligibility for government entitlements. Care managers can also assist in directing and supervising hands-on care or accompany the patient to physician visits.

Environmental modifications and strengthening exercises might prevent falls in this patient. Exercises which would benefit her overall health, might engage her, might improve her sleep, and could be prescribed with caregivers instructed to assist the patient in doing them. Medicare will pay for some of these services, for durable medical equipment, and, during this period of "skilled care," a home health aide may be reimbursable for a short period of time to assist with personal care and light housekeeping.

Despite the daughter's promises to avoid nursing home placement, practical limitations or a sentinel event – such as injury or serious medical illness – would make care at home increasingly difficult to provide. It is important to discuss all available options with the daughter and prepare her to accept her mother's likely further decline.

6. A primary care office should have printed resources available for the patient's family or should be able to supply phone numbers for local social service agencies, a local Agency on Aging, private geriatric care managers, or a consumer-oriented, non-profit group, such as the Alzheimer's Association, which has many local chapters throughout the United States. The Alzheimer's Association provides education, caregiver support groups, and assistance with temporary nursing home placement to provide respite for weary caregivers. It also has a "Safe Return Program" which consists of a tracking system through an identification bracelet worn by the patient. Each county in the United States has an area Agency on Aging, which is a good referral source for senior programs, home help, home-delivered meals, and other services for the aged. National professional organizations like the American Geriatrics Society, British Geriatrics Society, and others have websites with links to consumer-oriented resources, and can be accessed by the primary care provider or by the patient's caregiver (see references).

A supportive, ongoing relationship with the primary care provider is key to the health of the caregiver, which has a direct impact on the well being of the patient. Time should be allotted during each visit and phone call to ask not only how the patient is doing but also how the caregiver is doing. The visit should be arranged, if possible, to permit time to speak privately with the caregiver – e.g. while the nurse is with the patient.

REFERENCES

Alzheimer's Association. www.alz.org.
American Geriatrics Society. www.americangeriatrics.org.
British Geriatrics Society. www.bgs.org.uk.

BIBLIOGRAPHY

Burke, J. R. and Morgenlander, J. C. (1999). Managing common behavioral problems in dementia. *Postgraduate Medicine*, **106**, 131–40.

Burton, L. C., German, P. S., Gruber-Baldin, A. L. *et al.* (2001). Medical care for nursing home residents: differences by dementia status. Epidemiology of Dementia in Nursing Homes Research Group, *Journal of American Geriatrics Society*, **49**, 142–7.

Doody, R. S., Stevens, J. C., Beck, C. *et al.* (2001). Practice parameter: management of dementia (an evidence based review). Report of the Quality Standards Subcommittee of the American Academy of Neurology. *Neurology*, **56**, 1154–6.

Eng, C., Pedulla, J., Eleazer, G. P. *et al.* (1997). Program of All-inclusive Care for the Elderly (PACE): an innovative model of integrated geriatric care and financing. *Journal of the American Geriatrics Society*, **45**, 223–32.

Fick, D. M., Agostini, J. V., and Inouye, S. K. (2002). Delirium superimposed on dementia: a systematic review. *Journal of the American Geriatrics Society*, **50**, 1723–32.

Mace, N. L. and Rabins, P. V. (2001). *The 36-Hour Day: A Family Guide to Caring for Persons with Alzheimer's Disease, Related Dementing Illnesses, and Memory Loss in Late Life*, revised edn. New York: Warner Books.

Montauk, S. L. (1998). Home health care. *American Family Physician*, **58**, 1608–14.

Netting, F. E. and Williams, F. G. (1999). Geriatric case managers: integration into physician practices. *Care Management Journals*, **1**, 3–9.

Oldenquist, G. W., Scott, L., and Finucane, T. E. (2001). Home care: what a physician needs to know. *Cleveland Clinic Journal of Medicine*, **68**, 433–40.

Parks, S. M. and Novielli, K. D. (2000). A practical guide to caring for caregivers. *American Family Physician*, **62**, 2613–20, 2621–2.

Perry, R. J. and Miller, B. L. (2001). Behavior and treatment in frontotemporal dementia. *Neurology*, **56** (Suppl 4), S46–51.

Robinson, J. and Karon, S. L. (2000). Modeling Medicare costs of PACE (Program of All inclusive Care for the Elderly) populations. *Health Care Finance Review*, **21**, 149–70.

Ross, M. E. and Wright, M. F. (1998). Long-term care for elderly individuals and methods of financing. *Journal of Community Health Nursing*, **15**, 77–89.

Steffens, D. C. and Morgenlander, J. C. (1999). Initial evaluation of suspected dementia. *Postgraduate Medicine*, **106**, 72–83.

Strauss, P. J. and Lederman, N. M. (2003). The Complete Retirement Survival Guide, 2nd edn. New York: Checkmark Books.

Teri, L., Logsdon, R. G., Peskind, E. *et al.* (2000). Treatment of agitation in Alzheimer's Disease: a randomized, placebo-controlled clinical trial. *Neurology*, **55**, 1271–8.

U.S. Department of Health and Human Services. Centers for Medicare and Medicaid Services. (2005). *Medicare and You.* http://www.medicare.gov/publications/pubs/pdf/10050.pdf; accessed February 10, 2005.

Van Doorn, C., Gruber-Baldini, A. L., Zimmerman, S. *et al.* for the Epidemiology of Dementia in Nursing Homes Research Group. (2003). Dementia as a risk factor for falls and fall injuries among nursing home residents. *Journal of the American Geriatrics Society*, **51**, 1213–18.

Volicer, L., Harper, D. G., Manning, B. C. *et al.* (2001). Sundowning and circadian rhythms in Alzheimer's disease. *American Journal of Psychiatry*, **158**, 704–11.

▶▶ Severe dementia

Mrs. N, whom we met in Cases 4 and 5, eventually moved in with her daughter, who has hired a part-time home attendant to assist while she is at work. Mrs. N's granddaughter also assisted in her care. In the past 18 months, the patient's memory continued to decline, and she became incontinent of bladder and bowel. However, paranoia and delusions were initially much improved with risperidone, and lately she has done well without this medication.

Although Mrs. N does not know the name of the home attendant and believes that her daughter is her mother, she is calm and generally cooperative with care at home. She can no longer dress or bathe herself and eats only when prompted, and sometimes requires spoon feeding. She walks with assistance, but, while attempting to get out of bed, she tumbled to the floor, broke her hip, and was admitted to the hospital.

The hip is surgically repaired. The postoperative course is complicated by delirium, pneumonia, catheter-associated urinary tract infection, and a stage 2 sacral pressure ulcer. Her food intake was poor during her acute illnesses but family members brought food from home and fed her patiently in the evening. She eventually recovers and is evaluated for rehabilitation. Because of her dementia and increasing frailty, she is not considered a candidate for an acute rehabilitation hospital stay and is admitted to a local skilled nursing home for "subacute" rehabilitation. She makes some progress for about 2 weeks, gaining strength to transfer from the bed to the chair with assistance, but does not remember that her hip was repaired and often tries to get out of bed by herself. After 1 month, she stops making progress and the social worker informs the daughter that the Medicare will no longer pay for rehabilitation. She may remain in the nursing home, but will receive the monthly $5000 bill directly. The daughter bursts into tears and sobs, "How long can she last like this? I can't afford that much money! How can I take her home? I just can't take care of her anymore."

Case Studies in Geriatric Medicine, Judith C. Ahronheim *et al.* Published by Cambridge University Press.
© J. C. Ahronheim, Z.-B. Huang, V. Yen, C. M. Davitt, and D. Barile

Currently, the patient is alert and follows commands. She has poverty of speech, and answers some questions with short phrases, but does not hold a meaningful conversation. Her affect is flat, she has increased tone of her upper extremities, and requires assistance to stand and take a few steps. Her skin is intact. On a chair scale, the patient weighs 103 pounds.

Questions

1. What accounts for the social worker's admonition?
2. How can Mrs. N continue to pay for nursing home care?
3. What has caused Mrs. N's 25-pound weight loss over the past few years?
4. What can we tell the daughter regarding her mother's prognosis and life expectancy?

Answers

1. Like care at home, nursing home care is reimbursed by Medicare only when there is a skilled need (see Case 5), only for a limited period, and only in certain restricted circumstances. Unfortunately, this patient cannot understand or retain instructions, has therefore stopped making progress in her physical therapy, and will not be able to take advantage of the 100 days of rehabilitation reimbursed by Medicare. Since she has no other skilled needs (such as treatment of a pressure ulcer), she will no longer be deemed by Medicare to be benefiting from skilled care services. She could still remain in the nursing home, but, unless she had long-term care insurance or Medicaid, the high monthly bill would have to be paid out of pocket. As of this writing, the average cost of nursing home care in the United States is $50 000 per year with regional variations in rural and metropolitan areas.

2. The patient and not the daughter is responsible for the bill. Once Mrs. N's funds have been depleted (whether by nursing home costs or by expenses living at home), she may become eligible for Medicaid (see Case 5). States vary greatly in the amount of funds set aside for nursing home care and other benefits, and the number of Medicaid nursing home beds is limited. Medicaid covers nursing home expenses but at a low rate, with the difference absorbed by the nursing home's overall budget. Still, once a patient is in a nursing home, it is illegal for a Medicaid licensed facility to discharge a patient, even if he or she initially paid out of pocket and "spent down." However, patients who enter private nursing homes that do not have Medicaid

licenses can be discharged once their funds are spent, either to a Medicaid-licensed facility or home.

"Spending down" refers to an intentional or unintentional use of personal funds to levels low enough to qualify for Medicaid. Patients "spend down" by paying for help at home, for medical or living expenses, or for personal items, but many older Americans have taken advantage of the opportunity to spend down by planning in advance. Money may be set aside in a burial trust fund account to pay for funeral services, and gifts can be given to children and others, as long as each gift remains within the current allowable limit of $10 000 per year. Individuals often make larger transfers of funds specifically for this purpose, but these must be made well in advance. When an application is made for Medicaid, the government may examine up to 36 months of financial documents, such as bank statements and Social Security check records. If an illegal ("nonqualifying") transfer of funds occurred, such as an unusually large gift or withdrawal, then the patient could qualify for Medicaid only when those funds have been paid back and spent on health care. An attorney who specializes in elder law can be of assistance in financial planning for Medicaid eligibility.

As discussed in Case 5, private long-term care insurance covers nursing home care, but, even then, restrictions may exist.

Entitlements and other strategies for advance planning are discussed in detail in the references (see Strauss and Lederman, 2003).

3. Weight loss in dementia can be caused by multiple factors, including an inability to obtain food, forgetting to eat, failure for caregivers to address food preferences, or coexisting medical problems. Dementia itself may be associated with factors that can cause or promote weight loss. Alzheimer's disease is associated with marked changes in the olfactory lobe, and loss of sense of smell may precede dementia by many years, possibly leading to a reduction in appetite. Cytokines such as interleukin-6 (IL-6) and tumor necrosis factor (TNF) are elevated in dementia, and there is evidence that these may be involved in weight loss in dementia, perhaps by direct actions on the gastrointestinal system or indirectly via the central nervous system, affecting eating behaviors or altering metabolism. Abnormalities in specific parts that are associated with feeding behavior (the mesiotemporal cortex and anterior cingulate cortex) have been correlated with a greater likelihood of weight loss. Patients with dementia who carry the apoE epsilon 4 allele, which is associated with medial temporal lobe atrophy, are more likely to lose weight than are patients without this allele. These biologic issues are discussed in detail in the references (see Grundman *et al.*, 1996; Vanhanen *et al.*, 2001; Yeh *et al.*, 2001).

Advanced neurologic deterioration in late-stage dementia is associated with "aversive feeding behaviors," in which patients bite the spoon or push the feeder away, are unable to use utensils, or fail to distinguish between food and inanimate objects, such as a napkin or dish. Ultimately, patients develop progressive oral dyspraxia, impairing the oral preparatory phase of swallowing. Swallowing itself (pharyngeal and esophageal phase) is unimpaired in the absence of specific lesions as might be seen in stroke, but the patient fails to prepare the bolus and pass it back to the posterior pharynx. Since such patients require much assistance and often eat only small amounts at a time, frequent small feeds may be required. Caregivers busy with other responsibilities often cannot manage this, and staffing in nursing homes and hospitals is insufficient to provide the time to feed patients adequately. Caregiver burden has been identified as an independent risk factor for weight loss in patients with dementia.

Finally, normal aging is associated with a change in set point for food intake following overfeeding and underfeeding; this could well account for the delay in this patient's return of appetite following her acute illness. Fortunately, her family was permitted to feed the patient in the hospital and amplify her food intake.

4. Unless other life-threatening medical problems occur, the patient's cognitive and motor functions will continue to decline. The patient has already shown signs of late-stage dementia, such as poverty of speech, limited ambulation, and feeding problems. Patients who survive to the end stage cannot speak at all and are bed bound (see Case 7). It will be important to discuss sensitively with the daughter and other family members the expected course of the patient's disease, because accurate information presented in a nonthreatening way will assist them in making medical decisions about life-sustaining treatments or other invasive procedures. Patients with severe dementia who have been hospitalized have, on the average, approximately a 6-month survival (Meier *et al.*, 2001); the immediate cause of death is usually infection, and most often pneumonia, rather than the dementing illness per se. It may be helpful to introduce the concept of "terminal illness," which applies to patients like the present one. The range of survival is wide and the prognosis unpredictable in individual cases, making it important to assist family members in dealing with the uncertainty that lies ahead.

REFERENCES

Grundman, M., Corey-Bloom, J., Jernigan, T. *et al.* (1996). Low body weight in Alzheimer's disease is associated with mesial temporal cortex atrophy. *Neurology*, **46**, 1585–91.

Meier, D. E., Ahronheim, J. C., Morris, J. *et al.* (2001). High short-term mortality in hospitalized patients with advanced dementia: lack of benefit of tube-feeding. *Archives of Internal Medicine*, **161**, 594–9.

Strauss, P. J. and Lederman, N. M. (2003). *The Complete Retirement Survival Guide*, 2nd edn. New York: Checkmark Books.

Vanhanen, M., Kivipelto, M., Koivisto, K. *et al.* (2001). APOE-epsilon 4 is associated with weight loss in women with AD: a population-based study. *Neurology*, **56**, 655–9.

Yeh, S., Wu, S., Levine, D. M. *et al.* (2001). The correlation of cytokine levels with body weight after megestrol acetate treatment in geriatric patients. *Journal of Gerontology: Medical Sciences*, **56A**, M48–54.

BIBLIOGRAPHY

Ahronheim, J. C., Morrison, R. S., Morris, J. *et al.* (2000). Palliative care in advanced dementia: a randomized controlled trial and descriptive analysis. *Journal of Palliative Medicine*, **3**, 265–73.

Borenstein, G. A., Bowen, J. D., Rajaram, L. *et al.* (1999). Impaired olfaction as a marker for cognitive decline. Interaction with apolipoprotein E epsilon 4 status. *Neurology*, **53**, 1480–7.

Hu, X., Okamura, N., Arai, H. *et al.* (2002). Neuroanatomical correlates of low body weight in Alzheimer's disease: a PET study. *Progress in Neuropsychopharmacology and Biologic Psychiatry*, **26**, 1285–9.

Katz, S., Downs, T. D., Cash, H. R. *et al.* (1970). Progress in development of the index of ADL. *Gerontologist*, **10**, 20–30.

Kaufer, D. I. (2001). Long-term care in dementia: patients and caregivers. *Clinical Cornerstone*, **3**, 52–62.

Roberts, S. B., Fuss, P., Heyman, M. B. *et al.* (1994). Control of food intake in older men. *Journal of the American Medical Association*, **272**, 1601–6.

Schulz, R., Beach, S. R., Lind, B. *et al.* (2001). Involvement in caregiving and adjustment to death of a spouse: findings from the Caregiver Health Study. *Journal of the American Medical Association*, **285**, 3123–9.

Tariot, P. N., Ryan, J. M., Portsteinsson, A. P. *et al.* (2001). Pharmacologic therapy for behavioral symptoms of Alzheimer's disease. *Clinics in Geriatric Medicine*, **17**, 359–79.

Taylor, D. H., Jr., Schenkman, M., Zhou, J. *et al.* (2001). The relative effect of Alzheimer's disease and related dementias, disability, and comorbidities on cost of care for elderly persons. *Journals of Gerontology Series B: Psychological Sciences and Social Sciences*, **56**, S285–93.

Case 7

 Two women with advanced dementia

Miss. C

Miss. C is an 84-year-old woman who lives in a nursing home. She has hypertension, heart disease, diabetes, and peripheral vascular disease. She suffers from progressive dementia and is now bedridden, incontinent, and has severe contractures and necrotic ulcers and gangrenous areas of her left foot, leg, and hip. She is unable to take in food and water to maintain herself, and tube feeding is initiated.

Miss. C has never been married. Her only surviving blood relative is a nephew who has known her for 50 years, and who was appointed her legal guardian when she was deemed incompetent. He had refused to allow amputation 2 years before, stating that it would have been counter to his aunt's wishes, and she survived. Now, he feels that tube feeding would be of no long-term benefit and requests that it be discontinued and she be allowed to die. He cites the fact that she has always mistrusted doctors and, in the past, had expressed the desire to die in her own home.

Mrs. O

Mrs. O, a 77-year-old woman with a history of several strokes, has lost the ability to eat when fed. She is bedridden, incontinent, and suffers from advanced dementia.

Mrs. O worked for many years as a clerk in a hospital, and cared for two relatives while they died of cancer. On many occasions, she expressed her feelings opposing artificial life support, saying that she did not ever want to be a burden to anyone and felt that being kept alive by machines was "monstrous." Her physician wants to insert a feeding tube, but her two daughters, both nurses, refuse, stating that doing so would be contrary to their mother's wishes.

Case Studies in Geriatric Medicine, Judith C. Ahronheim *et al.* Published by Cambridge University Press.
© J. C. Ahronheim, Z.-B. Huang, V. Yen, C. M. Davitt, and D. Barile

Questions

1. What would these patients experience if tube feeding were withheld or withdrawn?
2. What effect would tube feeding have on Miss. C's skin ulcers or nutritional state, or risk of developing pneumonia?
3. What impact does tube feeding have on dementia?
4. Is it legal or ethical to withhold or withdraw tube feeding in either case? Why or why not?
5. Do the cases of Miss. C and Mrs. O differ from one another?
6. How are these patients similar or different from patients in a persistent vegetative state (PVS)?
7. Would the presence of a formal, written advance directive, such as a living will, change matters?

Answers

1. Concerns are often raised by family members and even health care providers that withholding or withdrawing tube feeding will lead to a painful death, or will cause a painful "death by starvation." However, no evidence exists to support this contention. The experience of competent hospice patients provides direct evidence that dying patients eat and drink very little at the end of life and can have any existing hunger, thirst, or dry mouth relieved with small amounts of food, water, or mouth care, and it would seem appropriate to extrapolate these observations to a dying patient who cannot communicate. In debilitated elderly, dehydration rapidly results in hyperosmolarity because of an impaired ability of the kidney to conserve salt and water, and coma occurs early on, probably because of severe underlying neurologic impairment.

   The term "starvation" is misleading and should be avoided because it conveys frightening images of otherwise healthy people who suffer from hunger and become increasingly debilitated as the result of protein calorie malnutrition. This contrasts sharply with sick or dying patients who are unable or who do not wish to eat or drink. Feeding tubes or other forms of artificial nutrition and hydration (ANH) can actually increase their discomfort. In dementia, invasive treatments such as feeding tubes may be painful or frightening, and patients often require restraints to prevent them from pulling out the tube. Complications of feeding tubes, such as cellulitis, tube trauma, peritonitis, and others, can produce pain or lead to additional painful treatments. Finally, susceptible patients who receive ANH sometimes develop pulmonary edema or other signs of fluid overload, which are less likely to occur in patients not receiving ANH. Complications of ANH are reviewed in the references (see Ahronheim, 1996; Huang and Ahronheim, 2000).

2. Wound healing can be impaired by deficiencies of certain nutrients, such as zinc, vitamin C, and protein. For this reason, tube feeding is sometimes recommended in patients with pressure sores and other skin ulcers. The premise that tube feeding can improve ulcer healing has not been adequately tested in clinical trials, but it is unlikely that artificially supplied nutrients alone would be sufficient to heal or prevent skin ulcers. Skin ulcers require rigorous nursing attention, including removal of pressure, friction, moisture, sometimes surgical debridement, and, above all, sufficient time for healing. Skin ulcers are discussed in further detail in Case 29.

Hypoalbuminemia in advanced dementia is often assumed to be the result of nutritional deficiency, which should therefore be corrected. Serum albumin, which does not decline in normal aging, can decline rapidly during illness and with poor oral intake; this is due to an age-associated decline in protein synthesis, compounded by marginal protein reserves due to age-related organ and muscle atrophy. Hypoalbuminemia is also seen in inflammatory states. In dementia, low albumin may exist in the absence of obvious impaired intake (or renal or gastrointestinal loss), and has been speculatively associated with cytokine production in dementia and mediated through the action on protein-producing hepatocytes. Likewise, weight loss in dementia can be multifactorial (see Case 6).

Feeding tubes are often recommended in patients who have developed aspiration pneumonia, under the assumption that pneumonia develops as the result of impaired swallowing. However, there is no evidence that gastrostomy tubes and even jejunostomy tubes prevent pneumonia, including that associated with aspiration. Neurologically impaired, bedridden patients have an extremely high incidence of pneumonia; this heightened risk is due to multiple factors, including age-related immunologic defects and susceptibility to extrinsic infection, abnormalities in the mucociliary clearance within the tracheobronchial tree, pooling of oropharyngeal secretions, and reflux of gastric as well as jejunal contents into the lung. This topic is reviewed in detail in the references (see Ahronheim, 1996; Finucane and Bynum, 1996).

3. There is no evidence that hydration or nutrient repletion can forestall or reverse the progressive neurologic degeneration of dementia. Although antioxidant vitamins have been proposed to ameliorate this process, there is no convincing evidence of benefit at this time. Likewise, no evidence of reversal exists from observations of innumerable patients who have been maintained on tube feeding for many years. Overall, tube-fed patients with advanced dementia survive on the average

approximately 6 months, approximately as long as those who are not tube fed (see Meier *et al.*, 2001); however, comparison data do not come from randomized controlled trials. If a patient with dementia cannot eat or drink at all and does not receive hydration, death will occur after approximately 3–14 days.

4. There is a consensus among ethicists and numerous organizations of health professionals that ANH may be withheld or withdrawn like other medical treatments if this is consistent with the patient's wishes. This is based on the ethical principle of patient autonomy – the right of a patient to determine his or her own medical treatment. When patients lack the ability to make their own health care decisions ("lack decisional capacity"), autonomy can be maintained through an authorized decision maker.

   This stance has generally been reflected in the courts and legislatures, but there has been longstanding controversy about ANH compared with other life-sustaining treatments, presumably because of the symbolic meaning attributed to food and water or perhaps because of misunderstanding among law makers about the medical aspects of tube feeding. In 1990, the United States Supreme Court, in the case of Nancy Cruzan (Cruzan v. Director, 1990), ruled that tube feeding was medical treatment that could be refused like other medical treatments. However, because the Court defined ANH as a medical treatment, separate, more stringent standards for ANH would seem illegal and the constitutionality of such statutory provisions has been questioned (see Sieger *et al.*, 2002).

5. The patients in these two cases both have advanced dementia, and, although Miss. C might have a poorer medical prognosis than Mrs. O, their precise outcomes were dependent on more than their medical conditions. In both cases, there was disagreement between parties that could only be resolved in court. In both cases, the family members felt that tube feeding would be against the patient's wishes, while the health providers felt the procedure was required and these disagreements could only be resolved in court. Both eventually were decided in appellate courts and became landmark "right-to-die" cases. Figure 4 serves as a "clue" regarding an important difference.

   Miss. C was Claire Conroy, an elderly New Jersey woman, whose case was ultimately heard by the New Jersey Supreme Court, and was one of the first cases in which it was ruled that there is no difference between artificial feeding and other forms of life support (In re. Conroy, 1985). This was also the first "right-to-die" case involving an adult who lacked decisional capacity because of dementia. Previous appellate cases dealt with patients who could not make medical decisions because of PVS, mental retardation, or other impairments. This case also reaffirmed the notion that there is no legal distinction between withholding or withdrawing treatment. Subsequent court cases have generally reaffirmed this stance, and extended these protections to patients whose lifespan was uncertain.

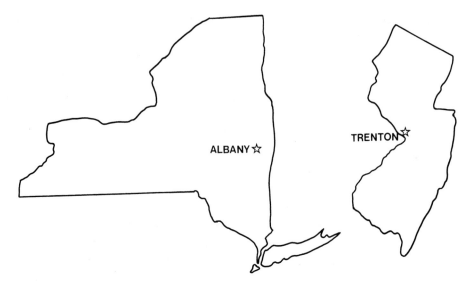

Figure 4 Jurisdictional differences led to disparate decisions about tube feeding in two patients with end-stage dementia.

Mrs. O, whose name was Mary O'Connor, lived in a different jurisdiction (New York State), and her case was decided quite differently (Matter of O'Connor, 1988). In Mrs. O'Connor's case, the state's highest court reversed two lower court decisions, and mandated that tube feeding be given. The Court held there was not "clear and convincing evidence" that she was opposed to artificial feeding in advanced dementia, despite her numerous statements regarding the abhorrence of artificial life support. The Court did not rule on the basis of prognosis, but on evidence of the patient's previously articulated wishes, which her family members were not allowed to interpret. The "clear and convincing" standard of New York, Missouri (where Ms Cruzan resided), and certain other states is more stringent than the standard of "substituted judgment" applied in states, such as New Jersey, in which a spokesperson is able to assert, in his or her best judgment, what an incompetent patient would have wanted. Thus, cases that were clinically similar, with evidence as to the patient's wishes comparable (perhaps even weaker for Miss Conroy than for Mrs. O'Connor), were decided quite differently in courts of law. The courts were acting to protect patient autonomy, and medical details were secondary.

Occasionally, the "best interests" standard is applied in court, as in one Arizona case, in which no one knew the patient – an elderly woman with multiple neurologic impairments – but tube feeding was stopped because it was found to be consistent with her best interests. "Best interests" are generally determined by weighing the benefits of a treatment against its burdens. If the burdens outweigh the benefits, then the treatment is considered not to be in the patient's best interests. This standard can be problematic, given the subjective nature of individual wants and desires, although generally a benefits–burdens analysis is based on what a "reasonable person" would want. Another point of view considers life itself as the highest good, never as a burden, and would therefore not consider ending life-sustaining treatment in most cases. The "best interests" standard is legally permissible in some, but not all, states.

6. PVS is a state of permanent eyes-open unconsciousness that results from complete and irreversible damage to the cerebral cortex. Brainstem functions such as respiration, pupillary responses, heartbeat, and pharyngeal–esophageal swallowing reflexes are maintained, and patients have been known to survive in this state for prolonged periods of time, the longest duration reported being 37 years. PVS must be distinguished from whole brain death, in which brainstem functions are also lost. When brainstem death occurs, respiration and heart beat soon cease.

   Patients with advanced dementia can sometimes progress to PVS but dementia can also be misdiagnosed as PVS. The distinction is important because patients with advanced dementia can experience pain, whereas a correctly diagnosed PVS patient is believed to be unable to experience anything, including pain.

   Legally, PVS and dementia may be governed by different legal standards in a few states, despite the fact that the difference is not always so vast from a neurologic point of view that clinical decisions must arbitrarily rest on these differences.

7. An advance directive such as a living will ("health care declaration"), proxy designation (also called "durable power of attorney for medical treatment" or "medical power of attorney"), executed while the individual has decisional capacity, provides written proof of the person's wishes regarding medical treatment, if the time comes that the patient loses the capacity to make these decisions. A living will delineates these wishes, while a durable power of attorney or proxy designation appoints an individual to make health care decisions. An advance directive may be oral, as opposed to written; conversations or oral instructions by a patient with capacity are considered to be evidence of the person's wishes. Likewise, written instructions may be informal – e.g. conveyed in a letter.

   As a practical matter, physicians and hospitals do not require written advance directives in all cases, and doing so would not only be unrealistic but would impose unacceptable burdens on patients. However, advance directives can be very important in cases in which there is controversy between surrogates and physicians, or among family members or other surrogate decision makers. Likewise, formal directives can be helpful in tube-feeding cases, which more often generate controversy than do other end-of-life decisions.

   Many states now have surrogate decision-making statutes, which delineate a hierarchy of people who are authorized to make decisions for patients who lack capacity but who have not executed formal advance directives. As in the case of written advance directives, surrogate decision-making statutes sometimes restrict decisions about tube feeding as compared with other treatments, such as demanding a higher level of evidence of the patient's wishes or specific preauthorization by the patient to refuse tube feeding. Whether such provisions are constitutional is debatable.

Caveats

1. In nursing homes, federal regulations motivate efforts to ascertain the patient's wishes and to encourage residents with capacity to execute formal advanced directives. However, a health care institution is permitted to refuse to withhold or withdraw ANH. Nursing homes are required to inform potential residents of such a policy ("conscience clause") upon admission, so the person could decide to go elsewhere. As a practical matter, however, patients or their family members may not understand this information or may not feel it is important enough to consider; if the issue of long-term feeding arises later on, it is difficult if not impossible to find another facility who would take the patient for the sole purpose of withdrawing tube feeding.

2. Disagreement on termination of treatment is sometimes due to a lack of communication rather than a difference in philosophy. Patients or their spokespersons may misunderstand the medical situation, and may change their position when the medical facts are clarified. The physician or the hospital may misunderstand the law, which, if clarified, may dispel fear of liability. For example, a physician may refuse to honor a living will in a state with only a proxy statute, or may refuse to honor a document from another state, thinking it would not apply in the state where care was being rendered. The absence of an actual statute does not mean that the document has no meaning, and many state statutes contain language explicitly permitting the use of appropriate documents from other jurisdictions. If not, such documents can be used as evidence of the person's wishes, if providers are unwilling to consider nonwritten statements as evidence of the person's wishes.

3. An instruction on an advance directive not to resuscitate (DNR) does not automatically ensure a person will have a DNR order in an institution or at home. Resuscitation decisions demand split-second action, and, unless emergency medical personnel or other health professionals have information to the contrary, they are required to resuscitate a person with impending cardiorespiratory arrest. For this reason, DNR discussions should occur as soon as possible for patients who are at risk for cardiorespiratory arrest.

REFERENCES

Ahronheim, J. C. (1996). Artificial nutrition and hydration in the terminally ill patient. *Clinics in Geriatric Medicine*, **12**, 379–91.

Cruzan v. Director, Missouri Department of Health, 497 U.S. 261 (1990).

Finucane, T. E. and Bynum, J. P. (1996). Use of tube feeding to prevent aspiration pneumonia. *Lancet*, **348**, 1421–4.

Huang, Z. B. and Ahronheim, J. C. (2000). Artificial nutrition and hydration in terminally ill patients: an update. *Clinics in Geriatric Medicine*, **16**, 313–25.

In re. Conroy, 98 NJ 321, 486 A.2d 1209 (1985).

Matter of O'Connor, 72 NY 2d 517 (1988).

Meier, D. E., Ahronheim, J. D., Morris, J. *et al.* (2001). High short-term mortality in hospitalized patients with advanced dementia: lack of benefit of tube feeding. *Archives of Internal Medicine*, **161**, 594–9.

Sieger, C. E., Arnold, J. F., and Ahronheim, J. C. (2002). Refusing artificial nutrition and hydration: does statutory law send the wrong message? *Journal of the American Geriatrics Society*, **50**, 544–50.

BIBLIOGRAPHY

American Academy of Neurology (1989). Position of the American Academy of Neurology on certain aspects of the care and management of the persistent vegetative state. *Neurology*, **39**, 125–6.

Childs, N. L., Mercer, W. N., and Childs, H. W. (1993). Accuracy of diagnosis of persistent vegetative state. *Neurology*, **43**, 1465–7.

Ciocon, J. O., Silverstone, F. A., Graver, M. *et al.* (1988). Tube feeding in elderly patients. Indications, benefits, and complications. *Archives of Internal Medicine*, **148**, 429–33.

Epstein, M. and Hollenberg, N. K. (1976). Age as a determinant of renal sodium conservation in normal man. *Journal of Laboratory and Clinical Medicine*, **87**, 411–17.

Finucane, T. E. (1999). Tube feeding in patients with advanced dementia: a review of the evidence. *Journal of the American Medical Association*, **282**, 1365–70.

Gillick, M. R. (2000). Rethinking the role of tube feeding in patients with advanced dementia. *New England Journal of Medicine*, **342**, 206–10.

McCann, R. M., Hall, W. J., and Groth-Juncker, A. (1994). Comfort care for terminally ill patients. The appropriate use of nutrition and hydration. *Journal of the American Medical Association*, **272**, 1263–6.

Rowe, J. W., Shock, N. W., and DeFronzo, R. A. (1976). The influence of age on the renal response to water deprivation in man. *Nephron*, **17**, 270–8.

Case 8

▶▶ Occupational deterioration

A 69-year-old woman has worked as a secretary for many years, and is about to become your patient. You receive a call from a concerned supervisor at her place of employment that the patient is no longer functioning well at work, where she is responsible for typing, payroll function, and signing checks. The office staff have been assisting her, but her function has deteriorated so much that action is called for. The supervisor wants to know what to expect, and whether there is anything she can do to help.

On physical examination, the patient's face is expressionless. She walks slowly, without swinging her arms, and has a slightly stooped posture. She has a resting, to-and-fro tremor of both hands, and her lips and legs are noted to tremble slightly. Upper extremities exhibit increased tone, suggestive of muscle rigidity. The patient says things are going well at work, but she appears and sounds depressed. Grossly, her memory appears intact; she is able to discuss her work, mentions her colleagues by name and talks about them warmly, and is able to discuss current events.

Levodopa–carbidopa (Sinemet) has been prescribed for her condition, but she takes it erratically, saying she can't remember to take it so often. She denies falls and dizziness and has not been treated with any psychiatric medications.

The patient lives alone, is unmarried, and has no children or close friends.

Questions

1. What disease does the physical examination suggest? How can this be ascertained?
2. Why might she be depressed?
3. What are some reasons that she is not functioning well at work?

Case Studies in Geriatric Medicine, Judith C. Ahronheim *et al.* Published by Cambridge University Press.
© J. C. Ahronheim, Z.-B. Huang, V. Yen, C. M. Davitt, and D. Barile

> 4. What can be done to maximize her occupational function?
> 5. What other symptoms may occur in the future?
> 6. What potential side effects of pharmacologic treatment are likely to occur?

Answers

1. The patient has classic idiopathic Parkinson's disease (PD), characterized in her case by signs such as "pill-rolling" tremor, bradykinesia (slowness of movement), rigidity, and mask-like facies. Sophisticated neuroimaging techniques may be able to identify a preclinical state, and are useful in research, but the clinical examination currently remains the "gold standard" in the diagnosis of this condition.

    Idiopathic PD must be distinguished from Parkinson-like symptoms that can be produced by drugs with dopamine antagonist activity, such as antipsychotic agents and metoclopramide, because this "drug-induced parkinsonism" is generally reversible with discontinuation of the drug. It is also important to distinguish parkinsonian tremor from other types of tremor that occur commonly in the elderly. Benign essential ("senile") tremor differs in that it may be familial, is not associated with symptoms of PD, such as rigidity or bradykinesia, and worsens on intention. Parkinsonian tremor improves on intention. Nervousness, agitation, and hyperthyroidism can worsen or unmask all of these tremors, and sleep suppresses them.

    Other neurologic conditions share features of PD in their early stages; these include progressive supranuclear palsy (PSP), multisystem atrophy, and dementia with Lewy bodies (DLB). Idiopathic PD can usually be differentiated from these conditions, which more often present without tremor, with truncal as opposed to limb rigidity, atypical symptoms such as dysarthria, or poor response to levodopa–carbidopa. In multisystem atrophy, autonomic dysfunction is prominent. These "Parkinson plus" syndromes are discussed in detail in the references (see Mark, 2001).

2. Depression is extremely common in PD, and occurs out of proportion to the severity of the disease. Depression is at least twice as common in PD than in other chronic diseases. Depression in PD is believed to be due to neurohormonal alterations, such as deficiencies in the dopaminergic and serotonin systems, although "exogenous" factors are likely to play a role, as would be expected in any patient who has to cope with loss. In this case, the patient is experiencing waning occupational function, difficulty learning new office techniques efficiently, lack of social supports outside the work place, and concerns about loss of income.

3. Bradykinesia refers not merely to slowness of gait, but to a generalized diminution in the rate and extent of movement. Certainly, the manual dexterity of a typist–payroll worker could be impaired by the disease. Handwriting characteristically deteriorates and not only shows the signs of a tremor, but may diminish in size ("micrographia"). Generalized symptoms such as fatigue and weakness are common and, along with depression, would certainly impair her stamina. The voice may become soft, making it difficult for others to understand the patient. Slowness of verbal response may give the appearance of dementia where none exists. This, combined with drooling that affects some patients, mask-like facies, and other symptoms, may interfere with personal interactions in the work setting. Finally, although the patient's memory does not seem overtly impaired, she might have subtle cognitive and visuomotor impairments, along with mood and personality derangements that may occur early on in the disease, sometimes before the onset of motor symptoms.

4. Although the long-term prognosis for her career is not good, much can be gained from a multipronged approach, including optimization of her medical regimen, physical therapy, treatment of depression, and advanced care planning. Fortunately, this woman works in a situation where others are patient and willing to help.

Drug selection must be carefully tailored to the needs of individual patients. Levodopa–carbidopa (Sinemet), at the lowest possible dose, is considered first-line treatment for most elderly. It is common practice to withhold levodopa–carbidopa until later in the disease, because levodopa metabolism produces oxidative radicals that have the potential to produce neuronal damage and accelerate disease progression. Dopamine agonists, such as bromocriptine (Parlodel) and pramipexole (Mirapex), are believed to confer neuroprotection by promoting the scavenging of free radicals. These, and other agents with neuroprotective potential, such as selegiline (Eldeprel), have therefore been promoted as initial therapy, with levodopa–carbidopa added later on to enhance control of motor symptoms. However, this approach has been a source of great controversy because evidence that neuroprotective agents retard progression and that levodopa accelerates it is inconclusive. In any case, this strategy may not be possible in elderly patients, who often fail to tolerate those medications.

This patient is a good candidate for levodopa–carbidopa at this time because her disease is impairing her function. Levodopa exerts its pharmacologic effect through its chief metabolite, dopamine. Since most ingested levodopa is rapidly converted to dopamine, which does not pass the blood–brain barrier, levodopa is given in combination with carbidopa, a peripheral inhibitor of this conversion. This combination enables more levodopa to pass into the brain before degradation, enhancing its efficacy and preventing nausea from excess peripheral dopamine.

Amantadine, and dopamine agonists such as bromocriptine and pramipexole, though often given as first-line therapy in younger patients with mild disease, in the elderly are generally reserved for adjunctive treatment, such as control of drug-induced dyskinesia or smoothing out dose response of levodopa–carbidopa. Anticholinergic agents such as benztropine (Cogentin) and trihexyphenidyl (Artane), and the anticholinergic antihistamine diphenhydramine (Benadryl), are used to ameliorate drooling and tremor. These anticholinergic agents are not always well tolerated in the elderly (see below). Treatment approaches are discussed in detail in the references (see Guttman *et al.*, 2003).

Treatment of motor symptoms often reduces depression in PD, but appropriate antidepressant medications and supportive psychotherapy are generally needed. Selective serotonin reuptake inhibitors (SSRIs) are generally better tolerated than other antidepressants in the elderly, although concern has been raised over their use in PD because of a slightly increased risk of extrapyramidal symptoms from SSRIs as compared with other antidepressants. Still, overall, SSRIs are the logical first-line treatment owing to their generally better overall tolerability.

Since exercise is important in maintaining function in the face of muscle rigidity, a regular exercise program should be suggested. Daily walks during lunchtime or coffee breaks might be effective, especially if there are others in the office to reinforce the regimen. A physical therapy program would probably be beneficial and should include gait training because postural instability and inability to maintain balance during change of position increase the risk of falls.

5. Over time, the effect of medications will wane. Many patients eventually experience the "on–off" phenomenon, a form of symptom fluctuation characterized by rapid improvement shortly after a dose of levodopa–carbidopa is given ("on"), followed by rapid deterioration ("off") at unpredictable intervals. This may be more than an end-of-dose phenomenon, but rather related to disease progression, which is associated with a decreased ability of the brain to store dopamine, and, possibly, enhanced production of toxic drug metabolites.

If the patient survives into the late stages of the disease, she will likely develop "dopa-resistant" symptoms including motor deterioration, worsening gait, loss of ambulation, and poverty of speech. Autonomic dysfunction may occur, leading to symptoms such as orthostatic hypotension, excessive sweating, and impaired thermoregulation. Urinary incontinence and constipation have been linked to neurologic changes in PD, although in older patients these symptoms may be due to coexisting pathology. Sleep disturbances, dementia, and hallucinations are common late in the disease. Dementia is progressive, and in severe cases resembles late-stage Alzheimer's disease and other neurodegenerative dementias (see Cases 6 and 7).

6. Dopaminergic agents themselves may produce psychiatric symptoms such as paranoia and hallucinations, and may also produce choreiform movements. These drug-related symptoms are generally reversible and tend to be dose related, but

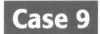

▸▸ Atypical dementia

A 77-year-old woman comes to your office at the urging of her family, who report that the patient has memory loss and personality change. She occasionally uses "vulgar language," has lapses in grooming, and sometimes seems to have a "blank stare." The patient has otherwise been healthy, lives independently since her husband died several years ago, and spends a lot of time with her adult children and grandchildren when she can. Her son lives in a nearby suburb and visits often.

The patient arrives at your office on time and is not accompanied by any family member. She is well groomed and dressed in stylish clothes. She is friendly and interactive, and her affect appears normal. She reports laughingly that her son wanted her to be seen because her "memory is not as good as it used to be," and she agrees, stating, "after all, I am 77." On physical examination, blood pressure and pulse are normal. Neurologic examination reveals normal deep tendon reflexes, downgoing plantar response, and no focal neurologic signs. There is no tremor. Gait seems slightly stereotypic.

Folstein Mini-Mental State Examination (MMSE) is administered. The patient knows the exact day and date and is able to recall three of three objects. She is unable to draw intersecting pentagon shapes and makes errors when subtracting serial 7s. Total score on the MMSE is 27 out of a possible 30 points.

Laboratory tests including blood chemistries, serum B12 level, thyroid-stimulating hormone (TSH), and serologic test for syphilis are all normal. Given the absence of focal findings, computed tomography (CT) scan is deferred.

Case Studies in Geriatric Medicine, Judith C. Ahronheim *et al.* Published by Cambridge University Press.
© J. C. Ahronheim, Z.-B. Huang, V. Yen, C. M. Davitt, and D. Barile

Questions

1. How would you interpret the MMSE results?
2. What would the CT scan be expected to reveal?
3. Given the family's observations, what might be going on?

Answers

1. Using the standard cut-off score (23 or less signifying dementia), this patient's overall score is within the normal range. However, the MMSE, as well as other instruments developed for screening or evaluation of dementia, have a limited sensitivity, depending on the characteristics of the screened population (see Case 4). The family has already observed changes, while the patient's impairment has not prevented her from appearing normal to a new observer. The importance of information from a reliable informant has led to informant-based instruments, such as the Informant Questionnaire in Cognitive Decline in the Elderly (IQCODE) (Jorm, 1994), which assess the patient's ability to perform certain functions and can enhance the sensitivity of other screening tests.

   Furthermore, the MMSE, which emphasizes memory parameters, is less sensitive in the diagnosis of nonAlzheimer's dementias, which may present with subtle symptoms such as personality change, mental slowing, or changes in other complex cognitive processes. Unlike most patients with early Alzheimer's disease, this patient has retained the ability to recall three objects and knows the exact date, but has made errors in nonmemory domains. The ability to draw a simple shape requires only basic visual–spatial skills, and her inability to do this in the context of retained orientation and object recall may imply some degree of impaired executive function. Although the ability to concentrate usually permits a normal person to subtract serial 7s, one could argue that someone who was "bad in arithmetic" might have great difficulty with this test. An alternate measure of concentration includes spelling a word backwards or reciting the months backwards. Additional neuropsychologic testing would be needed to delineate her cognitive deficits, but these do not accurately distinguish one form of dementia from another.

2. As discussed in Case 4, structural brain imaging often demonstrates abnormalities, such as atrophy or white matter changes, but these findings are present in many cognitively normal elderly and their detection does not aid the differential diagnosis. Moreover, this patient's lack of focal neurologic findings and the nature and onset of her symptoms make it very unlikely that neuroimaging would reveal a discrete

lesion. Functional neuroimaging, such as positron emission tomography (PET), may be capable of detecting abnormalities at an early stage in certain brain diseases, but currently these methods do not augment the value of clinical evaluation in differentiating one form of dementia from another.

3. Concerns about memory loss in a highly functioning individual suggests mild cognitive impairment (MCI) (see Case 2). However, there is little objective confirmation of memory loss on her interview or on screening with MMSE. MCI as currently defined, is believed to be a precursor to a "typical" dementia, such as Alzheimer's disease, whereas this patient's subtle reported changes are more consistent with the early stages of a nonAlzheimer's dementia.

It is possible that this patient is developing dementia with Lewy bodies (DLB), the second most common form of neurodegenerative dementia, in which parkinsonian signs are prominent, memory is spared early on, and delusions and deficits in attention and visual–spatial function occur. The frontotemporal dementias (classically, Pick's disease) present with a predominance of behavioral aberrations, including disinhibition and impulsiveness, or with language difficulties and personality change. Creutzfeld–Jakob disease (spongiform encephalopathy) increases in incidence with age but is a very rare disease overall. In this disease, ataxia and myoclonus are usually the presenting signs; dementia and motor dysfunction are rapidly progressive, and death usually occurs within 1–2 years. As discussed in Case 4, HIV dementia and Lyme disease should also be considered in certain circumstances, although, when asked, this patient and her family denied risk factors.

Eight months later, the patient is brought in by her son, who reports that her memory and ability to care for herself have gotten worse. They also note that the patient has seen "children's faces" in her bedroom at night, but rather than being troubled by them she has stated that "they are rather cute." On examination, she appears slightly disheveled – her clothes are clean but her dress is not stylish, and her grey hair roots are visible. The "blank stare" previously described by her son is clearly apparent to the physician, which she interprets as "parkinsonian facies." Her gait is now frankly parkinsonian. There is no tremor. MMSE is done; the patient knows the day and date and is able to recall three objects, but cannot spell "world" backwards or name the months backwards. The son has taken the patient to a neurologist who ordered a CT scan of the brain which shows cortical atrophy "appropriate for age."

Questions

1. How does this information change the differential diagnosis?
2. What treatment can be offered?

Answers

1. The presence of parkinsonism does not necessarily indicate idiopathic Parkinson's disease (PD). Many patients with PD develop dementia during the course of the disease, the incidence increasing with age at the onset of PD. Although subtle cognitive defects are common early on, the patient usually comes to attention because of typical motor symptoms, as described in Case 9. The present patient came to attention because of cognitive and behavioral changes, and, although the family had noted a "blank stare," the physician did not appreciate that subtle change when she met the patient for the first time. It is likely that this patient has DLB, which is part of a spectrum of disorders histologically associated with Lewy bodies. The clinical spectrum of these disorders includes PD, PD with dementia, DLB, and autonomic failure without parkinsonian motor features. Idiopathic PD usually presents with motor symptoms out of proportion to or in the absence of psychiatric or cognitive impairments, while DLB presents with cognitive or behavioral signs earlier than or out of proportion to parkinsonism. In addition to parkinsonian gait and facies, which this patient has, many other typical signs of PD may be present in DLB, but tremor is typically absent, as in this case.

   There is some overlap between the clinical features of DLB and Alzheimer's disease, but, in Alzheimer's disease, parkinsonian features are uncommon and memory loss is prominent earlier on. Frontotemporal dementias are associated with disinhibition, but parkinsonian features are not prominent.

   Other dementing illnesses associated with parkinsonian features are noted in Case 9 and discussed in the references (see Mark, 2001). In these diseases, dementia may be a late finding and motor abnormalities may overshadow cognitive problems early in the disease.

2. Although antiparkinsonian drugs, such as levodopa–carbidopa, may improve motor function in some patients with DLB, benefit is usually limited and often occurs at the expense of cognitive function. Delusions and hallucinations, which occur commonly in DLB, can be exacerbated by levodopa and dopamine agonists. Likewise, neuroleptic agents, which can control delusions and hallucinations, generally worsen parkinsonism and must be used with extreme caution. Even "atypical" neuroleptics, which preferably block D3, D4, and D4 receptors, such as olanzapine (Zyprexa) and quetiapine (Seroquel) may worsen parkinsonism in these patients. Clozapine (Clozaril) has been most consistently shown to reduce psychiatric symptoms while sparing motor function, although irreversible leukopenia can occur in rare circumstances.

   Cholinesterase inhibitors, such as donepezil and rivastigmine, may improve cognitive and behavioral symptoms in some patients with DLB. Improvements occur in apathy, delusions, attention, and, to a lesser extent, hallucinations. These improvements contrast with minimal observable benefit in memory among patients with Alzheimer's disease.

As with other progressive dementias, nonpharmacologic approaches should be employed whenever possible (see Case 5).

Caveat

Depression, hallucinations, and delusions occur in 30–50% of patients with DLB, often at the time of presentation. For this reason, such patients may often lead to psychiatric referral and misdiagnosis. Use of a neuroleptic in these situations can worsen the motor symptoms of the disease, often to a marked degree.

REFERENCES

Jorm, A. F. (1994). A short form of the Informant Questionnaire in Cognitive Decline in the Elderly (IQCODE): development and cross-validation. *Psychological Medicine*, **24**, 134–53.

Mark, M. H. (2001). Lumping and splitting the parkinson plus syndromes. Dementia with Lewy bodies, multiple system atrophy, progressive supranuclear palsy, and cortical-basal ganglionic degeneration. *Neurologic Clinics*, **19**, 607–27.

BIBLIOGRAPHY

Brown, P. (1997). The risk of bovine spongiform encephalopathy ("Mad Cow Disease") to human health. *Journal of the American Medical Association*, **278**, 1008–11.

Chui, H. and Zhang, Q. (1997). Evaluation of dementia: a systematic study of the usefulness of the American Academy of Neurology's practice parameters. *Neurology*, **49**, 925–35.

Folstein, M. F., Folstein, S. E., and McHugh, P. R. (1975). "Mini-Mental State." A practical method for grading the cognitive state of patients for the clinician. *Journal of Psychiatric Research*, **12**, 189–98.

Heyman, A., Fillenbaum, G. G., Gearing, M. *et al.* (1999). Comparison of Lewy body variant of Alzheimer's disease with pure Alzheimer's diease: consortium to Establish a Registry for Alzheimer's Disease, Part XIX. *Neurology*, **52**, 1839–44.

Knopman, D. S., DeKosky, S. T., Cummings, J. L. *et al.* (2001). Practice parameter: diagnosis of dementia (an evidence-based review). Report of the Quality Standards Subcommittee of the American Academy of Neurology. *Neurology*, **56**, 1143–53.

McKeith, I., Del Ser, T., Spano, P. *et al.* (2000). Efficacy of rivastigmine in dementia with Lewy bodies: a randomised, double-blind, placebo-controlled international study. *Lancet,* **356**, 2031–6.

McKeith, I. G. and Burn, D. (2000). Spectrum of Parkinson's disease, Parkinson's dementia, and Lewy body dementia. *Neurologic Clinics,* **18**, 865–83.

McKeith, I. G., Galasko, D., Kosaka, K. *et al.* (1996). Consensus guidelines for the clinical and pathologic diagnosis of dementia with Lewy bodies (DLB): report of the consortium on DLB international workshop. *Neurology,* **47**, 1113–24.

McKeith, I. G., Perry, E. K., and Perry, R. H. (1999). Report of the second dementia with Lewy body international workshop. *Neurology,* **53**, 902–5.

Neary, D., Snowden, J. S., Gustafson, L. *et al.* (1998). Frontotemporal lobar degeneration: a consensus on clinical diagnostic criteria. *Neurology,* **51**, 1546–54.

Petersen, R. C., Stevens, J. C., Ganguli, M. *et al.* (2001). Practice parameter: early detection of dementia: mild cognitive impairment (an evidence-based review). Report of the Quality Standards Subcommittee of the American Academy of Neurology. *Neurology,* **56**, 1133–42.

Small, J. B., Viitanen, M., and Backman, L. (1997). Mini-Mental State Examination item scores as predictors of Alzheimer's disease: incidence data from the Kungsholmen Project, Stockholm. *Journals of Gerontology,* **52A**, M299–304.

Tierney, M. C., Herrmann N., Geslani, D. M. *et al.* (2003). Contribution of informant and patient ratings to the accuracy of the mini-mental state examination in predicting probable Alzheimer's disease. *Journal of the American Geriatrics Society,* **51**, 813–18.

Case 10

▸▸ "Pseudodementia"

A 79-year-old retired teacher is brought to you by her son, who is worried that she has Alzheimer's disease. She is forgetful, requires assistance with most activities of daily living (ADL), has difficulty in sleeping, and spends her day in aimless behavior and complaining. The son reports that his mother had been "difficult," tending to be upset by trivial issues, and has withdrawn from many of her usual activities in the past year, since her 85-year-old husband had a stroke. The family was forced to hire a 24-hour home attendant, and the cost has been very burdensome. The son admits that the patient has seemed depressed, but says, "that's nothing new." She recently had a medical evaluation, which included blood tests, and everything "checked out."

The patient is slender and appears restless. Her affect is depressed but she answers questions and follows commands. Her blood pressure is 120/80; pulse is 70 and regular. She can walk unassisted and her gait is steady. She needs a lot of encouragement to complete the Mini-Mental State Examination (MMSE), scoring 24 out of 30. She recalls only two of three objects, is unable to give the exact date, and says it's spring although it is still winter. She first refused to spell "world" backward, but, after being encouraged, she tried and was able to do this correctly. When asked where she is, she shakes her head, saying, "oh, I don't know." She refuses to complete all items and frequently during the interview, she says, "why can't I go home?" Other than the MMSE, the neurologic examination is normal.

Questions

1. What is the cause of the patient's memory loss and decline in her ADL?
2. What treatment is indicated?
3. What alternate treatments exist for elderly patients?

Case Studies in Geriatric Medicine, Judith C. Ahronheim *et al.* Published by Cambridge University Press.
© J. C. Ahronheim, Z.-B. Huang, V. Yen, C. M. Davitt, and D. Barile

> 4. What impact will treatment have on her memory in the short term and in the long term?

Answers

1. Patients with dementia may develop behavioral problems and dependence in ADL, but this usually happens in the later stages. Although a MMSE score may be higher than a patient's function would predict, the patient's performance on the MMSE makes it difficult to attribute her ADL dependence to dementia alone. Likewise, there is no apparent evidence of a significant medical problem. Her ability to spell backwards suggests that she can focus her attention if she wants to, which makes delirium unlikely. Although the patient "acts" demented at home, her memory problem could be the result of depression, as her affect suggests, and this is consistent with the onset of symptoms following a major stressor (her husband's illness and associated financial strain), and with the possibility that she has had depression in the past. Alternatively, this patient might have early dementia or mild cognitive impairment with concurrent or associated depression.

   Depression in the elderly can present with cognitive deficits such as inattention, memory impairment, and slowness of mental processing. Physicians often fail to diagnose depression in elderly patients, who might focus on somatic symptoms, and underreport emotional ones. Declining cognitive function, medication side effects, or physical symptoms due to chronic disorders may all prevent the patient from describing depressive symptoms or may divert the patient's or the health care provider's attention from a mood disorder.

   The depression is best confirmed with a formal psychiatric interview, but several tools exist that can assist primary care providers to identify patients with depression (see Case 11). These scales can be used in patients with dementia if their cognitive function is adequate to comprehend the questions. The patient completed a 15-item version of the Geriatric Depression Scale (GDS) and scored 10 of 15, suggesting depression.

2. Whether the patient has depression affecting memory and behavior, or early dementia with depression, antidepressant medication should be given. Symptom relief will improve her function and will help to clarify the diagnosis. Although psychotherapy is useful in certain circumstances, especially as adjunctive therapy (see below), it is insufficient as initial treatment in severe depression, especially if cognitive dysfunction is present. Selective serotonin reuptake inhibitors (SSRIs) have mostly replaced tricyclic antidepressants (TCAs) as the first-line agents for elderly

patients with depression, with or without dementia, because they are generally as effective as TCAs but much better tolerated. However, SSRIs sometimes cause gastrointestinal disturbances, especially diarrhea, and, despite their paucity of constitutional symptoms, have, like TCAs, been associated with an increased risk of falls in nursing home patients. Among the SSRIs, sertraline (Zoloft), citalopram (Celexa), and perhaps the newest agent escitalopram (Lexapro) are the least likely to interact with other medications. Currently, this patient is not taking medications, so paroxetine (Paxil) would be an alternative. Fluoxetine (Prozac), which has a very long half-life, is usually reserved for patients who may not adhere to a daily regimen.

Bupropion (Wellbutrin) is also well tolerated by elderly patients and is "activating" and may be useful in patients who tend to be withdrawn. Other antidepressants, such as nefazodone (Serzone), mirtazapine (Remeron), and venlafaxine (Effexor), are more sedating and may be especially useful in patients with agitated depression or severe chronic insomnia, or when other antidepressants fail. In the elderly, especially those with dementia, sedating antidepressants are preferable to cotherapy with benzodiazepines which increase the risk of falls and mental confusion. Psychostimulants, such as methylphenidate or dextroamphetamine, are sometimes used in the management of depression when a rapid response is needed and are usually well tolerated in older individuals.

TCAs may still be important options in older patients with depression, but they must be used cautiously because of their anticholinergic properties, which can produce dry mouth, constipation, urinary retention, confusion, blurred vision, and orthostatic hypotension. TCAs can also cause sedation and slow cardiac conduction. Among TCAs, doxepin (Sinequan), amitriptyline (Elavil), and imipramine (Tofranil) are not recommended for older persons, while the less anticholinergic TCAs, nortriptyline (Pamelor) and desipramine (Norpramin), are preferred if a TCA is needed.

3. Psychotherapy may be effective in late-life depression, alone or in combination with antidepressant medication, as long as patients have adequate cognitive function. Standardized approaches, such as cognitive–behavioral therapy and interpersonal therapy, have demonstrated benefit. These are important alternatives in patients who do not want to take medication, cannot tolerate drug therapy, or need additional help dealing with stressful situations. In the long-term treatment of depression, psychotherapy can prolong the depression-free period.

Electroconvulsive therapy (ECT) is well tolerated by elderly patients and should be considered in major depression that does not respond to medications. Other indications include an inability to tolerate antidepressants, or when there is a life-threatening complication such as severe anorexia, weight loss, or catatonia. Elderly depressed patients with neurovegetative symptoms seem to respond better to ECT than to medication, while those with dementia may not adequately respond. The most common adverse effects of ECT are transient delirium or memory problems, and transient cardiac arrhythmias. ECT is discussed in detail in the references (see Kelly and Zisselman, 2000).

4. It is very likely that, when this patient's depression is adequately treated, her cognitive function might also improve. Nevertheless, depressed elderly patients with cognitive impairment often remain demented following antidepressant treatment and despite improvement in mood. Prospective observational studies have shown that many depressed patients with mild cognitive impairment later develop Alzheimer's disease (see van Reekum *et al.*, 1999; Visser *et al.*, 2000). Such patients tend to be older and have more severe memory impairment than those whose cognitive impairment is solely due to depression. Therefore, the term "*pseudo*dementia" (referring to patients whose cognitive function improves after treatment of depression) may be misleading, since some cases may actually represent preclinical dementia. After this patient is treated for depression, her cognitive function should be re-evaluated.

Caveat

The risk of suicide increases markedly with age among white men, with those older than 65 years having a suicide rate five times higher than the general population.

REFERENCES

Kelly, K. G. and Zisselman, M. (2000). Update on electroconvulsive therapy (ECT) in older adults. *Journal of the American Geriatrics Society*, **48**, 560–6.

van Reekum, R., Simard, M., Clarke, D. *et al.* (1999). Late-life depression as a possible predictor of dementia: cross-sectional and short-term follow-up results. *American Journal of Geriatric Psychiatry*, **7**, 151–9.

Visser, P. J., Verbey, F. R. J., Ponds, R. W. H. M. *et al.* (2000). Distinction between preclinical Alzheimer's disease and depression. *Journal of American Geriatric Society*, **48**, 479–84.

BIBLIOGRAPHY

Amenian, H. K., Pratt, L. A., Gallo, J. *et al.* (1998). Psychopathology as a predictor of disability: a population-based follow-up study in Baltimore, Maryland. *American Journal of Epidemiology*, **148**, 269–75.

Conwell, Y., Duberstein, P. R., Cox, C. *et al.* (1996). Relationships of age and axis I diagnoses in victims of completed suicide: a psychological autopsy study. *American Journal of Psychiatry*, **153**, 1001–8.

Dennis, M. S. and Lindesay, J. L. (1995). Suicide in the elderly: the United Kingdom Perspective. *International Psychogeriatrics*, **7**, 263–74.

Lebowitz, B. D., Pearson, J. L., Schneider, L. S. *et al.* (1997). Diagnosis and treatment of depression in late life. Consensus statement update. *Journal of American Medical Association*, **278**, 1186–90.

Meehan, P. J., Saltzman, L. E., and Sattin, R. W. (1991). Suicides among older United States residents: epidemiologic characteristics and trends. *American Journal of Public Health*, **81**, 1198–200.

Mulsant, B. H. and Ganguli, M. (1999). Epidemiology and diagnosis of depression in late life. *Journal of Clinical Psychiatry*, **60** (suppl 20), 9–15.

Parmelee, P. A., Katz, I. R., and Lawton, M. P. (1989). Depression among institutionalized aged: assessment and prevalence estimation. *Journal of Gerontology*, **44**, M22–9.

Reifler, B. V. (2000). A case of mistaken identity: pseudodementia is really predementia. *Journal of the American Geriatrics Society*, **48**, 593–4.

Reynolds, C. F. 3rd, Alexopoulos, G. S., Katz, I. R. *et al.* (2001). Chronic depression in the elderly: approaches for prevention. *Drugs and Aging*, **18**, 507–14.

Ritche, K., Touchon, J., and Ledesert, B. (1998). Progressive disability in senile dementia is accelerated in the presence of depression. *International Journal of Geriatric Psychiatry*, **13**, 459–61.

Solai, L. K., Mulsant, B. H., and Ploolck, B. G. (2001). Selective serotonin reuptake inhibitors for late-life depression: a comparative review. *Drugs and Aging*, **18**, 355–68.

Steffens, D. C., Skoog, I., Norton, M. C. *et al.* (2000). Prevalence of depression and its treatment in an elderly population: the Cache County Study. *Archives of General Psychiatry*, **57**, 601–7.

Thapa, P. B., Gideon, P., Cost, T. W. *et al.* (1998). Antidepressants and the risk of falls among nursing home residents. *New England Journal of Medicine*, **339**, 875–82.

Yousef, G., Ryan, W. J., Lambert, T. *et al.* (1998). A preliminary report: a new scale to identify the pseudodementia syndrome. *International Journal of Geriatric Psychiatry*, **3**, 389–99.

Case 11

▶▶ Chest pain

An 88-year-old woman comes in to your office and complains of "soreness in the chest." She seems distressed and clutches a bottle of pills in each hand. She tells you these are her friend's medications and asks, "Should I take this (nitroglycerin)? Should I take this (lorazepam)? Should I go out? Should I stay in? What should I do?"

The chest pain is not related to meals or exertion. Nothing seems to make it better or worse. Her physical examination, electrocardiogram (EKG), labs, chest X-ray, and abdominal ultrasound yield no clues. An investigation of the patient's life stressors is begun.

The patient's husband died 4 years ago of a myocardial infarction. She lives alone but has a lot of friends, and, since her husband's death, has resumed an active social life. She does, however, admit to a recent onset of anxious and depressed mood and worries about having a heart attack. She is reluctant to discuss more.

Questions

1. What information does the patient's EKG contribute to the diagnosis of ischemic heart disease?
2. What could be troubling an 88-year-old woman?
3. What further testing or treatment should be offered to this patient?

Answers

1. About 50% of elderly individuals have abnormalities of the resting EKG – most commonly, intraventricular conduction abnormalities, PR and QT prolongation,

Case Studies in Geriatric Medicine, Judith C. Ahronheim *et al.* Published by Cambridge University Press.
© J. C. Ahronheim, Z.-B. Huang, V. Yen, C. M. Davitt, and D. Barile

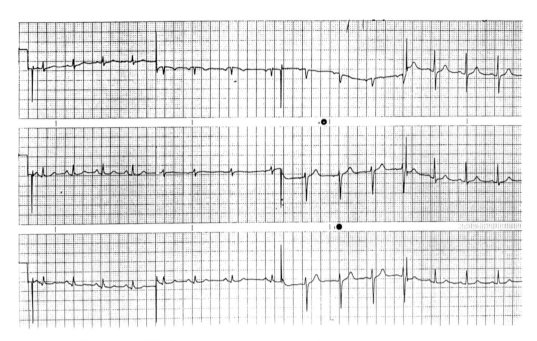

Figure 5   The patient's EKG showing poor R-wave progression.

and reduction in QRS voltage, as well as a more superior and leftward orientation of the QRS vector. This patient's EKG revealed poor R-wave progression (see
Figure 5); although suggestive of underlying cardiac disease, it is a nonspecific finding and neither rules in nor rules out cardiac disease. Change in body position
appears to affect the precordial leads much more in the elderly than in others,
perhaps because of alterations in thoracic anatomy or because of changes in elasticity of the great vessels. Thus, the information available on this patient is quite
nonspecific.

2. Although cardiac disease can present atypically in the elderly (see Case 15), the
patient's symptoms seem noncardiac in nature and could well be related to stress,
as her frustrated affect suggests. Somatic symptoms are a common manifestation
of depression and often mask depression in the elderly. Many elderly patients who
deny depression will present with somatic complaints rather than classic symptoms
of dysphoric mood. Physicians should evaluate and treat these patients based on
their particular clinical presentations, while maintaining a suspicion for depression.

Disease itself, and the inability to cope with the involution of health at the end of
life, can precipitate depression, but older individuals suffer repeated personal losses
as well. Death of a spouse is the most obvious major loss that should be inquired
about, but very elderly people often outlive siblings, close friends, and sometimes
their children. It is very important to inquire whether a distressed patient has

recently experienced the death of any of these important people. This particular patient had functioned well for the 4 years following the death of her husband, to whom she had been married since the age of 18, but she had recently started to date again. As a pitfall of her new lifestyle, she had been jilted by a regular gentleman visitor in favor of a younger woman, who herself was over 80 years of age. She did not volunteer this information, and it was not elicited immediately, perhaps because of the embarrassment that such behavior caused her. She may have viewed dating at her age as unseemly or may have felt guilt over renewed sexuality.

Other underrecognized stressors in late life can contribute to depressive symptoms, including loss of employment, especially among men 60–75 years of age. Other aspects of depression in the elderly are discussed in Case 10.

3. Although cardiac disease can present atypically in the elderly, further cardiac testing may not be warranted in this patient at this time. It would be very important to question her about any symptoms during future visits, but a cardiac workup at this point might cause her undue worry and could be counterproductive. Rather, attention to her stressors would take precedence, and this would represent a worthwhile effort by the primary care physician.

Tests to screen for depression might be revealing, since psychiatric consultation is often strongly resisted by patients who seek care for their symptoms from a primary care physician, and is not always necessary. Simple screening tests for depression in older adults can be effectively employed in primary care. The 30-item Geriatric Depression Scale (GDS) is widely used, but 15- and 5-item GDS instruments do not sacrifice accuracy and reduce administration time. Two questions or even one (e.g. "Do you often feel sad and depressed?") may be equally effective in uncovering depression (see Williams *et al.*, 2002).

Management of more severe depression is discussed in Case 10. In the present case, supportive psychotherapy, reassurance that her distress over the loss of her gentleman friend would pass, and emphasis of the importance of maximizing her social supports were of immense help. The patient's chest pain syndrome resolved and she resumed an active social life.

Caveats

1. Somatic complaints in depression differ from "somatization," which is a disorder consisting of multiple somatic complaints that recur over many years. These complaints cannot be explained by appropriate diagnostic tests, and patients who somatize are thought to have altered sensations of bodily functions that may be amplified with anxiety or life stressors. The "sick role" may also have particular rewards for the patient, such as attention from family members or their physician.

Somatization disorder manifests in younger adulthood and is unlikely in this patient whose first symptoms appeared late in life, and in seeming isolation.

2. Many people who commit suicide have visited their primary care provider in the month preceding their suicide. According to one large review, 43–70% of adults 55 years of age and older had made such a visit, compared with 10–36% of persons aged 35 and younger. Far fewer had made a recent visit to a mental health professional (see Luoma *et al.*, 2002).

REFERENCES

Luoma, J. B., Martin, C. E., and Pearson, J. L. (2002). Contact with mental health and primary care providers before suicide: a review of the evidence. *American Journal of Psychiatry*, **139**, 909–16.

Williams, J. W., Noel, P. H., Cordes, J. A. *et al.* (2002). Is the patient clinically depressed? *Journal of the American Medical Association*, **287**, 1160–70.

BIBLIOGRAPHY

Gallo, J. J. (1999). Depression without sadness: alternative presentations of depression in late life. *American Family Physician*, **60**, 820–6.

Hoyl, M. T., Alessi, C. A., and Harker, J. O. (1999). Development and testing of a five-item version of the geriatric depression scale. *Journal of the American Geriatric Society*, **47**, 873–8.

Mahoney, J., Drinka, T. J., and Abler, R. (1994). Screening for depression: single versus GDS. *Journal of the American Geriatric Society* **42**, 1006–8.

Servan-Schreiber, D., Kolb, R., and Tabas, G. (1999). The somatizing patient. *Primary Care.* **26**, 225–42.

Sinoff, G. (2002). Does the presence of anxiety affect the validity of a screening test for depression in the elderly? *International Journal of Geriatric Psychiatry*, **17**, 309–14.

Snyder, A. G. (2000). Measures of depression in older adults with generalized anxiety disorder: a psychometric evaluation. *Depression and Anxiety*, **11**, 114–20.

Wijeratne, C. and Hickie, I. (2001). Somatic distress syndromes in later life: the need for a paradigm change. *Psychological Medicine*, **31**, 571–6.

▶▶ Clearance for surgery

Mrs. F, your 91-year-old patient, comes to the office because she has noted small amounts of blood on the toilet tissue when she moves her bowels. She is healthy, cognitively intact, and lives independently. She walks about 2 miles per day when she does her errands, does not use a cane, and has not fallen. She is socially active and is in touch with family and friends who live nearby.

Approximately 9 years ago, the patient underwent abdominal hysterectomy for nonmalignant vaginal bleeding, and tolerated the procedure well. She has no history of cardiovascular disease.

On physical examination, Mrs. F looks well and is not pale. She is alert and interactive, with obvious normal mental status. Blood pressure is 150/80, pulse is 72 and regular. Lungs are clear. She has a grade II/VI systolic ejection murmur in the aortic area. She has no peripheral edema. Rectal examination reveals guaiac positive stool; no masses are palpable.

Colonoscopy is performed and reveals a large mass in the proximal sigmoid colon, which cannot be removed colonoscopically. Abdominal computed tomography (CT) scan demonstrates no metastatic disease.

Surgery is recommended but the patient demurs, saying she is afraid to have such a major procedure at her age.

Questions

1. How should Mrs. F's concerns be addressed?
2. What preoperative considerations should determine her surgical risk?
3. What kind of preoperative evaluation should she undergo and why?
4. What kind of postoperative issues will be important?

Case Studies in Geriatric Medicine, Judith C. Ahronheim *et al.* Published by Cambridge University Press.
© J. C. Ahronheim, Z.-B. Huang, V. Yen, C. M. Davitt, and D. Barile

Answers

1. The benefits and potential risks of this surgery should be explained to Mrs. F. In particular, she should be made aware that age alone does not determine whether surgery can be performed safely. Surgical risk depends more on the seriousness of the surgery and on the existence of underlying disease.

   Elderly patients who are otherwise well and have a high degree of function have an operative risk that is nearly as low as younger age groups when surgery is nonemergent. Reported series of very old adults undergoing various types of nonemergency surgery suggests that they tolerate the surgery or anesthesia well (see Hosking *et al.*, 1989; Warner *et al.*, 1998). Published series suggesting good outcomes in the oldest age groups, however, may reflect very careful selection of patients, or less invasive surgical procedures. Thus, the patient should be made aware that her overall health and function are high and that a careful risk assessment will precede any proposed surgery.

   It is important to emphasize to the patient that she has a potentially curable lesion. Limited study reveals that older patients undergoing resection of carcinoma of the colon do not have significantly higher postoperative mortality than younger adults (Irvin, 1988). As with other types of surgery, baseline physical and neurologic function, as well as underlying medical problems, seem more important predictors of survival and complication rate. Patients with advanced stage of disease have shorter survival postoperatively, as would be expected, but even if Mrs. F's cancer proved to be locally invasive, it would be entirely possible, given her advanced age, that she might still die of an unrelated cause before the cancer had a chance to metastasize and impair her quality of life.

2. Numerous risk assessment indices have been developed to predict patient outcomes following surgery, and widely used indices focus on cardiovascular or general morbidity and mortality. Degree of risk is determined by patient factors and whether the type of surgery is inherently low, intermediate, or high risk. Although advanced age is generally considered an independent risk factor, the weight given to age in these indices does not alone confer increased surgical risk; patients as old as Mrs. F, and even centenarians, may do well if carefully selected. However, older patients do tend to have a higher complication rate than expected, even if they are preoperatively determined to be at "low" risk. This may reflect a high rate of silent disease, especially cardiac disease, in the older age group.

   Morbidity and mortality are also related to the type of surgery. High or intermediate risk procedures, such as vascular, thoracic, or abdominal surgery, or hip arthroplasty, might pose a greater risk than a "low risk" (superficial) procedure such as cataract extraction or mastectomy. The apparent innate risk of specific procedures may be further enhanced by the common comorbidities that exist in patients who require them – for example, patients undergoing vascular procedures would be expected to have a higher burden of atherosclerotic risk factors, and abdominal surgery for potentially invasive colon carcinoma would be associated with a higher inherent risk of infection.

Another determinant of risk is whether the surgery is emergent or elective. In elective surgery, patients can be carefully selected and prepared. The inherent risks of emergency surgery are enhanced in the elderly, often because atypical presentations lead to delayed diagnosis (see Case 31) or because concerns over outcome lead to indecision and temporizing until the patient has clinically deteriorated. Thus, although this patient's surgery is not yet an emergency, it would be important to avoid unnecessary delay.

Although risk indices address the most common forms of perioperative morbidity, they do not address the risk of postoperative cognitive decline, which is a concern of many patients and their families. It is difficult to identify the risk factors for poor cognitive outcome following surgery because those with baseline cognitive impairment are more likely to deteriorate in the long term even if they have not undergone surgery.

3. In assessing the elderly for surgery, overall function and general health are very important, but cardiovascular, renal, and brain function deserve special attention.

   Mrs. F's systolic blood pressure is mildly elevated and, because she has no known history of hypertension, it is possible that her systolic blood pressure is labile and not sustained (see Case 14). Whereas careful preoperative evaluation and treatment are generally recommended if blood pressure exceeds 180/110, treatment of mild, labile systolic hypertension could theoretically worsen outcome by increasing the risk of intraoperative hypotension.

   Of greater concern is the increased prevalence of silent cardiac disease in late life. Although asymptomatic at this time, Mrs. F has a cardiac systolic murmur. A systolic murmur in the elderly could indicate aortic stenosis, which increases in incidence with age. Severe aortic stenosis (valve area less than approximately 0.8 mm^2) is the main type of valvular heart disease associated with perioperative cardiac complications, including heart failure, myocardial infarction, and death. Although aortic stenosis (AS) may be asymptomatic until very late and significant AS can be missed, significant AS is very unlikely in this physically active patient.

   As discussed in Case 2, murmurs of aortic origin in asymptomatic patients can be due to aortic sclerosis or mild stenosis, which should not themselves affect surgical outcome, although they are markers of silent coronary artery disease. According to existing guidelines, Mrs. F, who does not have symptoms of severe valvular heart disease, and who would be undergoing an intermediate risk procedure (intraperitoneal surgery), does not technically require preoperative cardiac evaluation, since intervention would only be justified if it were indicated regardless of whether she were having surgery (see Eagle *et al.*, 2002). One could, however, justify an evaluation to identify specific problems that would lead to recommendations for perioperative care. For example, diagnosis of aortic stenosis would lead to the avoidance of spinal anesthesia in certain surgeries, or, since auscultation may be misleading in the elderly due to thoracic and other anatomic changes, delineation of a "moderate risk" valve abnormality might prompt endocarditis prophylaxis a few hours before surgery.

Certain general caveats bear mentioning in the elderly, and would be pertinent to this patient. Although evidence does not support that "routine" preoperative testing adds to information recently gleaned, certain baseline information is helpful in perioperative management because of the high rate of overt and silent comorbidity. For example, a preoperative electrocardiogram (EKG) may be important because previously asymptomatic elderly may develop new EKG changes postoperatively. Laboratory evaluation helps to identify diseases such as diabetes and anemia, which are manageable, and liver disease, which require specific perioperative precautions. Baseline hemoglobin determination is important since drops in blood count can lead to ischemic events, and this requires extra attention in elderly patients for whom any "standard" threshold for transfusion might not apply. Although the presence of renal disease is predictive of postoperative renal failure, a normal baseline serum creatinine determination often masks renal insufficiency in the elderly. It is not necessary for the patient to undergo a 24-hour urine collection because this is cumbersome and would not change the need for vigilance. Rather, it is important to assume, based on the patient's age, that renal function may be lower than expected, and doses of renally eliminated medications (or hepatically metabolized medications with active metabolites) would need to be determined judiciously (see Case 20). Several important perioperative medications for which geriatric dosing precautions are often not considered include opioid analgesics, aminoglycoside antibiotics, and enoxaparin. Meperidine (Demerol; pethidine) is an opioid that should be avoided in the elderly because one renally eliminated metabolite can produce seizures.

Preoperative urinalysis may be useful if bladder catheterization is intended, to establish a baseline, because of the high prevalence of asymptomatic urinary tract infections in the elderly and because of the high risk of catheter-associated urinary tract infection.

4. Barring any unpredictable event, Mrs. F's high physical and cognitive function make her – on the surface – an excellent surgical candidate for her age. Postoperatively, it would be very important to monitor her for problems that cannot be predicted by her preoperative evaluation. These would include drug toxicity (owing to occult renal dysfunction or altered sensitivity), delirium (due to preclinical brain disease

and brought on by drug toxicity, infection, or other medical insults), and cardio-vascular events (owing to silent coronary artery disease, especially in the event of blood loss).

Thoracic and upper abdominal surgery and prolonged anesthesia are associated with a risk of pneumonia, and this risk is greater in older adults. This patient would otherwise be at lower risk because she is a nonsmoker and does not have a history of pulmonary disease. Nonetheless, it would be prudent to encourage her to perform incentive spirometry, and to be out of bed to chair, and to ambulate, as soon as possible. The physician should prescribe adequate analgesia to encourage cough, while being mindful of the increased risk in older adults of fecal impaction, confusion, and falling. If opioids are given around the clock, the patient must be re-evaluated frequently because active drug metabolites will accumulate and oversedation may occur in a delayed fashion. Despite her baseline ambulatory capability, opioid analgesics and delayed effects of anesthesia might increase her risk of falling and appropriate precautions should be instituted.

Prophylaxis for deep vein thrombosis should be given as in any postoperative patient, with careful attention to dosing (see Case 26).

Delirium is a common postoperative problem in the elderly. Controversy exists as to whether this is more likely in those with impaired cognitive function. Peri- and postoperative delirium are very common, and permanent postoperative decline in cognitive function sometimes occurs, although the risk of this is uncertain. Delirium (as well as persistent cognitive impairment) may occur in elderly patients with no documented history of dementia, possibly because they have preclinical dementia, or because of age-related factors affecting drug disposition. Infection, which is common following abdominal surgery, is a common cause of delirium in frail elderly. Perioperative delirium can be minimized with careful attention to medication regimens, avoidance of restraints, optimization of sensory stimuli, early recognition of delirium, and prompt treatment of medical comorbidities. Delirium is discussed further in Case 20.

REFERENCES

Eagle, K. A., Berger, P. B., Calkins, H. *et al.* (2002). ACC/AHA guideline update for periop-erative cardiovascular evaluation for noncardiac surgery. Executive summary: a report of the American College of Cardiology/American Heart Association Task Force on Practice Guidelines. *Circulation*, **105**, 1257–67.

Hosking, M. P., Warner, M. A., Lobdell, C. M. *et al.* (1989). Outcomes of surgery in patients 90 years of age and older. *Journal of the American Medical Association*, **261**, 1909–15.

Irvin, T. T. (1988). Prognosis of colorectal cancer in the elderly. *British Journal of Surgery*, **75**, 419–21.

Warner, M. A., Saletel, R. A., and Schroeder, D. R. (1998). Outcomes of anesthesia and surgery in people 100 years of age and older. *Journal of the American Geriatric Society*, **46**, 987–92.

BIBLIOGRAPHY

American College of Physicians (1997). Guidelines for assessing and managing perioperative risk from coronary artery disease associated with major noncardiac surgery. *Annals of Internal Medicine*, **127**, 309–28.

Dajani, A. S., Taubert, K. A., Wilson, W. *et al.* (1997). Prevention of bacterial endocarditis. Recommendations of the American Heart Association. *Circulation*, **96**, 358–66.

Das, P., Pocock, C., and Chambers, J. (2000). The patient with aortic stenosis: severe aortic stenosis may be missed during cardiovascular examination. *Quarterly Journal of Medicine*, **93**, 685–8.

Detsky, A. S., Abrams, H. B., McLaughlin, J. R. *et al.* (1986). Predicting cardiac complications in patients undergoing non-cardiac surgery. *Journal of General Internal Medicine*, **1**, 211–19.

Fick, D. M., Agostini, J. V., and Inouye, S. K. (2002). Delirium superimposed on dementia: a systematic review. *Journal of the American Geriatrics Society*, **50**, 1723–32.

Keller, S. M., Markovitz, L. J., Wilder, J. R. *et al.* (1987). Emergency and elective surgery in patients over age 70. *American Surgeon*, **53**, 636–40.

Macpherson, D. S., Snow, R., and Lofgren, R. P. (1990). Preoperative screening: value of previous tests. *Annals of Internal Medicine*, **113**, 969–73.

Murkin, J. M., Newman, S. P., Stump, D. A. *et al.* (1995). Statement of consensus on assessment of neurobehavioural outcomes after cardiac surgery. *Annals of Thoracic Surgery*, **59**, 1289–95.

Payne, J. E. and Meyer, H. J. (1995). The influence of other diseases upon the outcome of colorectal cancer patients. *Australian and New Zealand Journal of Surgery*, **65**, 398–402.

Raymer, K. and Yang, H. (1998). Patients with aortic stenosis: cardiac complications in non-cardiac surgery. *Canadian Journal of Anaesthesiology*, **45**, 855–9.

Thomas, D. R. and Ritchie, C. S. (1995). Preoperative assessment of older adults. *Journal of the American Geriatric Society*, **48**, 811–21.

Torsher, L. C., Shub, C., Rettke, S. R. *et al.* (1998). Risk of patients with severe aortic stenosis undergoing noncardiac surgery. *American Journal of Cardiology*, **84**, 448–52.

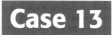

▸▸ Type 2 diabetes

Mr. G, a 75-year-old man, comes to you for the first time, as his new primary care physician. He has hypertension and diabetes, and has been taking atenolol and glyburide for the last 12 years. He has a history of myocardial infarction 6 months ago, but refused an angioplasty at that time. He describes some fatigue, as well as polyuria and blurred vision. He denies chest pain or shortness of breath. He has pains in his legs, especially when walking, and numbness in his feet. He states his cholesterol has "always been a little high," but he thinks he is taking "enough pills already," and he heard that lowering cholesterol doesn't do much good at his age. He does not smoke, does not follow any diet, and leads a sedentary lifestyle. One of the patient's sisters has had diabetes since age 60. His mother was diagnosed with diabetes at age 78, when she became comatose and was found to have an extremely high blood sugar level. Unlike the patient and his sister, his mother was considered "slim."

The patient is 5 feet 8 inches tall, and weighs 235 pounds. Blood pressure is 160/90 and heart rate is 68 and regular. Fundoscopic examination reveals silver wiring and exudates in the retinae. He has a left carotid bruit, but no cardiac murmur. His abdomen is obese. He has trace pedal edema with diminished dorsalis pedis pulses and diminished sensation to pinprick and vibration.

Pertinent laboratory values include hemoglobin A1c of 10% (<6.0% is nondiabetic range), HDL cholesterol 31 mg/dl, LDL cholesterol 155 mg/dl, triglycerides 298 mg/dl, and serum creatinine 1.9 mg/dl. Urinalysis revealed 2+ protein by dipstick, but no cells or casts.

Case Studies in Geriatric Medicine, Judith C. Ahronheim *et al.* Published by Cambridge University Press.
© J. C. Ahronheim, Z.-B. Huang, V. Yen, C. M. Davitt, and D. Barile

Questions

1. What argument should be made regarding cholesterol lowering and the use of lipid-lowering agents?
2. What long-term morbidity can result if Mr. G's diabetes management does not improve?
3. Based on the pathophysiology of type 2 diabetes, how should the patient be treated in order to improve outcomes and to avoid risks of treatment?
4. What age-related changes accounted for the acute syndrome in Mr. G's mother?
5. What practical obstacles in the elderly have an impact on diabetes management?

Answers

1. Despite Mr. G's misgivings, and ongoing debates about cholesterol lowering in his age group, recent trials involving individuals with ischemic heart disease including elderly patients have revealed that mortality risk reduction is greater among older patients than younger ones, presumably because of the high incidence of atherosclerotic heart disease deaths in the older cohort. Clinical trials have involved hydroxy methylglutaryl coenzyme A reductase inhibitors ("statins"), and benefits have been demonstrated in patients even in the eighth decade of life. Furthermore, treatment of older adults with a history of myocardial infarction may also reduce stroke. It is possible that anti-inflammatory effects of statins rather than cholesterol lowering per se produce the observed clinical benefits; however, earlier trials of nonstatins, such as bile acid sequestrants, have also demonstrated reduced coronary heart disease, albeit in nonelderly subjects.

   Although statin trials demonstrate statistically significant benefit, the rate of ischemic events and death is still high with treatment, as would be expected in elderly, high-risk patients, so Mr. G's concerns are not completely without logic. Also, he may be correct that lowering cholesterol (or even measuring it), at least in the very old, is unnecessary. For example, in one study in the Netherlands (Weverling-Rijnsburger *et al.*, 1997), 772 patients aged over 85 had their cholesterol measured; after 10 years of follow up, 89% had died, with the group with the highest cholesterol surviving the longest (4.3 years median) and those with the lowest cholesterol having the shortest survival (average 2.5 years). It is possible that low cholesterol was a marker for serious illness in that cohort. However, there is ample reason to recommend active treatment in a high-risk patient like Mr G, even if he were 10 years older, an important factor being his diabetes, which alone is considered an atherosclerotic equivalent. If Mr. G agrees to take a statin, it will be important to follow him carefully for adverse effects, because advanced age, frailty, multisystem disease, and diabetes itself increase the risk of developing statin-induced myopathy.

2. Contrary to some earlier beliefs, the presence of diabetes even after age 75 leads to excess mortality and functional decline compared with age-matched nondiabetics. Suboptimal control of type 2 diabetes, like type 1 diabetes, can result in microvascular complications (retinopathy, neuropathy, and nephropathy) and macrovascular complications (peripheral vascular, carotid artery, and atherosclerotic heart disease), and this risk can be reduced by good control. Of additional concern, diabetes is associated with cognitive decline among older patients, as compared with those without diabetes, possibly because of neurotoxicity associated with hyperglycemia, hypoglycemia, insulin, or perhaps glycosylation end products.

3. This patient requires active treatment to lower HgbA1c. Likewise, he requires control of blood pressure and lipid levels, since decreases in macrovascular disease appear to be even more closely linked to blood pressure and lipid control. Common phenotypes of type 2 diabetes are associated with an underlying insulin resistance, and, early in the disease, weight loss and exercise may be sufficient because they improve insulin resistance. However, pharmacologic treatment becomes necessary at some point, as insulinopenia inevitably develops in this progressive illness, and poor control may promote this deterioration ("glucotoxicity"). Mr. G has had diabetes for at least 12 years, which is currently uncontrolled, and he already has evidence of vasculopathy, so, although diet and exercise should be encouraged, intensive pharmacologic treatment will be needed.

    Ideally, drugs that stimulate insulin secretion (such as glyburide) should be combined with those that lower insulin resistance, such as metformin, which lowers blood glucose without increasing insulin levels. Metformin has the added benefit of being the only antidiabetes medication associated with weight loss rather than weight gain. However, it should not be given in renal insufficiency because it is eliminated by the kidney and can cause dose-related lactic acidosis. The thiazolidinedione drugs, rosiglitazone and pioglitazone, also decrease Hgb A1c, without raising insulin levels.

    Pharmacologic treatment that targets insulin resistance may also ameliorate other manifestations of this patient's disease. Mr. G has a complex of symptoms termed "Syndrome X," the so-called visceral adiposity metabolic syndrome, consisting of elevated body mass index (BMI) and waist circumference, hypertriglyceridemia, hypertension, and fasting hyperglycemia. This syndrome is associated with metabolic factors beyond hyperglycemia that contribute to vasculopathy through inflammation, endothelial dysfunction, a prothrombotic state, highly atherogenic lipid particles, and hyperlipidemia, and some of these effects can be ameliorated to a degree by thiazolidinediones. These agents may also contribute to beta cell preservation as well as adipose tissue redistribution. The beneficial effects of these agents on glycemic control and serum lipids in the elderly appear to be similar to the effects seen in younger patients. They may occasionally cause liver damage and are contraindicated in settings of liver disease. More commonly, they can produce edema and, in some patients, cause fluid overload and congestive heart failure.

The use of aspirin confers additional cardioprotective effect. Angiotensin-converting enzyme (ACE) inhibitors, and also angiotensin II receptor blockers, reduce proteinuria and delay the onset of renal insufficiency in older adults.

Despite the potential benefits of insulin resistance drugs, progressive insulinopenia will necessitate insulin treatment at some time in Mr. G's disease, perhaps very soon. It can be initiated in conjunction with oral agents to improve glycemic control, but, at some point, may be the only treatment that is effective.

Tighter control often carries an increased risk of hypoglycemia, and this risk is greatest among the elderly. With aging, there is a decreased counter-regulatory response in levels of glucagon and growth hormone. In addition, normal, nondiabetic elderly have decreased and delayed epinephrine and norepinephrine responses to hypoglycemia. Furthermore, some elderly diabetic patients mount epinephrine responses at higher glucose levels, similar to those seen in younger, type I diabetics with poor control. Additional changes in elderly diabetics include a decreased ability of the liver to store and release glycogen, decreases in the hunger response to hypoglycemia, and decreased perception of symptoms ("hypoglycemic unawareness"). It is widely believed, though poorly documented, that a single episode of severe hypoglycemia can have a much more deleterious outcome, such as myocardial infarction or stroke, in an elderly patient than in a younger patient, and one study suggested that hypoglycemic coma may occur at higher levels of blood sugar as well (Ben-Ami H et al., 1999). Despite lack of convincing evidence, vigilance is required in elderly diabetics, who more often have additional risk factors for hypoglycemia and its consequences, such as diminished cardiac output and cerebral circulation at baseline.

4. The patient's mother was not diagnosed as diabetic until she became comatose at the age of 78. Whether or not his mother was actually "slim," it is true that many elderly type 2 diabetics are not obese. Age is often accompanied by changes in carbohydrate metabolism, such as decreases in beta cell insulin release and

postreceptor decrease in glucose uptake. Hyperglycemia may result in such individuals because of the decrease in lean body mass and relative increased adiposity that occurs with aging. Diabetes in such "nonobese" patients may be more related to insulinopenic responses to glucose than to the elevated hepatic glucose production and resistance to insulin-mediated glucose disposal seen in the obese elderly and nonelderly diabetic. Decreased physical activity may be an additional factor.

Most elderly diabetics who present with coma have a hyperosmolar state, which develops when the patient has hyperglycemic osmotic diuresis, leading to dehydration. Because thirst response to dehydration is impaired with aging, polydipsia often does not occur in patients with significant hyperglycemia, and a cognitive or functionally impaired patient may be unable to ask for or obtain sufficient fluids. In such situations, the patient may present with nonspecific symptoms such as confusion, depression, failure to thrive, or urinary incontinence. Alternatively, the diabetes may be first discovered during hospitalization for myocardial infarction, stroke, sepsis, or hyperosmolar, nonketotic coma. The mortality of hyperosmolar coma is much higher in the elderly than in younger adults.

Some "ketosis-prone" type 2 diabetics may develop ketoacidosis under severe medical stress. Under ordinary conditions, their insulin levels may be sufficient, but, under the stress of serious illness, the ratio of counter-regulatory hormones to insulin is elevated and ketosis supervenes.

5. Older diabetics who have functional impairments – whether due to diabetes or unrelated comorbidity – may have difficulty managing many aspects of their care. They may lack knowledge about or be unable to comprehend information that they need, such as need for regular food intake or recognition and management of hypoglycemia. They may be unable to act on hypoglycemia, or make medication errors, such as drawing up excess insulin. Decreased mobility due to physical impairments, decreased vision, cognitive disorders (which can themselves be worsened by hyperglycemia), depression, social problems, and increased threat of, and susceptibility to, hypoglycemia, as well as limited access to nutritionally balanced meals, all can contribute to difficulties with diabetes management in the elderly. Aging and neurologic disease can impair the thirst response to dehydration and, when ill, patients may exhibit hypodipsia when hyperglycemia should physiologically lead to polydipsia and maintenance of hydration.

Elderly patients with diabetes use almost twice as many inpatient and outpatient resources as those without diabetes. Attention should also be paid to caregivers, who need to be involved far more frequently when the patient is diabetic. Close management by an interdisciplinary team is essential for the functionally impaired elderly diabetic.

REFERENCES

Ben-Ami, H., Nagachandran, P., Mendelson, A. *et al.* (1999). Drug induced hypoglycemic coma in 102 diabetic patients. *Archives of Internal Medicine*, **159**, 281–4.

Weverling-Rijnsburger, A. W., Blauw, G. J., Lagaay, A. M. *et al.* (1997). Total cholesterol and the risk of mortality in the oldest old. *Lancet*, **350**, 1119–23.

BIBLIOGRAPHY

Beebe, K. and Patel, J. (1999). Rosiglitazone is effective and well tolerated in patients over 65 years with type 2 diabetes. *Diabetes*, **42** Suppl 1, A111.

Carlsson, C. M., Carnes, M, McBride, P. E. *et al.* (1999). Managing dyslipidemia in the elderly. *Journal of the American Geriatrics Society*, **47**, 1458–65.

Coscelli, C., Lostia, S. A., Lunetta, M. *et al.* (1995). Safety, efficacy, acceptability of a pre-filled insulin pen in diabetic patients over 60 years old. *Diabetes Research and Clinical Practice*, **28**, 173–7.

DeFronzo, R. A. (1999). Pharmacologic therapy for type 2 diabetes mellitus. *Annals of Internal Medicine*, **131**, 281–303.

Groop, L. C., Bottazzo, G. F., and Doniach, D. (1986). Islet cell antibodies identify latent type 1 diabetes in patients aged 35–75 years at diagnosis. *Diabetes*, **35**, 237–41.

Grundy, S. M., Cleeman, J. I., Rifkind, B. H. *et al.*, for the Coordinating Committee of the National Cholesterol Education Program (1999). Cholesterol lowering in the elderly population. *Archives of Internal Medicine*, **159**, 1670–8.

Heart Outcomes Prevention Evaluation Study Investigators (2000). Effect of ramipril on cardiovascular and microvascular outcomes in people with diabetes mellitus: results of the HOPE study and MICRO-HOPE substudy. *Lancet*, **22**, 253–9.

Hunt, D. H., Young, P. Y., Simes, J. *et al.*, for the LIPID investigators (2001). Benefits of pravastatin on cardiovascular events and mortality in older patients with coronary heart disease are equal to or exceed those seen in younger patients: results from the LIPID trial. *Annals of Internal Medicine*, **134**, 931–40.

Lewis, S. J., Moye, L. A., Sacks, F. M. *et al.* (1998). Effect of pravastatin on cardiovascular events in older patients with myocardial infarction and cholesterol in the average range: results of the Cholesterol and Recurrent Events (CARE) trial. *Annals of Internal Medicine*, **129**, 681–9.

Mahler, R. J. and Adler, M. L. (1999). Type 2 diabetes mellitus: update on diagnosis, pathophysiology and treatment. *Journal of Clinical Endocrinology and Metabolism*, **84**, 1165–71.

Meneilly, G. S. and Tessier, D. (2001). Diabetes in elderly adults. *Journals of Gerontology: Medical Sciences*, **56A**, M5–13.

Parulkar, A. A., Pendergrass, M. L., Granda-Ayala, R. L. *et al.* (2001). Nonhypoglycemic effects of thiazolidinediones. *Annals of Internal Medicine*, **134**, 61–71.

Pasternak, R. C., Smith, S. C., Bairey-Merz, C. N. *et al.* (2002). ACC/AHA/NHLBI clinical advisory on the use and safety of statins. *Circulation*, **106**, 1024–8.

Saito, I., Folsom, A. R., Brancati, F. L. *et al.* (2000). Nontraditional risk factors for coronary heart disease incidence among persons with diabetes: the Atherosclerosis Risk in Communities (ARIC) Study. *Annals of Internal Medicine*, **133**, 81–91.

Shepherd, J., Blauw, G. J., Murphy, M. B. *et al.* (2002). Pravastatin in elderly individuals at risk of vascular disease (PROSPER): a randomized controlled trial. *Lancet*, **360**, 1623–30.

Shorr, R. I., Ray, W. A., Daughterty, J. R. *et al.* (1997). Incidence and risk factors for serious hypoglycemia in older persons using insulin or sulfonylureas. *Archives of Internal Medicine*, **157**, 1681–6.

Stratton, I. M., Adler, A. I., Neil, H. A. *et al.*, for the UKPDS Study Group. (2000). Association of glycemia with macrovascular and microvascular complications of type 2 diabetes (UKPDS 35): prospective observational study. *British Medical Journal*, **321**, 405–12.

Turner, R. C., Cull, C., Frighi, V. *et al.*, for the UKPDS study group (1999). Glycemic control with diet, sulfonylurea, metformin, or insulin in patients with type 2 diabetes mellitus: progressive requirement for multiple therapies (UKPDS 49). *Journal of the American Medical Association*, **281**, 2005–12.

UKPDS Study Group (1998). Intensive blood-glucose control with sulphonylureas or insulin compared with conventional treatment and risk of complications in patients with type 2 diabetes (UKPDS 33). UK Prospective Diabetes Study (UKPDS) Group. *Lancet*, **352**, 837–9.

Case 14

▸▸ Two patients with hypertension

Mr. G

Mr. G, whom we met in Case 13, has been coming regularly to your office and has agreed to most of your recommendations. His current daily medications include amlodipine (Norvasc) 10 mg, enalapril (Vasotec) 10 mg, glipizide (Glucotrol) 10 mg, rosiglitazone (Avandia) 8 mg, enteric-coated aspirin 325 mg, and a multivitamin. Today, his blood pressure is 164/80 and heart rate is 72 beats per minute and regular. His weight is 186 pounds, a 4 pound reduction since his first visit with you 6 months ago. Jugular veins are not distended, lungs are clear, and heart examination is unremarkable. He has mild bilateral ankle edema. Significant laboratory values include HbA1c 7.5%, BUN 24 mg/dl, serum creatinine 1.8 mg/dl, total cholesterol 224 mg/dl, triglyceride 180 mg/dl, HDL 30 mg/dl, and LDL 151 mg/dl.

Mrs. K

Mrs. K is a 90-year-old woman who has moved to the community recently. She feels well except for pain in both knees while walking, for which she takes acetaminophen. She has also taken baby aspirin once daily for many years. She denied a history of hypertension, diabetes, or heart disease, and has never smoked. On physical examination, she is a slender, healthy appearing woman. Her blood pressure is 165/80, heart rate is 78 beats per minute, and regular, respiratory rate is 12; lung, heart and abdominal examinations are unremarkable. Examination of the lower extremities reveals strong peripheral pulses and no edema. Blood tests including blood count, creatinine, glucose, and thyroid-stimulating hormone (TSH) are all normal. Electrocardiogram shows left ventricular hypertrophy (LVH) by voltage criteria, without other abnormalities. You tell her that her blood pressure is high and she expresses doubt, saying, "I have never had high blood pressure!"

Case Studies in Geriatric Medicine, Judith C. Ahronheim *et al.* Published by Cambridge University Press.
© J. C. Ahronheim, Z.-B. Huang, V. Yen, C. M. Davitt, and D. Barile

Questions

1. What criteria should be used in elderly patients to determine if blood pressure is high enough to be treated?
2. How should you approach the management of blood pressure in Mr. G and Mrs. K?
3. What pharmacologic agents should be used in older adults with hypertension?
4. What lifestyle modifications should be recommended?

Answers

1. Hypertension (HTN) is generally defined as systolic blood pressure (SBP) ≥140 mm Hg or diastolic blood pressure (DBP) ≥90 mm Hg. Isolated systolic hypertension (ISH) is defined as SBP 140 mm Hg or greater and DBP less than 90 mm Hg. According to recent guidelines, these criteria apply to all adults, regardless of age (Chobanian *et al.*, 2003), and, using these criteria, about two-thirds of hypertensive patients between the ages of 65 and 89 have isolated systolic hypertension. These guidelines are based on a doubling of cardiovascular mortality risk for each 20/10 increment in blood pressure over 115/75, labeling systolic pressure greater than 120 as "prehypertension." Before treating or counseling and possibly unnecessarily upsetting a 90-year-old patient, it would be important to place these recommendations in perspective.

   SBP elevation in late life has long been considered an inevitable consequence of advancing age, due to decreased compliance of the arterial wall, and was considered unimportant, in contrast to diastolic hypertension, which was thought to reflect increased peripheral vascular resistance and to be harmful. The differing age distribution of ISH and diastolic hypertension is illustrated in Figure 6. Longitudinal and prospective data have demonstrated clearly that SBP is a better independent predictor for cardiovascular events than DBP, even in subjects with mildly elevated SBP. More recently, large, double-blind, controlled studies of people 65 years of age and older with SBP ≥160 mm Hg demonstrated that lowering SBP significantly reduces the incidence of stroke, cardiovascular events, and all-cause of mortality. The mean age of "elderly" subjects in most clinical trials is about 70, and, official guidelines notwithstanding, the benefits of treatment in elderly patients with SBP between 140 to 159 are yet to be proved.

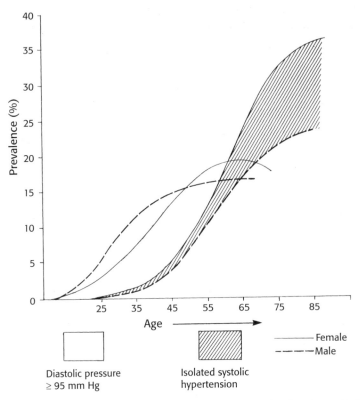

Figure 6   Differing age distribution of diastolic hypertension and isolated systolic hypertension (ISH) is the basis for the traditional view that ISH is "normal" and therefore not harmful. Chart adapted from data in Hutchison (1981) and Wilking *et al.* (1988).

Both of our patients satisfied the criteria for ISH. However, official criteria can only be used as a general guide. The approach to a patient meeting the criteria of hypertension, especially those older than 80 years with SBP between 140 and 160 without evidence of target organ damage, requires careful consideration (see below).

2. Mr. G's blood pressure is elevated, despite antihypertensive medications, and he has several additional cardiac risk factors. There is ample evidence that blood pressure lowering delays and prevents nephropathy and reduces cardiovascular events, even in patients over 65, and a target blood pressure less than 130/85 is recommended in diabetes. Because the patient also has proteinuria, the target might be even stricter (≤125/75). Although these recommendations are based on data in patients younger than 70 years, there is currently no evidence that this target should not be applied to Mr. G., who has compelling reasons for aggressive treatment. However, successful treatment will depend on his ability to adhere to and tolerate the recommended regimen.

There are additional caveats to consider before treating Mrs. K, who is 90 years old. Information on people in their nineties is sparse, and it is legitimate to ask if reducing this woman's SBP would benefit her in any way. Her projected life span is about 4–5 years. In two major studies of hypertension in the elderly (see SHEP Cooperative Research Group, 1991; Staessen JA *et al.*, 1997), the average age of subjects was almost 20 years younger than Mrs. K. In these studies, 100 patients with ISH (SBP $\geqslant$160 in both studies) need to be treated with antihypertensive medications for 2–5 years in order to achieve a reduction of stroke and major cardiovascular events by three and five episodes, respectively. Pharmacologic treatment of hypertension can reduce the severity of or reverse LVH, which is an independent factor for congestive heart failure. Even if Mrs. K's LVH were confirmed by echocardiography, any projected benefit of treatment would still be based on the extrapolation of data from younger individuals.

It will also be important to confirm whether Mrs. K has sustained hypertension. Systolic pressure is more labile than diastolic pressure. Blood pressure in general varies from day to day, at different times during the day, and from minute to minute. The "white coat effect," an elevation in blood pressure associated with measurement in the doctor's office, occurs in adults of all ages but the difference between office and ambulatory blood pressure may increase with age (see Wiinberg *et al.*, 1995). "Pseudohypertension," or elevated cuff pressure in the face of normal intra-arterial pressure, is another problem that should be considered in elderly patients whose blood pressure seems hard to control. Falsely elevated cuff pressure occurs when arteries lack distensibility or are calcified, requiring greater extrinsic pressure before they can be compressed. The frequency of this problem is uncertain because confirmation requires monitoring that is invasive or impractical. Nonetheless, it should be considered, especially when patients undergoing treatment seem to develop symptoms of hypotension in the face of normal or elevated cuff pressure.

Despite these caveats, Mrs. K's general good health and functional status makes her an appropriate candidate for treatment. However, vigilance is required for symptoms that might occur if blood pressure were lowered to youthful target levels. Mrs. K preferred not to receive any antihypertensive medication, but she continued to take coated baby aspirin and wanted to hear more about lifestyle modification. She comes to the office periodically and her SBP has varied between 145 and 170.

3. Most antihypertensive drugs, alone or in combination, are effective in reducing SBP and decreasing cardiovascular morbidity and mortality in elderly patients with ISH. There is no "drug of choice" for the elderly hypertensive. Rather, the initial drug choice should be based on the patient's profile, comorbidity, potential side effects, and physician's experience. Recommendations to initiate treatment with thiazide diuretics or beta-blockers in combination with thiazides are based on the earliest studies of ISH that used these agents and not others (SHEP Cooperative Research

Group, 1991), and more recent studies do not consistently demonstrate the benefit of one agent over another. In fact, many geriatric patients cannot tolerate diuretics because of bladder problems (see Case 33).

Specific agents should be selected when common comorbid conditions exist for which these agents are known to be effective – e.g. angiotensin-converting enzyme (ACE) inhibitors in diabetes or heart failure, and beta-blockers or ACE inhibitors in myocardial infarction. Conversely, elderly patients commonly experience certain symptoms with specific agents, such as constipation or leg edema with calcium channel blockers (CCBs); when these effects occur, they may sometimes be mistakenly attributed to other causes and lead to unnecessary evaluation and erroneous treatment.

Owing to pharmacokinetic changes that occur in late life (see Case 20), an increased incidence of adverse drug reactions, and occasional heightened sensitivity to blood pressure-lowering effects, the starting dose should be lower than, usually about one-half of, the dose for younger patients, and the dose gradually increased if necessary. Delayed elimination of renally eliminated drugs, such as ACE inhibitors, can sometimes be harnessed so shorter-acting agents, such as captopril, can be given less often.

4. Like younger adults, elderly patients with hypertension should attempt lifestyle modification, such as weight loss if obese, exercise, smoking cessation, and avoidance of excessive alcohol use, because the benefits of these interventions are broader than merely blood pressure reduction. High dietary potassium intake may improve blood pressure control and an adequate intake of potassium in foods like fruits and vegetables are recommended along with other lifestyle modifications. Salt restriction remains somewhat controversial for elderly hypertensives, however. Controlled studies have shown the effectiveness of dietary sodium restriction in reducing blood pressure in hypertensive and normotensive adults. However, before recommending a salt-restricted diet for an elderly patient, several caveats should be considered. First, evidence of benefit comes from studies of community residing "older" adults (e.g. Johnson *et al.*, 2001), but not in very old or frail patients, who may already be malnourished and would possibly be harmed rather than helped by enforced dietary restriction. Second, nonmodifiable genetic factors may determine whether hypertensive patients are salt sensitive or salt insensitive. Third, most studies of the effects of salt restriction employed very severe restriction of sodium, which is difficult to achieve in clinical practice. Finally, there is a decline in renal solute conservation with age; the clinical implications of this physiologic change with regard to salt restriction, blood pressure, or intravascular volume are not known.

Many exercises are impractical in patients with physical limitations who are unable to increase aerobic physical activity sufficiently, if at all. In these cases, creative interventions should be considered, including movement therapy, or a physical therapy program tailored to the needs of the particular patient. Mrs. K should be counseled to participate in moderate exercise, such as walking, because of overall benefits to her well being. Mr. G requires more intensive intervention and counseling regarding the importance of controlling blood glucose, hypertension, lipids, and weight, and might benefit from progressive resistance training if aerobic exercises are difficult or impractical.

REFERENCES

Chobanian, A. V., Bakris, G. L., Black, H. R. *et al.*, for the National Heart, Lung, and Blood Institute Joint National Committee on Prevention, Detection, Evaluation, and Treatment of High Blood Pressure; National High Blood Pressure Education Program Coordinating Committee (2003). The seventh report of the Joint National Committee on Prevention, Detection, Evaluation, and Treatment of High Blood Pressure: the JNC 7 report. *Journal of the American Medical Association*, **289**, 2560–72.

Hutchison, B. (1981). Hypertension in the elderly. *Canadian Family Physician*, **27**, 1579–86.

Johnson, A. G., Nguyen, T. V., and Davis, D. (2001). Blood pressure is linked to salt intake and modulated by the angiotensinogen gene in normotensive and hypertensive elderly subjects. *Journal of Hypertension*, **19**, 1053–60.

SHEP Cooperative Research Group (1991). Prevention of stroke by antihypertensive drug treatment in older persons with isolated systolic hypertension: final results of the Systolic Hypertension in the Elderly Program (SHEP). *Journal of the American Medical Association*, **265**, 3255–64.

Staessen, J. A., Fagard, R., Thijs, L. *et al.*, for the Systolic Hypertension in Europe (Syst-Eur) Trial Investigators (1997). Randomized double-blind comparison of placebo and active treatment for older patients with isolated systolic hypertension. *Lancet*, **350**, 757–64.

Wiinberg, N., Hoegholm, A., Christensen, H. R. *et al.* (1995). 24-hour ambulatory blood pressure in 352 normal Danish subjects, related to age and gender. *American Journal of Hypertension*, **8**, 978–86.

Wilking, S. V. B., Belanger, A., Kannel, W. B. *et al.* (1988). Determinants of isolated systolic hypertension. *Journal of the American Medical Association*, **260**, 3451–5.

BIBLIOGRAPHY

Dahlof, B., Lindholm, L. H., Hansson, L. *et al.* (1991). Morbidity and mortality in the Swedish trial in old patients with hypertension (STOP-Hypertension). *Lancet*, **338**, 1281–5.

Epstein, M. and Hallenberg, N. K. (1976). Age as a determinant of renal sodium conservation in normal men. *Journal of Clinical Laboratory Medicine*, **87**, 411–17.

Fagard, R. H. (2002). Epidemiology of hypertension in the elderly. *American Journal of Geriatric Cardiology*, **11**, 23–8.

Gueyffier, F., Bulpitt, C., Boissel J. P. *et al.*, for the INDANA Group (1999). Antihypertensive drugs in very old people: a subgroup meta-analysis of randomised controlled trials. *Lancet*, **353**, 793–6.

Liu, L., Wang, J. G., Gong, L. *et al.*, for the Systolic Hypertension in China (Syst-China) Collaborative Group (1998). Comparison of active treatment and placebo in older Chinese patients with isolated systolic hypertension. *Journal of Hypertension*, **16**, 1823–9.

MacMahon, M., Sheahan, N. F., Colgan, M. P. *et al.* (1995). Arterial closing pressure correlates with diastolic pseudohypertension in the elderly. *Journals of Gerontology*, **50A**, M56–8.

Medical Research Council Working Party (1992). Medical Research Council trial of treatment of hypertension in older adults: principal results. *British Medical Journal*, **304**, 405–12.

Myers, M. E. (1996). Systolic hypertension and the white coat phenomenon. *American Journal of Hypertension*, **9**, 938–40.

Perry, H. M., Jr., Davis, B. R., Price, T. R. *et al.*, for the SHEP Cooperative Research Group (2000). Effect of treating isolated systolic hypertension on the risk of developing various types and subtypes of stroke: the Systolic Hypertension in the Elderly Program (SHEP). *Journal of the American Medical Association*, **284**, 465–71.

Staessen, J. A., Gasowski, J., Wang, J. G. *et al.* (2000). Risks of untreated and treated isolated systolic hypertension in the elderly: meta-analysis of outcome trials. *Lancet*, **355**, 865–72.

Staessen, J. A., Wang, J. G., Thijs., L. *et al.* (1999). Overview of the outcome trials in older patients with isolated systolic hypertension. *Journal of Human Hypertension*, **13**, 859–63.

Stamler, J., Stamler, R., and Neaton, J. (1993). Blood pressure, systolic and diastolic, and cardiovascular risks: US population data. *Archives of Internal Medicine*, **153**, 598–615.

Whelton, P. K., He, J., Culter, J. A. *et al.* (1997). Effects of oral potassium on blood pressure: meta-analysis of randomized controlled clinical trials. *Journal of the American Medical Association*, **277**, 1624–32.

Zuschke, C. A. and Pettyjohn, F. S. (1995). Pseudohypertension. *Southern Medical Journal*, **88**, 1185–90.

Case 15

▸▸ A fall

An 82-year-old woman is sent to the emergency department after she fell in her home and was unable to get up. She has no history of falls, but is being treated for chronic low back pain due to degenerative disc disease and for mild hypertension. Her medications include acetaminophen as needed and amlodipine 5 mg daily. In addition, she has chronic urinary urgency with occasional incontinence but has declined medications for this problem.

The patient has been experiencing increasing fatigue over the past 3–4 days. She admits that she has also experienced shortness of breath for some time. She denies chest pain, dizziness, palpitations, or loss of consciousness, and has no history of hypertension, asthma, or heart disease. She does not smoke or drink alcoholic beverages. She is a widow but lives near her daughter and has remained physically and socially active.

On physical examination, the patient is alert and oriented. Her blood pressure is 100/60, her heart rate is 102 and regular, and she has a respiratory rate of 24. Her oxygen saturation is 92% at room air. Jugular veins are not distended. Significant findings include a grade III/VI systolic murmur over the base and left sternal border, bilateral basilar rales, and trace ankle edema. There are no focal neurologic signs. She has no tenderness or bruising in the hips or buttocks.

Question

Based on the history and physical examination, what is the differential diagnosis of this patient's fall?

Case Studies in Geriatric Medicine, Judith C. Ahronheim *et al.* Published by Cambridge University Press.
© J. C. Ahronheim, Z.-B. Huang, V. Yen, C. M. Davitt, and D. Barile

Answer

Fatigue and falling are nonspecific and frequently experienced by elderly patients, but both symptoms are new in this patient. Although falls in the elderly are often related to musculoskeletal and other functional problems, as discussed in Case 24, this hypertensive patient's relatively low blood pressure and apparent weakness make it important to consider a serious medical condition. Systemic infections are common causes of changes in functional status in the elderly, and can present nonspecifically. Neurologic conditions such as stroke, transient ischemic attack (TIA), and seizure are also important considerations in an elderly patient who falls, but history and physical examination do not suggest a neurologic event in this patient. Although TIA by definition leaves no signs, it is also not typically followed by constitutional symptoms. Seizure in the elderly generally occurs if there is a prior history of stroke, an intracranial space-occupying lesion, or a medication known to cause seizures. Other considerations with this presentation might include metabolic disturbances, dehydration, or drug toxicity. Pulmonary embolism can present with tachypnea, tachycardia, lung rales, and syncope, but the patient has no obvious risk factors. Cardiovascular problems, such as an acute ischemic event or heart failure, should be considered in this patient, especially because of her shortness of breath and physical findings. Anemia is a common cause of this patient's presentation, and, in late life, anemia often comes to light when the patient develops signs of acute heart disease.

Blood count, blood glucose, and electrolytes are normal, and stool was negative for occult blood. Her electrocardiogram (EKG) showed sinus tachycardia at 104 beats per minute, Q wave in II, ST elevation in aVR, III, V1, and V2, and ST depression in I II, aVL, V5, and V6. Chest X-ray revealed increased interstitial markings, pulmonary vascular congestion, and small right pleural effusion.

The patient was given oxygen and chewable aspirin, and intravenous heparin was begun. Cardiac enzymes were elevated, confirming the diagnosis of acute myocardial infarction, and she was admitted to the coronary care unit (CCU). Echocardiogram was performed.

Six days later she is transferred to a general medical floor. Blood pressure was 120/70, heart rate 74 and regular. Heart failure resolved and cardiac enzymes normalized. Her total cholesterol level was 128 mg/dl, LDL-cholesterol 82 mg/dl, HDL-cholesterol 25 mg/dl, and triglyceride 105 mg/dl. Her medications at this time included aspirin 325 mg daily, metoprolol 50 mg bid, and captopril 6.25 mg tid.

Questions

1. What additional initial treatment could have been given?
2. What accounts for the patient's muted presentation?
3. What measures should be taken to prevent this problem from recurring?

Answers

1. If the patient were younger than 75 years of age, she might have been considered a good candidate for thrombolytic treatment on the basis of a confirmed myocardial infarction (minimum criterion ST elevation in at least two contiguous leads). She had no absolute contraindications, such as a previous hemorrhagic stroke or any stroke in the past year, or relative contraindications, such as severe uncontrolled hypertension, current use of anticoagulants or bleeding diathesis, or active peptic ulcer. Although patients aged 75 and older may be considered for thrombolytic treatment, the risk of hemorrhagic stroke may outweigh any benefit in individual patients. It would, nonetheless, be tempting to consider such treatment in a previously healthy and high functioning 82-year-old patient without contraindications; however, thrombolytic therapy is generally ineffective if given more than 12 hours after the onset of the ischemic event and, because of her atypical presentation, the duration would be difficult to determine. Atypical presentations are common reasons for delayed treatment of many serious conditions in the elderly (see Cases 31 and 38).

   Angioplasty is associated with a better outcome than thrombolytic treatment in patients this age. Patients over 80 years of age have a worse outcome following angioplasty than other adults, and this is likely to be due to associated comorbidity or a greater burden of cardiovascular disease (Wennberg et al., 1999).

2. The patient's muted presentation – notably, the absence of pain – is very common in elderly patients with acute myocardial infarction and may account for delayed diagnosis or misdiagnosis. Some patients have no symptoms at all. When there are symptoms, classic ones, such as precordial chest pressure or pain, diaphoresis, and nausea, are seen less often, whereas dyspnea, weakness, falling, confusion, dizziness, or exacerbation of heart failure are more common in the elderly. These phenomena have been explained by age-associated cardiac changes, including prolonged

diastolic relaxation of the myocardium, enhanced afterload due to increased arterial stiffness, and reduced beta-adrenergic response.

Variations of the classic presentations of angina occur as well. Dyspnea or fatigue may be the major manifestations, and "silent" or painless ischemia is highly prevalent in this age group. In the ischemic cascade, left ventricular contraction is impaired first, producing characteristic EKG changes, and then pain occurs. The left ventricle tends to stiffen with age and, when ischemic heart disease develops, symptoms of left ventricular dysfunction may occur early and dyspnea or fatigue will cause the patient to rest before pain actually begins. Decreased pain perception has been offered as another explanation offered for the atypical presentation (see Ambepitiya *et al.*, 1994), but this notion is controversial.

3. There is an increased risk of mortality in the first year following myocardial infarction, particularly in the first 6 months. This patient's echocardiogram revealed moderate left ventricular dysfunction, consistent with her clinical signs of congestive heart failure (CHF). Measures should be taken to reduce her risk of reinfarction and to continue treatment of her CHF. Aspirin, beta-blockers, and cholesterol-lowering agents reduce the risk of subsequent cardiac events and death, and risk reduction may be greater for older as compared with younger adults, presumably because of the high incidence of atherosclerotic disease in late life. Among patients with myocardial infarction and ventricular dysfunction, angiotensin-converting enzyme inhibitors decrease mortality, hospitalization for heart failure, and recurrent myocardial infarction in people 65 years of age and older.

Although her LDL-C level on admission was already under 100 mg/dl, this can be misleadingly low in the setting of acute coronary events. Because this level can soon return to baseline, lipid levels should be followed before or soon after discharge because early treatment with lipid-lowering agents may reduce cardiac mortality. Hyperlipidemia in the elderly is discussed in Case 13.

Strict attention should be paid to enabling this patient to regain her previous level of functioning. This is very important for elderly hospitalized patients, who can rapidly develop "deconditioning" with bed rest, and are subject to other "hazards of hospitalization" (see Creditor, 1993). Six days after admission, this patient was still at bed rest and had an indwelling catheter. Indwelling catheters are commonly used routinely and are frequently left in place because they have been "forgotten," or believed to be needed for the management of incontinence. However, they have been shown to increase mortality in hospitalized patients and are rarely, if ever, indicated in the management of incontinence (see Cases 33 and 34). Action at this point should include removal of the bladder catheter, use of a bedside commode and scheduled toileting, allowing the patient out of bed with assistance, and rehabilitation consultation.

REFERENCES

Ambepitiya, G., Roberts, M., Ranjadayalan, K. *et al.* (1994). Silent exertional myocardial ischemia in the elderly: a quantitative analysis of anginal perceptual threshold and the influence of autonomic function. *Journal of the American Geriatrics Society*, **42**, 732–7.

Creditor, M. C. (1993). Hazards of hospitalization of the elderly. *Annals of Internal Medicine*, **118**, 219–23.

Wennberg, D. E., Makenka, D. J., Sengupta, A. *et al.* (1999). Percutaneous transluminal coronary angioplasty in the elderly: epidemiology, clinical risk factors, and in-hospital outcomes. The Northern New England Cardiovascular Disease Study Group. *American Heart Journal*, **137**, 639–45.

BIBLIOGRAPHY

Aronow, W. S. (1998). Management of older persons after myocardial infarction. *Journal of American Geriatrics Society*, **46**, 1459–68.

De Boer, M. J., Ottervanger, J. P., van't Hof, A. W. *et al.* (2002). Reperfusion therapy in elderly patients with acute myocardial infarction: a randomized comparison of primary angioplasty and thrombolytic therapy. *Journal of the American College of Cardiology*, **39**, 1723–8.

Deedwania, P. C. (2000). Silent myocardial ischaemia in the elderly. *Drugs and Aging*, **16**, 381–9.

Ganz, D. A., Lamas, G. A., Orav, E. J. *et al.* (1999). Age-related differences in management of heart disease: a study of cardiac medication use in an older cohort. *Journal of the American Geriatrics Society*, **47**, 145–50.

Gregoratos, G. (2001). Clinical manifestations of acute myocardial infarction in older patients. *American Journal of Geriatric Cardiology*, **10**, 345–7.

Henkin, Y., Crystal, E., Goldberg, Y. *et al.* (2002). Usefulness of lipoprotein changes during acute coronary syndromes for prediction postdischarge lipoprotein levels. *American Journal of Cardiology*, **89**, 7–11.

Lakatta, E. G. (1999). Cardiovascular aging research: the next horizon. *Journal of the American Geriatrics Society*, **47**, 613–25.

Mehta, S., Urban, P., and Benedetti, E. D. (2001). Acute myocardial infection. *Clinical Evidence*, **6**, 8–30.

Ryan, T. J., Antman, E. M., Brooks, N. H. *et al.* (1999). 1999 update – ACC/AHA guidelines for the management of patients with acute myocardial infarction: executive summary and recommendations. *Circulation*, **100**, 1016–30.

Shlipak, M. G., Browner, W. S., and Noguchi, H. I. (2001). Comparison of the effects of angiotensin converting enzyme inhibitors and beta blockers on survival in elderly patients with reduced left ventricular function after myocardial infarction. *American Journal of Medicine*, **110**, 425–33.

Sudlow, C., Lonn, E., Pignone, M. *et al.* (1991). Secondary prevention of ischaemic cardiac events. *Clinical Evidence*, **6**, 114–43.

Tresch, D. D. (1998). Management of the older patient with acute myocardial infarction: differences in clinical presentations between older and younger patients. *Journal of the American Geriatrics Society*, **46**, 1157–62.

Tresch D. D. and Alla, H. R. (2001). Diagnosis and management of myocardial ischemia (angina) in the elderly patient. *American Journal of Geriatric Cardiology*, **10**, 337–44.

▸▸ Wheezing

An 85-year-old woman is brought to the emergency department by her home health aide because of shortness of breath and worsening cough for 1 week. She has a long history of hypertension, diabetes, chronic obstructive pulmonary disease (COPD), bronchiectasis, osteoporosis, and osteoarthritis. She had smoked heavily all her adult life but quit 20 years ago. Over the last 2 years, she has had several admissions for COPD exacerbation, which responded to antibiotics and corticosteroids.

The patient adheres carefully to her regimen of medications, which include inhaled corticosteroids and bronchodilators, lisinopril, rosiglitazone, calcium and vitamin D, and acetaminophen. Her blood pressure and blood sugar have been under good control. She lives by herself and is assisted by a home health aide 8 hours a day.

In the emergency room, her blood pressure is 170/90, pulse is 88 and regular, respiratory rate is 28 per minute, and temperature is 98 °F. Lung examination reveals basilar crackles (unchanged from previous examinations), diffuse rhonchi, and wheezing. No peripheral edema is noted. The electrocardiogram (EKG) reveals left ventricular hypertrophy (LVH). Chest X-ray shows poor inspiration, increased vascular markings, and a retrocardiac infiltrate. She is admitted and treated with intravenous methylprednisone, antibiotics, and nebulized bronchodilators. She feels better in a few hours.

The next morning, to your surprise, you find the patient's respiratory status has worsened. She is sitting upright in bed, has labored breathing, and wheezing can be heard without the stethoscope.

A repeat chest X-ray is performed.

Case Studies in Geriatric Medicine, Judith C. Ahronheim *et al.* Published by Cambridge University Press.
© J. C. Ahronheim, Z.-B. Huang, V. Yen, C. M. Davitt, and D. Barile

Questions

    1. What is the cause of the patient's worsening condition?
    2. What is the pathophysiology? How can the diagnosis be confirmed?
    3. What factors could have contributed to this patient's problem?
    4. How should this condition be treated?

Answers

1. When an elderly patient presents with cough, dyspnea, or wheezing, congestive heart failure (CHF) should always be in the differential diagnosis, even when there is a history of COPD. This is especially important when the patient has a history of hypertension, diabetes, or ischemic heart disease. This patient's medical history made COPD exacerbation the major consideration on admission. However, despite aggressive treatment, her wheezing and dyspnea eventually worsened. Wheezing is a common finding in elderly patients with CHF, even in those without a known history of bronchospastic disease. Patients with this "cardiac asthma" have a bronchospastic response to methacholine, compared with heart failure patients who do not have wheezing.

   A repeat chest X-ray showed small bilateral pleural effusions and pulmonary vascular congestion, in addition to the previous finding of a retrocardiac infiltrate. Intravenous furosemide and morphine were given and the patient improved. The dose of lisinopril was increased to 10 mg daily, with a plan to increase further, as tolerated. Repeat EKG showed no changes and cardiac enzymes were normal. Thyroid function tests and repeat complete blood count (CBC) were ordered, and an echocardiogram was performed.

2. The patient's echocardiogram revealed LVH, normal left ventricular (LV) function with an ejection fraction (EF) of 65%, and mild pulmonary hypertension. CHF with preserved left ventricular function suggests the patient has diastolic dysfunction – an important cause of CHF in the elderly.

   Heart failure can be associated with either reduced cardiac output (LV systolic dysfunction) or with normal cardiac output. If the maintenance of adequate cardiac output requires a higher than normal LV filling pressure, it is referred to as diastolic dysfunction. The patient may be asymptomatic or may experience only reduced exercise tolerance, or may have overt heart failure that is clinically identical to LV failure. Among patients with CHF, diastolic dysfunction accounts for fewer than

10% of cases under the age of 65, but the proportion increases with advancing age, accounting for more than 50% of cases after age 75.

Many factors may affect diastolic function, the most important being LV relaxation, LV stiffness, and left atrial function. LV relaxation, which occurs during early diastole, is an energy-dependent process and can be readily affected by ischemia. LV diastolic stiffness or compliance is affected by myocardial fiber distensibility, connective tissue elasticity, chamber size, wall thickness, and the condition of the pericardium. Left atrial contraction, which occurs in late diastole, accounts for less than 20% of filling volume in young, healthy persons, whereas, in patients with early diastolic dysfunction, the left atrium increases contractility to compensate for LV diastolic dysfunction and can contribute up to 50% of the filling volume.

Diastolic dysfunction can be caused by impaired energy-dependent ventricular relaxation, which occurs in ischemic heart disease, hypertrophy, tachycardia, and increased afterload such as in aortic stenosis, or it can be due to reduced passive elastic properties, which occur in hypertension with LVH or if there are increased myocardial connective tissue components, such as fibrosis, diabetes, or infiltrative diseases such as amyloidosis. Both mechanisms exist to a limited degree in normal aging. Diastolic dysfunction is more common in women than in men and is the cause of nearly two-thirds of all CHF cases in women over the age of 80. The reason for the gender difference is not clear, but it may be related to the greater frequency of systolic heart failure in the male cohort.

Accurate diagnosis of diastolic dysfunction requires simultaneous measurements of LV pressures and volumes to create pressure–volume curves, using cardiac catheterization. This is invasive and unpractical. Clinically, the diagnosis of diastolic heart failure relies on clinical criteria for CHF with documentation of preserved LV function by Doppler echocardiogram (i.e. EF >45%), and absence of other conditions that also cause CHF with normal LV systolic function, such as anemia and thyrotoxicosis. This patient's thyroid function tests and CBC were normal.

3. Long-standing hypertension, diabetes, and possible coronary artery disease, as well as aging, probably all contributed to this patient's diastolic dysfunction. Thiazolidinediones, such as rosiglitazone, may cause fluid retention and precipitate overt CHF in patients with underlying cardiac dysfunction. These drugs are believed to produce peripheral vasodilatation, which leads to decreased mean arterial pressure and consequent renal retention of sodium and water. Recently, in vitro evidence of pulmonary endothelial cell permeability has been reported (see Idris *et al.*, 2003), but more research is needed to confirm a cellular mechanism.

The exacerbation of COPD and the overnight intravenous fluid infusion might also have contributed to the rapid worsening of this patient's CHF. After alleviation of pulmonary congestion with diuretics, the dose of lisinopril was further increased to 20 mg and the patient tolerated it well. Her weight decreased by

6 pounds over 4 days. Her pneumonia and COPD improved and corticosteroids were tapered. Rosiglitazone was discontinued, glipizide was instituted, and the patient was discharged home.

4. Treatment of underlying or exacerbating conditions, such as hypertension, myocardial ischemia, and tachyarrhythmias, is important. In contrast to systolic heart failure, virtually no randomized controlled trials have been conducted of the treatment of diastolic heart failure. Clinical experience and limited evidence indicate that most treatments for systolic heart failure can also benefit patients with diastolic heart failure. Diuretics are useful for acute exacerbation of pulmonary congestion and fluid retention, such as in this case. However, since patients with diastolic dysfunction depend on an adequate preload to maintain normal cardiac output, overuse of diuretics should be avoided. There is some evidence that angiotensin-converting enzyme (ACE) inhibitors and angiotensin receptor blockers (ARBs) improve diastolic function. A possible mechanism might be their ability to affect beneficially the myocardial remodeling process in CHF. Beta-blockers may also be beneficial for patients with diastolic dysfunction. In addition to their antihypertensive and anti-ischemic properties, they improve diastolic filling by reducing heart rate in patients with tachycardia. Digoxin is not usually recommended in patients with CHF associated with diastolic dysfunction, but it has been used successfully and safely to control heart rate in patients with atrial fibrillation coexisting with diastolic dysfunction.

Caveat

A clinical diagnosis of CHF with preserved systolic function does not always mean the patient's heart failure was due to diastolic dysfunction. Heart failure can be due to secondary causes, such as anemia or thyrotoxicosis, despite preservation of systolic function. In fact, anemia is an important cause of heart failure in the elderly. The clinical diagnosis of CHF can be in error (e.g. confused with COPD exacerbation), the measurement of LVEF can vary depending on techniques, technician, and examination. Patient factors, such as obesity or emphysema, can impair the quality of echocardiogram examination and LVEF can be misleadingly high in mitral regurgitation.

REFERENCE

Idris, I., Gray, S., and Donnelly, R. (2003). Rosiglitazone and pulmonary oedema: an acute dose-dependent effect on human endothelial cell permeability. *Diabetologia*, **46**, 288–90.

BIBLIOGRAPHY

Benbow, A., Stewart, M., and Yeoman, G. (2001). Thiazolidinediones for type 2 diabetes. All glitazones may exacerbate heart failure. *British Medical Journal*, **322**, 236.

Campbell, R., Banner, R., Konick-McMahan, J. *et al.* (1998). Discharge planning and home follow-up of the elderly patient with heart failure. *Geriatric Nursing*, **33**, 497–513.

Dauterman, K. W., Massie, B. M., and Gheorghiade, M. (1998). Heart failure associated with preserved systolic function: a common and costly clinical entity. *American Heart Journal*, **135**, S310–19.

Garcia, M. (2000). Diastolic dysfunction and heart failure: causes and treatment options. *Cleveland Clinic Journal of Medicine*, **67**, 727–38.

Rich, M. W. (2001). Heart failure in the 21st century: a cardiogeriatric syndrome. *Journals of Gerontology*, **56A**, M88–96.

Tang, W. H. W., Francis, G. S., Hoogwerf, B. J. *et al.* (2003). Fluid retention after initiation of thiazolidinedione therapy in diabetic patients with established chronic heart failure. *Journal of the American College of Cardiology*, **41**, 1394–8.

Tecce, M., Pennington, J., Segal, B. *et al.* (1999). Heart failure: clinical implications of systolic and diastolic dysfunction. *Geriatrics*, **54**, 24–33.

Case 17

▶▶ Acute hemiparesis

Mrs. D, who is 84 years old, is having dinner with her daughter's family when, suddenly, some food drops out of her mouth. Her son-in-law notices that she is staring into space and asks her what is wrong but she cannot get the words out to explain. It appears as though she has dropped her fork and has begun to drool. The family grows alarmed and calls an ambulance, which takes her to the emergency room. Her neurologic symptoms resolve before she reaches the hospital and she is sent home, having been instructed to take one enteric-coated aspirin daily. Carotid doppler reveals diffuse atherosclerosis throughout both carotid systems and a large nonobstructive plaque in the left carotid bulb with "no hemodynamic significance."

Six months later, a similar episode occurs, but this time the symptoms do not resolve. On physical examination, Mrs. D is alert, her pulse is 108 and irregular, and her blood pressure is 180/80. She has a bruit over the left carotid artery and flattening of the right nasolabial fold. Her right upper and lower extremities are weak. When asked how she feels, she appears to be attempting an answer but cannot speak. She is unable to cooperate for a full sensory examination, but she appears to have slightly decreased sensation to pinprick on the right side. Stool is guaiac negative.

Computed tomography scan shows a cerebral infarct in the territory of the left middle cerebral artery. There is no apparent hemorrhage. Electrocardiogram shows atrial fibrillation.

Questions

1. What is the relationship between the patient's cardiac arrhythmia and the neurologic episode? Her carotid arterial disease and the episode?
2. What treatment should be given for the stroke at this time?

Case Studies in Geriatric Medicine, Judith C. Ahronheim *et al.* Published by Cambridge University Press.
© J. C. Ahronheim, Z.-B. Huang, V. Yen, C. M. Davitt, and D. Barile

3. How can further strokes be prevented?
4. What is the value of cardioversion for this patient?
5. What other deficits might this patient experience that are seen in middle cerebral artery strokes?

Answers

1. Mrs. D's arrhythmia suggests (but does not prove) that her stroke is due to a thromboembolism of cardiac origin. Patients with atrial fibrillation (AF) have nearly a 6-fold increased risk of stroke than those without AF (and more than 10-fold in the presence of rheumatic valvular disease). The incidence of stroke attributable to AF increases with age from 1.5% among patients aged 50–59 years to 23.5% among those aged 80–89 (see Wolf *et al.*, 1991). However, the preceding transient ischemic attack (TIA) in the same vascular territory, her carotid bruit, and abnormal carotid doppler examination suggest that either neurologic event could have been a consequence of carotid artery disease. This situation – comorbidity that increases stroke risk – commonly poses diagnostic dilemmas in elderly patients. Other cardiovascular stroke risk factors that increase with age include hypertension, left ventricular diastolic and systolic dysfunction, aortic arch calcification, and diabetes; in fact, advanced age alone is the strongest independent risk factor for stroke. Although TIA may occur in the setting of AF, the source of the transient event cannot be proven.

   It is generally not possible to prove that a stroke is cardioembolic in origin based on physical findings or neuroimaging. Although autopsy studies reveal a higher incidence of arterial emboli in stroke patients with AF than in those with sinus rhythm, this does not prove that the source of the embolus is the atrium, since atrial thrombi are not always demonstrated. (Conversely, one could argue that atrial thrombus might be absent because it had embolized.)

   Although it is theoretically possible that Mrs. D's stroke was not cardioembolic in origin, the association of AF is a compelling reason to treat the stroke as if it were. Echocardiographic findings in patients with AF often suggest stasis within the left atrial appendage, and such findings are associated with an elevated risk of stroke. Furthermore, warfarin is often effective in preventing stroke in patients with AF (see below) but is less likely to prevent lacunar stroke or "ischemic" stroke associated with carotid arterial disease when the latter are not associated with atrial fibrillation.

2. Acute nonhemorrhagic stroke is often treated with thrombolytic agents, such as recombinant tissue plasminogen activator, streptokinase, or urokinase, which, when

used promptly after a stroke, have been shown to reduce substantially death and disability. Unfortunately, too few subjects in clinical trials have been over the age of 80 to draw conclusions about the risk–benefit ratio in this age group. Since stroke rate, disability, and mortality increase with age, the absolute risk reduction should be greatest in the very elderly. However, elderly patients who receive thrombolytic agents in the setting of acute myocardial infarction have a higher rate of intracranial hemorrhage than do younger adults.

Anticoagulation, however, is frequently given in the setting of acute nonhemorrhagic stroke in the setting of AF. This approach is not without risk, though, since acute ischemic stroke may be associated with spontaneous petechial hemorrhage, which could turn into frank intracranial hemorrhage with or thrombolytic agents.

Attention to this patient's overall medical condition is important. Issues specific to acute stroke include metabolic factors such as electrolyte abnormalities, hypoglycemia in patients being treated for diabetes, and hyperthyroidism in patients with acute AF. Management of hypertension in acute stroke is problematic; except in extreme elevations (e.g. systolic pressure greater than 220 mmHg), lowering blood pressure in the setting of acute stroke may worsen rather than improve prognosis, by extending the area of infarct and by compromising blood flow to the "ischemic penumbra," a potentially viable area surrounding the ischemic core of a brain infarct. Acute stroke may itself elevate blood pressure, and, as the patient stabilizes, the blood pressure may normalize. Guidelines are given in the references (see McDowell et al., 1997).

It is important to be attentive to the early complications of stroke, such as shoulder subluxation, deep vein thrombosis, aspiration, and pressure ulcers. Shoulder subluxation is a common complication of acute hemiparesis. The paretic arm should be supported; this can be done by placing the affected arm in a sling. The sling must be fitted correctly and appropriate measures taken to prevent spasticity of the paretic arm, or contractures may result. Likewise, the patient should be turned frequently to avoid pressure on bony prominences, if she cannot maneuver on her own, in order to prevent pressure ulcers.

When stroke is complicated by altered mental status or dysphagia, there is an increased risk of aspiration pneumonia. Speech and swallowing therapy may be helpful for patients who can cooperate with therapeutic swallowing exercises. Patients who acutely lose the ability to swallow may need artificial nutrition and hydration; however, gastrostomy or jejunostomy feeding may not reduce the risk of aspiration pneumonia (see Case 7).

3. Statistically, there is approximately a 20% risk that Mrs. D will have another stroke within the next year because of the association with AF, whether or not it has "caused" her present stroke. The history of TIA itself is associated with a significant risk of stroke within the first year.

Anticoagulation with warfarin should be considered in the long term, unless there is an absolute contraindication – such as evidence of intracerebral bleeding or other serious bleeding disorder. Relative contraindications among the elderly include falling, recurrent gastrointestinal bleeding in the setting of unstable cardiac disease, and the inability to adhere to a strict medication regimen.

Warfarin is probably at least as effective in reducing stroke in the elderly patient with AF as it is in middle-aged adults. Being female and over 75 years of age places this patient at higher risk of stroke than other subgroups of patients with AF. Adjusted-dose warfarin is currently the most effective pharmacologic treatment for reducing the risk of cardioembolic stroke in such patients, but may be no more effective (and is possibly a riskier treatment) in reducing noncardioembolic stroke risk.

It is not surprising that aspirin failed to prevent Mrs. D's stroke. Although aspirin is often prescribed to prevent cardioembolic stroke in patients who cannot take warfarin, it has virtually no protective effect in "high-risk" subgroups of patients with AF, such as this patient – a women over 75 years of age, with prior TIA, and possible hypertension (Hart *et al.*, 1999). Other regimens for stroke prevention include combined treatment with aspirin and high-dose dipyridamole (Aggrenox), or clopidogrel with or without aspirin, but these antithrombotic agents are best used in the prevention of noncardioembolic strokes.

The patient's cholesterol profile should be assessed and treated if necessary. Cholesterol lowering with hydroxy methylglutaryl coenzyme A reductase inhibitors ("statins") may reduce the risk of stroke (see Case 13), although the risk reduction is less impressive than for cardiac events. Furthermore, clinical trials have not included substantial numbers of patients over 75 years of age, and the impact of statins in AF-associated stroke is not known. If statins are given to patients on warfarin, careful drug selection is needed to avoid potential interactions with the anticoagulant.

Once the patient's neurologic status has stabilized, blood pressure should be optimized, as discussed in Case 14.

Endarterectomy may be useful in reducing stroke in patients with high-grade (>70%) symptomatic carotid stenosis, including in carefully selected patients 75 years of age and older. However, it is difficult to gauge whether patients with coexisting AF would benefit from this procedure.

4. The use of cardioversion in AF to maintain sinus rhythm is controversial. The likelihood that someone of this patient's age will maintain sinus rhythm after successful cardioversion is low. Recent evidence indicates that patients with recurrent AF may do as well or even better with rate control than with efforts to restore and maintain sinus rhythm (see AFFIRM, 2000; Van Gelder *et al.*, 2002). In elderly patients, this may be partly related to the need for repeated cardioversion and the use of potentially toxic drugs such as amiodarone, which has an extremely long half-life and

may be poorly tolerated in the elderly. Furthermore, apparent restoration of sinus rhythm may be misleading, as many such patients continue to have undetected paroxysmal AF.

There may still be a place for attempting cardioversion in new-onset AF; however, restoration of sinus rhythm should not reduce vigilance or create a false sense of security that this will reduce stroke risk.

5. Mrs. D apparently has developed a feared and extremely troublesome deficit – aphasia (or "dysphasia," if the deficit is incomplete), a problem in the language centers of the brain. The mechanical apparatus of phonation (tongue, palate, and lips) are intact, but the brain is unable to create normal speech. Writing is generally impaired as well. The language centers are most often located on the left ("dominant") side of the brain, even in left-handed people. Aphasia differs from dysarthria, in which language centers are unaffected but there is damage to the neurologic or muscular supply to the organs of phonation; although speech and comprehension are normal, words are slurred and sometimes barely intelligible. Dysarthria is associated with a better general functional outcome than aphasia.

Aphasia is often classified as "expressive" and nonfluent, or "receptive" and fluent. Fluent (Wernicke's) aphasia is characterized by well-articulated speech that seems syntactical but does not make sense because it contains many paraphrasias – i.e. words or parts of words are often substituted with irrelevant words or syllables. In nonfluent (Broca's) aphasia, production of speech is sparse and patients often appear extremely frustrated by their inability to speak. Mrs. D has Broca's aphasia, which generally involves lesions in the territory of the middle cerebral artery, and is often associated with hemiparesis. In contrast, patients with Wernicke's aphasia seem unaware of their speech deficits and, because the territory of the inferior middle cerebral artery is generally involved, there may be little or no hemiparesis. These seemingly articulate patients may present a picture of a functioning individual but they fail to understand what is going on and require much care. The classic dichotomy of Broca's and Wernicke's aphasia persists, although the syndromes commonly overlap, probably because of the complexity of the neurologic structures involved and depending on the extent of neurologic damage. Complete or near-complete loss of expressive and receptive aspects is termed global aphasia.

Homonymous hemianopsia is another common feature of middle cerebral artery occlusion. Vision is impaired in visual space on the side opposite the lesion (the same side as the hemiparesis). This is a subtle finding, particularly in perceptually impaired patients with left-brain lesions, and can be mistaken for inattention. The stroke patient should be examined carefully for the presence of hemianopsia so that other deficits can be evaluated accurately. Other subtle findings include visual spatial deficits and neglect of the involved extremities, body, or left-half of space.

Caveats

1. Although most people with AF do not have hyperthyroidism, among adults over 65 years who have low thyroid-stimulating hormone levels or overt hyperthyroidism, approximately 12–14% have AF. Among very old people with thyrotoxicosis, as many as one-third may present with AF (see Tibaldi, 1986; Auer *et al.*, 2001).
2. An unusual cause of stroke in the elderly is temporal arteritis. This condition generally involves medium-sized arteries, but is unlikely to cause hemiparesis; rather, "strokes" most often cause visual loss when small retinal arteries are occluded.

REFERENCES

Atrial Fibrillation Follow-up Investigation of Rhythm Management (AFFIRM) Investigators (2002). A comparison of rate control and rhythm control in patients with atrial fibrillation. *New England Journal of Medicine*, **347**, 1825–33.

Auer, J., Scheibner, P., Mische, T. *et al.* (2001). Subclinical hyperthyroidism as a risk factor for atrial fibrillation. *American Heart Journal*, **142**, 838–42.

Hart, R. G., Pearce, L. A., McBride, R. *et al.* (1999). Factors associated with ischemic stroke during aspirin therapy in atrial fibrillation: analysis of 2012 participants in the SPAF I–III clinical trials. The Stroke Prevention in Atrial Fibrillation (SPAF) Investigators. *Stroke*, **30**, 1223–9.

McDowell, F. H., Brott T. G., Goldstein, M. *et al.* (1997). Stroke: the first hours, emergency evaluation, and treatment. National Stroke Association Consensus Statement. *Stroke Clinical Update (Special Edition)*, 1–14.

Tibaldi, J. M. (1986). Thyrotoxicosis in the very old. *American Journal of Medicine*, **81**, 619–22.

Van Gelder, I. C., Hagens, V. E., Bosker, H. A. *et al.*, for the Rate Control versus Electrical Cardioversion for Persistent Atrial Fibrillation Study Group (2002). A comparison of rate control and rhythm control in patients with recurrent persistent atrial fibrillation. *New England Journal of Medicine*, **347**, 1834–40.

Wolf, P. A., Abbott, R. D., and Kannel, W. B. (1991). Atrial fibrillation as an independent risk factor for stroke: the Framingham study. *Stroke*, **22**, 983–8.

BIBLIOGRAPHY

Albert, M. and Helm-Estabrooks, N. (1988). Diagnosis and treatment of aphasia. *Journal of the American Medical Association*, **259**, 1043–7, 1205–10.

Feinberg, W. M., Blackshear, J. L., Laupacis, A. *et al.* (1995). The prevalence of atrial fibrillation: analysis and implications. *Archives of Internal Medicine*, **155**, 469–73.

Gage, B. F., Fihn, S. D., and White, R. H. (2001). Warfarin therapy for an octogenarian who has atrial fibrillation. *Annals of Internal Medicine*, **134**, 465–74.

Hart R. G., Halperin, J. L., Pearce, L. A. *et al.* (2003). Lessons from the Stroke Prevention in Atrial Fibrillation Trials. *Annals of Internal Medicine*, **138**, 831–8.

Hart, R. G., Pearce, L. A., Miller, V. T. *et al.*, on behalf of the SPAF investigators. (2000). Cardioembolic vs. noncardioembolic strokes in atrial fibrillation: frequency and effect of antithrombotic agents in the Stroke Prevention in Atrial Fibrillation Studies. *Cerebrovascular Diseases*, **10**, 39–43.

Kannel, W. B., Abbott, R. D., Savage, D. D. *et al.* (1982). Epidemiologic features of chronic atrial fibrillation. *New England Journal of Medicine*, **306**, 1018–22.

Kanter, M. C., Tegeler, C. H., and Pearce, L. A. (1994). Carotid stenosis in patients with AF. Prevalence, risk factors, and relationship to stroke in the Stroke Prevention in Atrial Fibrillation Study. *Archives of Internal Medicine*, **154**, 1372–7.

Miller, V. T., Rothrock, J. F., Pearce, L. A. *et al.* (1993). Ischemic stroke in patients with atrial fibrillation: effect of aspirin according to stroke mechanism. Stroke Prevention in Atrial Fibrillation Investigators. *Neurology*, **43**, 32–6.

Muir, K. W. and Roberts, M. (2000). Thrombolytic therapy for stroke: a review with particular reference to elderly patients. *Drugs and Aging*, **16**, 41–54.

Rothwell, P. M., Eliasziw, M., Gutnikov, S. A. *et al.*, for the Carotid Endarterectomy Trialists' Collaboration (2003). Analysis of pooled data from the randomised controlled trials of endarterectomy for symptomatic carotid stenosis. *Lancet*, **361**, 107–16.

Stroke Prevention in Atrial Fibrillation Investigators (1996). Adjusted-dose warfarin versus low-intensity, fixed dose warfarin plus aspirin for high-risk patients with atrial fibrillation: Stroke Prevention in Atrial Fibrillation III randomised clinical trial. *Lancet*, **348**, 633–8.

Case 18

▸▸ Chronic hemiparesis

After 3 months of rehabilitation, Mrs. D, whom we met in Case 17, "plateaus." She has regained some speech but produces few words. Her right arm and leg are very weak. There is increased tone but no significant spasticity. Impaired plantar flexion in her paretic limb has left her with a foot drop. She has learned to transfer from chair to bed and toilet, can ambulate with a cane and contact guarding, but has difficulty getting to her feet without help. She seems to comprehend speech and follows commands regularly. She is able to feed herself if food is prepared, cut, and brought to her. She has difficulty dressing and grooming and requires assistance in handling her personal affairs. She has been living in a skilled nursing facility with a rehabilitation service, and wishes to live in her daughter's home. The family is eager to have her live with them, and is prepared to pay for a home attendant if necessary.

Hypertension and heart rate are well controlled on metoprolol, hydrochlorothiazide, and losartan, and her INR is controlled on warfarin 4 mg daily.

Questions

1. How can the devices pictured (Figure 7) be useful to her?
2. What are some of the late complications and sequelae of stroke, and what can be done about them?
3. How can the patient's activities of daily living be described? What can be done?

Case Studies in Geriatric Medicine, Judith C. Ahronheim *et al.* Published by Cambridge University Press. © J. C. Ahronheim, Z.-B. Huang, V. Yen, C. M. Davitt, and D. Barile

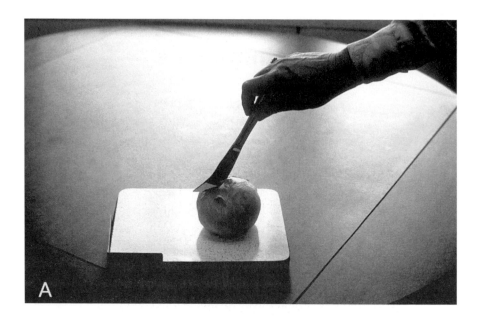

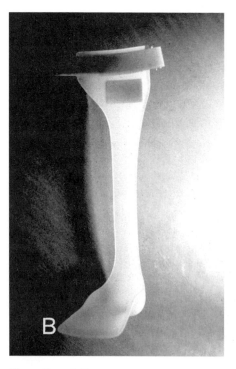

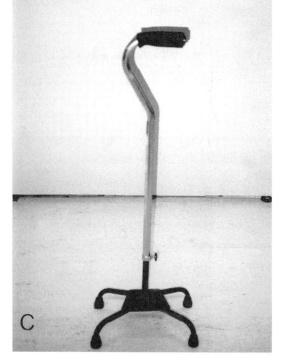

Figure 7   A–E, see text.

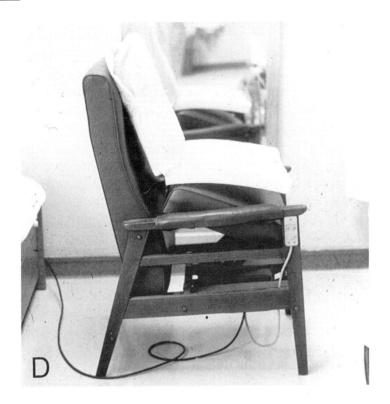

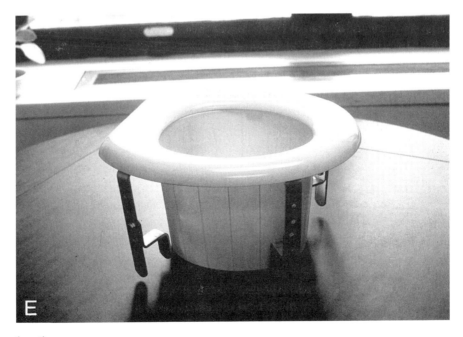

Figure 7   (cont.)

Answers

1. Unique utensils exist so that people with only one useful hand can prepare and eat food. The device pictured in Figure 7A can assist the patient to cut her food on her own. It is being demonstrated on a cutting board that is adherent to the counter and will be of additional help if she wishes to prepare her own food. A commercially made plastic nonslip mat (Dycem® and others) can be placed under the plates and cutlery to prevent slipping and make them easier to grip. This material can be cut and mounted on objects such as cups and pieces of cutlery. Numerous other devices are available to assist hemiparetic people in improving their independence, including Velcro closures for shoes and garments, long-handled shoehorns, stocking pulls, and zipper pulls. These devices and others are also useful to patients with limitations due to other disorders, such as Parkinson's disease, arthritis, fractures, and amputations.

   The posterior leaf splint (Figure 7B) is lightweight and well tolerated. It is constructed so that it will prevent involuntary plantar flexion and is a very useful "orthotic" in stroke patients whose hemiparesis includes weak dorsiflexion or ankle instability. If there is severe spasticity, this type of orthotic cannot be used. The posterior leaf splint is lightweight and better tolerated than a heavier metal brace.

   The four-pronged "quad" cane (Figure 7C) will confer greater stability than an ordinary cane, and, if adequate, is preferred by patients to the more cumbersome and conspicuous walker, especially outside of the home. However, patients must be able to use this aid properly; for example, a poorly taught or cognitively impaired patient may fail to rest all four prongs on the ground, or may hold it backwards and trip over the base. In general, a cane should be held on the side opposite the deficit and planted firmly ahead before moving the impaired limb. Then, the first step is taken by the impaired leg and weight is planted. The sequence is: cane, impaired leg, strong leg. The height of the cane should be adjusted so the top is at the level of the femoral trochanter and the elbow is flexed 15–30 degrees.

   Some patients will reserve a walker for inhome use, often preferring wheeled walkers which allow for more speedy ambulation. The wheeled walker is not as stable as a standard walker and patients with instability due to paretic limbs should generally avoid them.

   Pain, stiffness, or weakness in joints or muscles responsible for extension at the knee and hip make it extremely difficult for people with a variety of disorders to get out of low chairs. Straight-backed armchairs are the best standard chairs for such patients, but the pictured seat-lift chair (Figure 7D) gives the patient additional mechanical assistance, and may be particularly useful for a patient with a weak arm.

Toilet seats are even lower than standard chairs. The raised toilet seat (Figure 7E) will be very useful to this patient, and should be installed along with strategically placed arm rails. Independence in toileting is one of the most important parts of rehabilitation because being put on and off a toilet can be emotionally devastating.

2. Contractures and pain often occur in paretic extremities. Early institution of range-of-motion exercises, treatment of accompanying pain, and splinting to counteract an imbalance between agonist and antagonist muscle groups can prevent contractures. Antispasticity medications, such as baclofen and benzodiazepines, frequently exacerbate cognitive deficits in elderly patients, and must be used with extreme caution. Chronic pain in paretic extremities can also be due to lesions involving the thalamus, or from mechanical disturbances resulting from spastic or flaccid paralysis of the arm. Mechanical factors include traction or compression neuropathy, shoulder subluxation, or rotator cuff tear, which is sometimes caused when caregivers move or position the patient improperly. Incorrect or prolonged use of an arm sling may result in adduction and internal rotation contracture and adhesive capsulitis of the shoulder. The "shoulder–hand" syndrome is a painful sequela of hemiplegic stroke. It is an abnormality in the sympathetic nervous system, thought to be a "reflex sympathetic dystrophy" related to mechanical damage to the shoulder. Symptoms consist of progressive pain and decreased range of motion of the affected shoulder, along with swelling and coldness. The pain can be prevented with local steroids or systemic analgesia, accompanied by regular range-of-motion exercises.

Stroke patients are at a high risk of falling. The risk is due not only to weakness or spasticity in the leg, but also to visual field deficits, cognitive impairments, and spatial–perceptual deficits. Impaired dorsiflexion with foot drop commonly occurs in hemiparetic patients and can increase the risk of falls by causing tripping.

Immobilized patients are likely to develop skin ulcers at pressure points. Normal people shift position automatically, even during sleep, thereby preventing critical increases in capillary pressure that eventually lead to skin breakdown. Paralysis prevents this automatic protective shifting of position. The risk of pressure sores increases with age because of age-related skin changes, including thinning of the skin, decreased subcutaneous fat over bony prominences, and sluggish wound healing. The presence of contractures predisposes to pressure ulcers in unexpected sites. The mainstay in the prevention and treatment of pressure sores is the relief of pressure and avoidance of friction and excessive moisture. Although patients who must sit for prolonged periods or are bedbound often benefit from "waffle"-style, air-filled, or other cushions or mattresses that distribute pressure, it is imperative to assist the patient in frequent position changes as this is the best preventive maneuver and will promote comfort. Skin ulcers are discussed further in Case 29.

Poststroke depression occurs in 20–60% of patients, but may respond well to treatment with supportive therapy, medication, or electroconvulsive therapy. Unfortunately, it is often unrecognized or left untreated. Dementia often occurs at the time of major hemispheric stroke, but progressive dementia is generally due to coexisting Alzheimer's disease or other neurodegenerative disorder.

Deep vein thrombosis commonly develops in paralyzed legs and may produce pulmonary emboli. Nonparetic limbs may also be at risk in patients with spatial neglect of the affected side. They not only bump into objects in that side of space, but also fail to move the paretic limb passively. They sometimes lack insight into their deficits, which exacerbates the problem. Since speech is usually unimpaired in people with right-sided brain lesions, observers and caregivers tend to underestimate the patient's deficits.

Urinary incontinence is a common complication of stroke, but, in elderly stroke patients, the etiology is more commonly functional, related to immobility superimposed on pre-existing detrusor instability (see Case 33).

Seizures may develop at stroke onset or days to months later. Most poststroke seizures occur within the first 24 hours, and are more common in hemorrhagic than nonhemorrhagic stroke, but, among the latter, a second peak in incidence occurs 6–12 months later. When seizures develop late, they are more likely to be recurrent ("epilepsy"), probably because they are related to scarring and an established irritable focus. Poststroke seizures tend to be of the partial variety and, since those that occur early on are rarely recurrent, long-term anticonvulsant treatment is not always needed.

3. "ADL" is the expression used to refer to a patient's ability to perform activities of daily living. ADL assessment includes ability to toilet, dress, groom, bathe, ambulate, transfer, and feed. A more sensitive set of functional measures are the IADLs (instrumental activities of daily living), which include cooking, shopping, handling finances, keeping house, using the telephone, and ability to use transportation. The IADL scale is relevant to community-dwelling elderly, or recovering stroke or fracture patients that are being considered for discharge home, while the ADL scale would perhaps be more relevant for the patient who required institutionalization or around-the-clock home care.

The present patient should undergo physical therapy, in order to maximize physical function, occupational therapy, in order to become able to perform specific tasks, and speech therapy, in order to maximize verbal performance. When neurologic and functional return have leveled off, the patient is said to "plateau." At this point, rehabilitation goals are directed at the maintenance of physical and psychologic function.

This patient needs assistance with ADLs as well as IADLs. Although the family is willing to pay for a home attendant, government entitlements in the United States would make it prudent for the patient to pay for this out of her own savings (see Case 6). Care through a certified home care agency might be restricted (e.g. an aid could remind the patient to take medications but not administer them). Privately paid home attendants are not restricted in the type of care they can provide but are also not subject to standards of training.

Care could be augmented by one or more home visits by a geriatrician and a geriatric assessment team. Since she has limited mobility, it would be easier for the patient and her family if they did not have to transport her to the office. The team could see first hand how the patient manages in her own environment and assess the need for any further equipment or any environmental modifications. One could also review her medications and assess the interactions between the patient, the family, and the home attendant.

BIBLIOGRAPHY

Alexander, H., Bugge, C., and Hagen, S. (2001). What is the association between the different components of stroke rehabilitation and health outcomes? *Clinical Rehabilitation*, **15**, 207–15.

Bladin, C. F., Alexandrov, A. V., Bellavance, A. L. *et al.* (2000). Seizures after stroke. A prospective multicenter study. *Archives of Neurology*, **57**, 1617–22.

Cherney, L. R., Halper, A. S., Kwasnica, C. M. *et al.* (2001). Recovery of functional status after right hemisphere stroke: relationship with unilateral neglect. *Archives of Physical Medicine and Rehabilitation*, **8**, 322–8.

Gall, A. (2001). Post stroke depression. *Hospital Medicine*, **62**, 268–73.

Gilad, R., Lampl, Y., Eschel, Y. *et al.* (2001). Antiepileptic treatment in patients with early post ischemic stroke seizures: a retrospective study. *Cerebrovascular Disease*, **12**, 39–43.

Grant, J. S., Elliott, T. R., Giger J. N. *et al.* (2001). Social problem-solving telephone partnerships with family caregivers of persons with stroke. *International Journal of Rehabilitation Research*, **24**, 181–9.

Lo Faso, V. (2000). The doctor-patient relationship in the home. *Clinics in Geriatric Medicine*, **16**, 83–94.

Montauk, S. L. (1998). Home health care. *American Family Physician*, **58**, 1608–14.

Oldenquist, G. W., Scott, L., and Finucane, T. E. (2001). Home care: what a physician needs to know. *Cleveland Clinic Journal of Medicine*, **68**, 433–40.

Palmer, R. M. (1999). Geriatric assessment. *Medical Clinics of North America*, **83**, 1503–23.

Thomas, D. R. (2001). Prevention and treatment of pressure sores: what works? What doesn't? *Cleveland Clinic Journal of Medicine*, **68**, 704–22.

Case 19

▸▸ Lower gastrointestinal hemorrhage

> Mrs. D, whom we met in Cases 17 and 18, is discharged home where care
> is provided by family members and a paid home attendant. Her current
> medications include metoprolol 50 mg bid, warfarin 4 mg daily, losartan
> 50 mg daily, hydrochlorothiazide 25 mg daily, and laxatives as needed. She
> visited her primary care physician regularly and INR is monitored and main-
> tained between 2 and 3.
>
> Six months later, the patient was admitted to the hospital for weakness fol-
> lowing a lower gastrointestinal hemorrhage. On admission, her hemoglobin
> was 8.5 g and INR was 6.

Questions

1. What accounts for the patient's elevated INR?
2. What workup should be done?

Answers

1. Important causes of elevated INR in a patient on warfarin include nonadherence to
   the drug regimen, medical illness, particularly hepatic disease, nutritional problems
   leading to vitamin K deficiency, and drug interactions.

   Age alone has been associated with increased warfarin sensitivity. Warfarin clearance declines with age. This has been attributed to decreased liver size, but the precise
   mechanism has not been defined. It has been speculatively attributed to age-related
   changes in the vitamin K epoxide reductase system (see Loebstein *et al.*, 2001),

Case Studies in Geriatric Medicine, Judith C. Ahronheim *et al.* Published by Cambridge University Press.
© J. C. Ahronheim, Z.-B. Huang, V. Yen, C. M. Davitt, and D. Barile

which is involved in the formation of active vitamin K and which is inhibited by warfarin.

Among the elderly, nonadherence is a particularly important problem, and correlates directly with the number of pills prescribed, increasing when patients take as few as three or more pills per day. Memory disorders make safe prescribing extremely difficult and generally require close supervision. Visual disorders create problems as well, since labels are difficult to read and many pills look alike. Certain brands of pills look alike, including warfarin and hydrochlorothiazide, which Mrs. D is taking, and, unless a reliable method of medication administration or dispensing is in place, errors are common, even for patients with normal vision and cognition. This patient's caregivers assisted in giving her medications which were carefully placed in a reminder box every week.

The usual cause of altered sensitivity to warfarin is a drug–drug or nutrient–drug interaction. Mrs. D's caregivers must be queried closely about medications to see if new drugs, including over-the-counter agents, have been introduced since her last visit (see Case 32). This review should include queries about prescriptions by other physicians or providers (including consultants referred by the primary provider), and about drugs, herbals, or nutrients purchased without prescription, and, if possible, should include inspection of the medications in their bottles or dose dispenser. Over-the-counter medications that increase warfarin sensitivity include cimetidine and ranitidine, and, to a lesser extent, acetaminophen. Other over-the-counter medications that can increase bleeding in patients on warfarin include medications that can inhibit platelet function, like aspirin, clopidogrel, and nonsteroidal anti-inflammatory agents, such as ibuprofen and naproxen. Herbal remedies have also been noted to interact with warfarin, as noted in Case 21.

A very large number of medications interact with warfarin, most by inhibiting the enzymes that degrade it. This patient had been referred to a urologist for a workup of microhematuria. During the workup, a urine culture revealed bacterial infection and, 1 week ago, ciprofloxacin was prescribed. Quinolones, as well as sulfonamides and certain macrolide antibiotics, bind to cytochrome P450 enzymes, inhibiting warfarin metabolism and increasing warfarin sensitivity. Other antibiotics can increase warfarin sensitivity if they alter intestinal bacteria and deplete vitamin K.

Because geriatric patients are often referred to specialists, it is important to counsel any patient on warfarin closely regarding the risks of drug and nutrient interactions, and this counseling should include instructions to contact the primary care physician before taking a newly prescribed medication, even if the prescribing physician was consulted by the primary provider.

2. A colonoscopy should be performed. The elderly experience a greater number of bleeding episodes from anticoagulants than do younger adults, even when the INR

is in the therapeutic range. This increased danger is probably due to the presence of underlying bleedable lesions, usually in the gastrointestinal tract. This patient was found to have a large rectal polyp on colonoscopy, which was the source of the bleeding. Because of the frequent comorbidity in the elderly leading to anticoagulation-associated bleeding, endoscopic or other investigations to search for undiagnosed lesions are generally warranted even when bleeding is asymptomatic. This admonition should apply to nonelderly adults as well.

Caveat

Although COX-2 selective inhibitors, which are available only by prescription, do not impair platelet function, they may participate in pharmacokinetic interactions, inhibiting warfarin metabolism and increasing INR (Hylek, 2001).

REFERENCES

Hylek, E. M. (2001). Oral anticoagulants. Pharmacologic issues for use in the elderly. *Clinics in Geriatric Medicine*, **17**, 1–13.

Loebstein, R., Yonath, H., Peleg, D. *et al.* (2001). Interindividual variability in sensitivity to warfarin – nature or nurture? *Clinical Pharmacology and Therapeutics*, **70**, 159–64.

BIBLIOGRAPHY

Kane, G. C. and Lipsky, J. L. (2000). Drug-grapefruit juice interactions. *Mayo Clinic Proceedings*, **75**, 933–42.

Schaefer, M. G., Plowman, B. K., Morreale, A. P. *et al.* (2003). Interaction of rofecoxib and celecoxib with warfarin. *American Journal of Health-Systems Pharmacy*, **60**, 1319–23.

▶▶ Delirium

A 90-year-old woman is brought to the hospital because of severe back pain and an inability to walk. She had been taking ibuprofen, acetaminophen, and, most recently, celocoxib (Celebrex) 200 mg bid without relief.

Except for some difficulty walking, she has been in relatively good health and was living by herself in a one-bedroom apartment in a large metropolitan area. Neighbors and friends have been assisting her with shopping, cleaning, and other chores. The patient has never been married and has one niece who lives in a small town about 40 miles away.

Physical examination was consistent with paraspinal muscle spasm and she was admitted to the hospital. Magnetic resonance imaging of the spine is recommended but the patient says she is extremely anxious about feeling "claustrophobic" during the test. Her doctors reassure her that she will be properly sedated prior to the examination and lorazepam (Ativan) 1 mg was given.

That night, the patient became confused and the hospital bed rails were raised "for safety," but, when she tried to climb out of bed, wrist and vest restraints were applied. An oncall physician gave a telephone order for haloperidol (Haldol) 1 mg q 2 hours as needed for delirium.

The patient was still confused 24 hours later and the pain persisted. Cyclobenzaprine (Flexeril) 10 mg tid was administered and oxycodone–acetaminophen (Percocet) was ordered as needed. The patient continued to be confused, expecially at night. She repeatedly said she wanted to leave the hospital, stating the staff were "trying to kidnap" her, and she continued to try to climb out of bed. A psychiatry consultant was called, who diagnosed dementia complicated by paranoia and "sundowning." He discontinued haloperidol, ordered risperidone (Risperdal) 0.5 mg tid as needed, and suggested Flexeril be discontinued.

The patient's pain persisted and the medical staff prescribed amitryptyline (Elavil) 25 mg for a "potential neuropathic component." Orphenadrine (Norflex) was ordered for "breakthrough" pain and spasm.

Case Studies in Geriatric Medicine, Judith C. Ahronheim *et al.* Published by Cambridge University Press.
© J. C. Ahronheim, Z.-B. Huang, V. Yen, C. M. Davitt, and D. Barile

The patient's confusion and agitation persisted. A pain consultant was called; he stated that tricyclic antidepressants were "risky" in the elderly and recommended replacing it with gabapentin (Neurontin) beginning at the low dose of 200 mg tid, with gradual increases every 3 days to a maximum 24-hour dose of 1800 mg. He also recommended that the Percocet be given every 6 hours, stating that "around-the-clock" dosing regimens were more likely to provide pain relief.

A geriatric consultant was called.

Questions

1. What did the geriatrician recommend?
2. What role did medication play in this patient's altered mental status?
3. What age-related pharmacokinetic and pharmacodynamic changes have led to this problem?
4. What are the risk factors for delirium in hospitalized elderly?
5. What medications can be given for pain in elderly patients who do not respond to acetaminophen?

Answers

1. It is likely that the geriatrician would have inquired about the patient's baseline function, noting she ordinarily functioned at a high level. He would have recommended removal of restraints, drastic changes in her medication regimen, and use of interpersonal methods to improve her orientation. The acute change and the nature of the patient's behavior would have led to the diagnosis of delirium. However, early input would likely have prevented the cascade of events that was brought on by lorazepam and incorrect management of resulting delirium.

   Delirium is a disturbance in consciousness accompanied by a new change in cognition, and occurs very commonly in hospitalized elderly. Initially, the patient has difficulty maintaining attention and consciousness fluctuates; delirium can progress to stupor and coma, with the attendant complications, and is a medical (as opposed to a psychiatric) emergency. Thus, when there is a change in mental status, medical or drug-induced causes should be considered and evaluated by the medical staff before a psychiatry consult is called.

Delirium in hospitalized patients can be due to medical illness, impaired sensory input (usually in patients with underlying brain disease, visual, or hearing deficits), and medications. Delirium can be exacerbated by sensory deprivation, mechanical restraints, and, often, medications given to reduce delirium. In this case, the most likely cause was lorazepam, but a careful examination was called for, so all potential causes would be considered.

The mechanism of delirium is poorly understood, but is believed to be caused by aberrations in one or more neurotransmitter systems. Geriatric patients are at particularly high risk, owing to age-related structural changes in the brain, alterations in specific neurotransmitter systems, and the coexistence of overt or preclinical brain disease, such as dementia.

2. Medications that could have potentially affected this patient's cognition include lorazepam, cyclobenzaprine, oxycodone, amitriptyline, orphenadrine, gabapentin, and even ibuprofen. Although neuroleptics such as haloperidol and risperidone may be useful in reducing agitation or psychotic symptoms in delirium, they may worsen confusion in certain instances. In short, almost all of the medications prescribed for this patient could have individually produced these problems. Unexpectedly small doses may be poorly tolerated in the elderly, as exemplified by the effect of 1 mg of lorazepam on this 90-year-old patient.

Benzodiazepines are particularly problematic in older adults and should generally be avoided. Although they are indicated in delirium tremens, in which agitation and psychotic symptoms often predominate, they must be used with extra caution in the elderly in order to avoid stupor and drug-induced coma.

The range of medications that can cause delirium is very broad. These include obvious agents, such as sedatives, hypnotics, neuroleptics, and tricyclic antidepressants, as well as a variety of agents from many drug classes, including anticonvulsants, histamine-2 blockers, opioid analgesics, quinolone antibiotics, nonselective cyclo-oxygenase inhibitors (nonsteroidal anti-inflammatory agents or NSAIDs), and others. This patient was taking medications from many of these classes. Drugs causing cognitive impairment are reviewed in the references (see Moore and O' Keeffe, 1999).

3. Age-related changes that affect drug metabolism and disposition ("pharmacokinetic" changes) and changes altering the effect of drug at the tissue level ("pharmacodynamic" changes) may increase the risk of drug-induced delirium.

Renal function declines with age, on the average, delaying clearance of renally eliminated drugs such as gabapentin and many NSAIDs. This age-related decline has been demonstrated in cross-sectional studies, but one longitudinal study demonstrated that as many as one-third of patients followed for 15 years do not experience this decline (Lindeman *et al.*, 1985). Serum creatinine does not accurately reflect decreases in glomerular filtration rate late in life because muscle mass, the source of measured creatinine, declines with age.

Liver size and blood flow decline with age, so hepatic extraction declines, making metabolism less efficient overall. "Phase I" hepatic metabolism (oxidation–reduction) declines with age, so that drugs handled by these processes, such as tricyclic antidepressants, opioids, neuroleptics, and most other sedatives, may be metabolized more slowly. The issue of whether age-related decline is universal is complicated by the marked genetic variability in oxidative enzymes. More importantly, phase I metabolites often have the same pharmacologic activity as the parent drug, and are eliminated by the kidney. "Phase II" metabolism (conjugation) changes little with age. This group of reactions (e.g. glucuronidation and acetylation) involves attachment of the drug to a larger endogenous molecule, producing generally inactive metabolites. Lorazepam and certain other benzodiazepines, such as temezapem, are metabolized by glucuronidation to inactive metabolites so the half-life is not significantly prolonged; still, these drugs are poorly tolerated owing to enhanced pharmacodynamic effects (see below). Moreover, diazepam (Valium), chlordiazepoxide (Librium), and other "long-acting" benzodiazepines undergo phase I metabolism, yielding active metabolites with extended half-lives.

Although serum albumin does not decline in normal aging, it is typically depressed in chronically or acutely ill elderly (see Case 7). This increases the free fraction of highly bound drugs, such as phenytoin; toxic levels of this drug generally produce ataxia in younger adults but more often produce lethargy or altered mental status in the elderly. Free drug also undergoes metabolism and excretion more readily, so the effect may not be clinically significant on a chronic basis; however, therapeutic monitoring of highly protein-bound drugs can be affected by changes in serum protein levels. Most laboratories measure total drug levels (bound plus unbound drug). Because the bound fraction of highly bound drugs accounts for more than 95%, "total" drug levels may be misleadingly low, leading to an erroneous increase in dosing.

With advancing age, total body fat increases and lean body mass decreases as the percentage of total body weight. Therefore, the volume of distribution (V_D) of lipid-soluble drugs increases with age, while the V_D of drugs that distribute in water decreases with age. Many psychotropic drugs are highly lipid soluble and accumulate in tissues, resulting in delayed toxicity and compounding the problem of delayed hepatic and renal elimination. In contrast, drugs that distribute in water, such as alcohol, have a higher peak plasma level after a given initial dose, and may produce an exaggerated response (see Case 27). Still, fat soluble drugs enter the central nervous system rapidly and may produce confusion for that reason.

4. Important risk factors for delirium include advanced age, renal impairment, and use of multiple medications. Because a normal serum creatinine level often masks renal insufficiency in the elderly, dosing guidelines for renally eliminated drugs may not be followed and repeated dosing of certain drugs, such as opioid analgesics or long-acting benzodiazepines, might lead to progressive cognitive impairment over a period of hours or even days.

    "Polypharmacy," or the use of multiple medications, also plays a role in the development of delirium, as well as other adverse drug events. In this case, the patient was given several drugs that affect the central nervous system, albeit via differing mechanisms of action. Coadministration produces an additive effect at the tissue level.

    Specific factors, including serious illness and possibly the presence of dementia, increase the risk. Patients with dementia are at greater risk when delirium occurs because it may not be recognized by medical staff, and delirium in these patients may be associated with greater morbidity than when it occurs in patients without dementia. Frequently, a combination of predisposing factors interact to produce delirium, including dementia, serious illness, and visual or hearing impairment. Compounding these problems are hospital-related factors, such as the introduction of medications, bladder catheters, and mechanical restraints, and sleep deprivation.

5. While NSAIDs may be superior to acetaminophen in conditions associated with inflammation, such as herniated disc and inflammatory arthritis, they may not provide more analgesia than comparable doses of acetaminophen in other situations, and have greater toxicity. Although some data suggest NSAIDs are superior to acetaminophen in osteoarthritis (Case *et al.*, 2003), this may not be true for all patients. Regular (as opposed to casual) use of NSAIDs is associated with a high prevalence of gastrointestinal bleeding among the elderly, because of underlying atrophic gastritis and loss of cytoprotection. Central nervous system toxicity has been reported with NSAIDs, but is relatively uncommon. Cyclo-oxygenase 2 (COX-2) inhibitors, such as celocoxib, have a lower risk of gastrointestinal toxicity, but probably do not confer greater analgesia than older NSAIDs, and are more likely to produce fluid retention and to elevate blood pressure.

    Opioids are powerful analgesics, so small doses may produce marked improvement in symptoms. They lack gastric and renal toxicity, but commonly cause dose-related delirium. Doses must be initiated and titrated carefully and the patient re-evaluated frequently, as repeated doses may lead to progressive increases in blood levels of active metabolites as well as of parent drug. Side effects such as constipation can generally be managed with laxatives or other maneuvers. Tramadol, an analgesic with opioid-like activity, may be an acceptable alternative to opioids in some patients, and is less likely to cause constipation, but may produce central nervous system side effects and has the potential for producing some pharma-cokinetic drug interactions. In addition to inhibiting cytochrome P450 enzymes, tramadol can increase serotonin neurotransmission and has been reported to pro-duce the serotonin syndrome when used in conjunction with other serotoninergic drugs.

Centrally acting muscle relaxants, such as cyclobenzaprine and orphenadrine, may relieve symptoms in muscle spasm, but most of the effect may be mediated by central mechanisms and even sedation, so pain relief commonly occurs at the expense of mental status.

Tricyclic antidepressants (TCAs), such as amitriptyline, and anticonvulsants, such as gabapentin, may provide adjunctive treatment in a variety of pain syn-dromes and are sometimes more effective than opioids in neuropathic pain. TCAs often worsen confusion and can precipitate delirium or symptoms of dementia in patients with subclinical dementia; this has been attributed to their anticholiner-gic effect and worsening of the derangements in central cholinergic mechanisms in dementia. Amitriptyline has particularly potent anticholinergic action; if a TCA were desired, nortriptyline would be less likely to cause cognitive impairment. Like-wise, gabapentin can cause confusion. This drug is renally eliminated and has a long half-life in the elderly, so dose titrations have to be made carefully.

Nonpharmacologic management of pain, such as physical therapy modalities, may be highly effective and are reviewed in the references (see Smith *et al.*, 1999).

REFERENCES

Case, J. P., Galiunas, A. J., and Block, J. A. (2003). Lack of efficacy of acetaminophen in treating symptomatic knee osteoarthritis. *Archives of Internal Medicine*, **163**, 169–78.

Moore, A. R. and O'Keeffe, S. T. (1999). Drug-induced cognitive impairment in the elderly. *Drugs and Aging*, **15**, 15–28.

Lindeman, R. D., Tobin, J., and Shock, N. W. (1985). Longitudinal studies on the rate of decline in renal function with age. *Journal of the American Geriatrics Society*, **33**, 278–85.

Smith, B. H., Hopton, J. L., and Chambers, W. A. (1999). Chronic pain in primary care. *Family Practice*, **16**, 475–82.

BIBLIOGRAPHY

Fick, D. M., Agostini, J. V., and Inouye, S. K. (2002). Delirium superimposed on dementia: a systemic review. *Journal of the American Geriatrics Society*, **50**, 1723–32.

Flacker, J. M. and Lipsitz, L. A. (1999). Neural mechanisms of delirum: current hypotheses and evolving concepts. *Journals of Gerontology: Biological Sciences*, **54A**, B239–46.

Inouye, S. K. (1994). The dilemma of delirium: clinical and research controversies regarding diagnosis and evaluation of delirium in hospitalized elderly medical patients. *American Journal of Medicine*, **97**, 278–88.

Inouye, S. K., Bogardus, S. T., Charpentier, P. A. *et al.* (1999). A multicomponent intervention to prevent delirium in hospitalized older patients. *New England Journal of Medicine*, **340**, 669–76.

Inouye, S. K., van Dyck, C. H., Alessi, C. A. *et al.* (1990). Clarifying confusion: the confusion assessment method. *Annals of Internal Medicine*, **113**, 941–8.

O'Keefe, K. P. and Sanson, T. G. (1998). Elderly patients with altered mental status. *Emergency Medicine Clinics of North America*, **16**, 1–17.

Smith, M. J., Breitbart, W. S., and Meredith, M. P. (1995). A critique of instruments and methods to detect, diagnose, and rate delirium. *Journal of Pain and Symptom Management*, **10**, 35–77.

Verrico, M. M., Weber, R. J., McKaveney, T. P. *et al.* (2003). Adverse drug events involving COX-2 inhibitors. *Annals of Pharmacotherapy*, **37**, 1203–13.

▶▶ Herbal remedies

Mr. H is a 76-year-old man whom you have been following for several years. He has a history of transient ischemic attack (TIA) and chronic atrial fibrillation. He has been on warfarin 2.5 mg at bedtime for the past year, with INR in the therapeutic range. He has been increasingly depressed and anxious since the death of his wife 6 months ago. He says, "I think I'm losing my marbles like my father" and feels his sleep patterns have become "out of whack". When you question him further, he states that one reason that he can't sleep soundly is that he must get out of bed several times a night to urinate. His INR, which was previously 2.4, is now 0.9. You wonder about his compliance and re-emphasize the need to take his warfarin properly, which he insists that he does. You ask him if any of his other doctors have prescribed any new medicines, which he denies. In fact, he tells you he stopped taking oxybutinin, which a urologist prescribed for his bladder problems, because it "didn't work." You increase the daily dose of warfarin to 3 mg.

One week later, you see his name on a sign-in sheet for a "brown bag" day, sponsored by the medical center pharmacy. For this event, patients bring in all their medications, including vitamins and over the counter preparations. You see saw palmetto, St. John's Wort, echinacea, valerian root, ginkgo biloba, and glucosamine/chondroitin. When you confront him about these medicines at his next visit – saying, "Why are you taking this garbage?" – he becomes upset and does not return to your office.

Questions

1. For what reasons might Mr. H be taking these nonprescribed remedies?
2. What evidence exists regarding their efficacy?

Case Studies in Geriatric Medicine, Judith C. Ahronheim *et al.* Published by Cambridge University Press.
© J. C. Ahronheim, Z.-B. Huang, V. Yen, C. M. Davitt, and D. Barile

3. What possible harm could be caused by these remedies?
4. How can the issue of complementary/alternative medications best be addressed by the primary care provider?

Answers

1. In general, patients seem to seek alternative therapies for disease prevention, because of perceived side effects or lack of efficacy from conventional medicine, because conventional therapies for the patient's conditions are either ineffective or nonexistent, and because of perceived spiritual or emotional benefit from alternative therapies. The most common ailments leading to the use of herbal remedies include colds, burns, headaches, allergies, insomnia, premenstrual syndrome, depression, and menopause.

   Mr. H's choices are likely to be specific to his own concerns. For example, saw palmetto, which has been used for centuries for urogenital symptoms, is currently advocated for the treatment of benign prostatic hyperplasia (BPH). Active ingredients of saw palmetto include beta-sitosterol and other esterified sterols; the preparation may inhibit 5-alpha reductase (a finasteride-like effect) and it may have antiandrogen effects as well. St. John's wort is an extract from the *Hypericum perforatum* plant which may have some serotonergic effect; hence, it has been used as an antidepressant. Echinacea preparations are from the purple coneflower in the daisy family and have been used for centuries by Native Americans as antiseptics and analgesics; currently, they are popularly used to prevent or shorten the course of common colds. Valerian root has been used since the time of Hippocrates. It has been shown to influence gamma-aminobutyric acid (GABA) neurotransmission, may improve sleep latency and increase REM sleep, and is currently used as an anxiolytic and sleep aid. Ginkgo biloba, which has been promoted for memory enhancement, contains flavonoids and terpenoids among their active ingredients; these function as antioxidants to scavenge free radicals, which have been implicated in the pathogenesis of Alzheimer's disease and other neurodegenerative disorders. The terpenoids also have an inhibitory effect on platelet-activating factor. Glucosamine and chondroitin have been promoted for osteoarthritis, as glucosamine is a basic component of articular cartilage glycosaminoglycan, and chondroitin sulfate, a glycosaminoglycan itself, seems to maintain viscosity in joints, stimulate cartilage repair, and inhibit enzymatic breakdown of cartilage.

2. Saw palmetto has been shown to improve scores on urinary tract symptom scales and increase urinary flow rates; some studies show it to be more effective than placebo, and somewhat comparable to finasteride. In contrast to finasteride, which decreases prostate volume over time, saw palmetto has not been associated with a decrease in prostate volume. Also unlike finasteride, saw palmetto does not decrease prostate-specific antigen (PSA).

Some studies suggest that St. John's Wort is more effective than placebo in reducing symptoms of depression, but this has not been consistently demonstrated. Echinacea has not been shown to prevent colds, and evidence regarding its effect on the duration of colds is conflicting. Likewise, although a well-designed study of a specific extract of ginkgo in 327 dementia patients showed benefit (LeBars *et al.*, 1997), in a study of healthy older adults ginkgo was no more effective than placebo in improving memory (Solomon *et al.*, 2002).

A meta-analysis of studies that evaluated glucosamine and chondroitin in arthritis revealed reduction in symptom scores and increases in functional outcomes of up to 40% when compared with placebo. (McAlindon *et al.*, 2000). However, many of the studies were considered to have methodologic flaws that undermined the levels of evidence. In addition to flaws common to clinical trials in general (such as nonstandardized diagnostic methods or outcomes measurements, short duration of studies, or absence of a placebo arm), an important problem in most studies of herbal and nutrient preparations is that of nonstandardized doses without measurement of drug levels. In general, many studies of these unregulated substances use widely differing doses, often using preparations in which concentration varies from pill to pill or from bottle to bottle, or herbals that have been prepared from different parts of the raw plant or have undergone a different extraction process. This problem extends to real world use – e.g. ginseng contains at least 28 active ingredients with different pharmacologic actions. The source of this popular agent, *Panax ginseng*, is diverse, including dried root, leaves, and flowers. This could account for the great variability in observed actions and potential adverse effects. All of these factors would have to be taken into account in evaluating the validity of studies.

Overall, there appears to be scanty objective evidence showing benefit from many of these therapies, but insufficient data are available at present. This does not mean that active ingredients in these preparations lack the potential of beneficial therapeutic effect. However, proof of efficacy would require the same high standard of evidence demanded of orthodox treatments, including randomized, double-blind, controlled design and standardized, purified ingredients in the active arm of the trial.

These caveats must also be applied to nutrients that are considered to be "orthodox" treatments. For example, although the efficacy of vitamin D, calcium, and certain other constituents of vitamin preparations has been well established, these conventional treatments may be influenced by a lack of quality control because they are not subject to the same governmental oversight as non-nutrients. Under the 1994 Federal Dietary Supplement Health and Education Act, which was passed in response to consumer pressure for better access to nontraditional therapies, dietary supplements, including most herbal remedies, are exempt from stringent Food and Drug Administration (FDA) regulations and they are not required to meet FDA safety and efficacy standards. Herbal products have sometimes been found to be contaminated with toxins or other harmful ingredients, or to lack all or some of the active ingredients listed on the label. Marketing and labels are permitted to claim the supplement helps maintain a bodily function, but may not claim they treat, cure, or ameliorate a disease. The manufacturer is required to maintain quality, but the government can only intervene after a specific preparation is marketed *and* harm results. This semantic distinction exempts most herbal supplements from the research, oversight, postmarketing surveillance, and requirements for adverse outcome reporting that controls – but also thereby gives the patient a certain degree of confidence in – the pharmaceutical industry.

3. As would be expected from any agent that has a therapeutic effect, adverse effects have been reported with herbal and nutrient preparations. Because of a finasteride-like effect, saw palmetto may reduce libido. Whereas studies have shown that finasteride does not appear to affect adversely serum lipids or bone density, no long-term data exist regarding the effects of saw palmetto. Echinacea has been reported to cause allergic reactions. Discontinuation of valerian may produce withdrawal symptoms similar to those seen with benzodiazepines.

    Like approved antidepressants, St. John's wort has potential adverse effects. Specifically, it can cause photosensitivity, dry mouth, dizziness, and fatigue, as well as the serotonin syndrome, especially when used along with selective serotonin reuptake inhibitors (SSRIs). Unlike standard antidepressants, St. John's wort may induce CYP450 enzymes and has been reported to decrease levels of concurrently administered theophylline, cyclosporin, digoxin, oral contraceptives, and warfarin. Thus, it is possible that St. John's Wort played a role in Mr. H's newly subtherapeutic INR. Mr. H would also need to be advised about other potential interactions. For example, ginkgo has been reported to increase the risk of bleeding in patients on blood-thinning medications, including warfarin, and several herbs have been reported to have the potential to cause problems at surgery, including garlic, ginseng, ginkgo, and vitamin E. Ginkgo has platelet-activating factor antagonist activity, and subdural hematomas and anterior chamber bleeding have been reported in patients on ginkgo combined with other blood-thinning medications. Garlic and ginseng at high doses can inhibit platelet aggregation, ginger has inhibitory effects on thromboxane synthetase, and vitamin E at high doses can antagonize the function of other fat-soluble vitamins, resulting in coagulation disorders. It is recommended that all herbals be discontinued 2–3 weeks prior to surgery.

An illustration of the active ingredients in nutrients and other "natural" substances is the increasingly well-known effect of grapefruit juice, which contains furanocoumarins that inhibit intestinal CYP3A4 enzymes and increase circulating levels of a number of drugs, including warfarin. Drug–nutrient interactions have been recognized for many years and have been reviewed in detail (see Fugh-Berman, 2000).

5. Patients should be asked about herbal remedies and other "unapproved" treatments in a nonjudgmental fashion. Using the term "alternative" might even be considered judgmental by some patients. A judgmental approach can, after all, be countered with the argument that prescription drugs are also potential poisons. It is very important that the physician make an effort to become knowledgeable about the potential risks and benefits of these agents – alone and in combination with other medications – especially since there is clearly a belief by patients, and likely also by physicians, that since these are not prescription medications, there are less adverse effects. Not only will this effort help the patient to obtain accurate information, but it will enhance the physician's credibility and improve the patient–doctor relationship. The physician should also inform patients that there is a lack of standardization and quality control such that the purity and identity of ingredients cannot be guaranteed.

Since many complementary and alternative medicine (CAM) therapies appear to be associated with health promotion and disease prevention, the physician can ask about the patient's use of CAM in the context of lifestyle questions, and should specifically ask whether the patient takes nonprescribed nutrients or pharmaceuticals. Information about other CAM therapies, such as homeopathy and naturopathy, mind–body interventions, such as meditation, body-based methods, such as chiropractic manipulation and massage, and therapies which purport to harness energy fields, such as Qi gong and therapeutic touch, are reviewed in the references (see The National Center for Complementary and Alternative Medicine, 2004).

Caveats

As few as 25% of physicians routinely ask patients about their use of alternative therapies. However, 12–44% of the general population and, in one survey, 73% of patients over 65 used CAM, with only 35% of this usage documented in patients' chart (see Eisenberg *et al.*, 1998).

REFERENCES

Eisenberg, D. M., Davis, R. B., Ettner, S. L. *et al.* (1998). Trends in alternative medicine use in the US 1990–1997. *Journal of the American Medical Association*, **280**, 1569–75.

Fugh-Berman, A. (2000). Herb-drug interactions. *Lancet*, **355**, 134–8.

LeBars, P. L., Katz, M. M., Berman, N. *et al.*, for the North American Ginkgo Biloba Study Group (1997). A placebo controlled, double blind randomized trial of an extract of ginkgo biloba for dementia. *Journal of the American Medical Association*, **278**, 1327–32.

McAlindon, T. E., LaValley, M. P., Gulin, J. P. *et al.* (2000). Glucosamine and chondroitin for treatment of osteoarthritis: a systematic quality assessment and meta-analysis. *Journal of the American Medical Association*, **283**, 1469–75.

National Center for Complementary and Alternative Medicine. http://nccam.nih.gov/health/whatiscam; accessed February 21, 2005.

Solomon, P. R., Adams, F., Silver, A. *et al.* (2002). Ginkgo for memory enhancement. A randomized controlled trial. *Journal of the American Medical Association*, **288**, 835–40.

BIBLIOGRAPHY

Ang-Lee, M. K., Moss, J., and Yuan, C. S. (2001). Herbal medicines and perioperative care. *Journal of the American Medical Association*, **286**, 208–16.

Astin, J. A., Pelletier, K. P., Marie, A. *et al.* (2000). Complementary and alternative medicine use among elderly persons: one-year analysis of a Blue Shield Medicare supplement. *Journals of Gerontology: Medical Sciences*, **55A**, M1–6.

Cohen, R. J., Ek, K., and Pan, C. X. (2002). Complementary and alternative medicine (CAM) use by older adults: a comparison of self report and physician chart documentation. *Journals of Gerontology: Medical Sciences*, **57A**, M223–7.

Eisenberg, D. M. (1997). Advising patients who seek alternative medical therapy. *Annals of Internal Medicine*, **127**, 61–9.

Ernst, E. (2002). The risk-benefit profile of commonly used herbal therapies: gingko, St John's wort, ginseng, echinacea, saw palmetto, and kava. *Annals of Internal Medicine*, **136**, 42–53.

Flahery, J. H., Takahashi, R., Teoh, J. A. *et al.* (2001). Use of alternative therapies in older outpatients in the United States and Japan: prevalence, reporting patterns, and perceived effectiveness. *Journals of Gerontology Medical Sciences*, **56A**, M650–5.

Garges, H. P., Varia, I., and Doraiswamy, P. M. (1998). Cardiac complications and delirium associated with valerian root withdrawal. *Journal of the American Medical Association*, **280**, 1566–7.

Gaster, B. and Holroyd, J. (2000). St Johns wort for depression: a systematic review. *Archives of Internal Medicine*, **160**, 152–6.

Grimm, W. and Muller, H. (1999). A randomized controlled trial of the fluid extract of *E. purpurea* on the incidence and severity of colds and respiratory infections. *American Journal of Medicine*, **171**, 198–200.

Hypericum Depression Trial Study Group (2002). Effect of *Hypericum perforatum* (St John's Wort) in major depressive disorder. A randomized controlled trial. *Journal of the American Medical Association*, **287**, 1807–14.

Kane, G. C. and Lipsky, J. L. (2000). Drug-grapefruit juice interactions. *Mayo Clinic Proceedings*, **75**, 933–42.

Knudtson, M. L., Wyse, D. G., Galbraith, P. D. *et al.* (2002). Chelation therapy for ischemic heart disease. A randomized controlled trial. *Journal of the American Medical Association*, **287**, 481–6.

Lantz, M. S., Buchalter, E., and Giambanco, V. (1999). St Johns wort and antidepressant drug interactions in the elderly. *Journal of Geriatric Psychiatry and Neurology*, **12**, 7–10.

Matthews, M. K. (1998). Association of ginkgo biloba with intracerebral hemorrhage. *Neurology*, **50**, 1993–4.

Milan, F. (2001). An overview of herbal medicine for the primary care provider: an evidence based approach. *Primary Care Reports*, **7**, 105–16.

Rosenblatt, M. and Mindel, J. (1997). Spontaneous hyphema associated with ingestion of ginkgo biloba extract. *New England Journal of Medicine*, **336**, 1108.

Ruschitzka, F., Meier, P. J., Turina, M. *et al.* (2000). Acute heart transplant rejection due to St John's wort. *Lancet*, **355**, 548–9.

Wilt, T. J., Ishani, A., Stark, G. L. *et al.* (1998). Saw palmetto extracts for treatment of benign prostatic hyperplasia: a systematic review. *Journal of the American Medical Association*, **280**, 1604–9.

Yeh, G. Y., Eisenberg, D. M., Kaptchuk, T. J. *et al.* (2003). Systematic review of herbs and dietary supplements for glycemic control in diabetes. *Diabetes Care*, **26**, 1277–94.

Case 22

▸▸ Insomnia

A 78-year-old woman is being treated for congestive heart failure (CHF), hypothyroidism, atrial fibrillation, osteoarthritis, diabetes, and hypertension. She takes warfarin, atenolol, furosemide, ramipril, metformin, L-thyroxine (Synthroid), acetaminophen, and temazepam. You are her new doctor in a busy medical clinic at a large metropolitan hospital. The clinic clerk presents you with three large volumes of her chart.

The patient is accompanied by her live-in home attendant. On questioning, the patient admits to shortness of breath, fatigue, and difficulty sleeping. She is completely alert and able to recite her medication regimen correctly. She admits to a depressed mood that she attributes to "all of the medical problems" and also reports taking frequent naps during the day.

Her blood pressure is 130/90, and pulse is 60 and irregular. Pertinent findings on her physical examination include obesity, bibasilar rales, holosystolic murmur at the left sternal border, audible valve click, genu varum, and edema of her lower legs. You order blood and urine tests and rewrite all of her prescriptions, increasing the furosemide.

Laboratory evaluation is unrevealing. Blood sugar is 108 mg/dl. On follow up 1 week later, her pulmonary examination and lower extremity edema are improved. The patient, however, still complains of difficulty sleeping. She is often unable to fall asleep and sometimes wakes in the middle of the night, but she denies orthopnea. Although you have a good working relationship with this patient, she is reluctant to stop the temazepam because she believes she needs it for sleep. You reduce the furosemide to three times a week and increase the ramipril to maximize the treatment of her heart failure.

Case Studies in Geriatric Medicine, Judith C. Ahronheim *et al.* Published by Cambridge University Press.
© J. C. Ahronheim, Z.-B. Huang, V. Yen, C. M. Davitt, and D. Barile

Questions

1. What are the possible factors that could be disturbing her sleep?
2. What questions should you ask this elderly woman to shed light on the etiology of her insomnia?
3. How is temazepam affecting her sleep? What will happen if you discontinue it?
4. Would other pharmacologic agents have any advantages (or disadvantages)?
5. How should you treat this woman's insomnia?
6. When are sleep studies indicated?

Answers

1. Physiologic changes in sleep architecture occur with age. These include decreases in deep sleep (stages 3 and 4), increased numbers of nocturnal arousals (often unnoticed by the patient), and altered circadian rhythms with a tendency to "phase advance," with sleepiness occurring earlier in the evening and awakening earlier in the morning. Many patients are unable to adjust to altered circadian rhythms and may complain of insomnia, although their total sleep time may be normal. In other cases, nocturnal arousals may lead to daytime sleepiness and napping. These changes are not considered pathologic unless they interfere with daytime function. In this patient's case, daytime napping could increase her total sleep time and make it more difficult to go to sleep at night.

   Like many elderly, this patient has certain conditions that could predispose her to or exacerbate sleep problems. In addition to depression and anxiety, medical problems that contribute to insomnia include gastroesophageal reflux disease, pain syndromes, nocturia, dyspnea, hyperthyroidism, and CHF. Moderate to severe CHF can cause central sleep apnea (Cheyne Stokes respiration). Patients themselves do not usually associate this condition with insomnia symptoms; rather, a patient might complain of daytime somnolence or dyspnea, while periodic breathing might be apparent to a family member or live-in aide. Likewise, obstructive sleep apnea, which more commonly occurs in obese males, presents as daytime somnolence.

   Many medications can affect the sleep–wake cycle and sleep architecture, including beta-blockers, corticosteroids, theophylline, psychostimulants, and excess thyroid hormone. Certain hydroxy methylglutaryl coenzyme A reductase inhibitors ("statins") can produce bizarre dreams, disrupting sleep. Alcohol shortens sleep latency, but disrupts sleep by reducing REM sleep and increasing nocturnal and early morning awakening (see Case 27). Atenolol is less likely to enter the brain than more lipid-soluble beta-blockers and is unlikely to be causing this patient's problem. However, it would be important to ascertain that thyroid function tests were normal.

2. In order to determine the etiology of the sleep disorder, a careful history is essential. What are her sleep patterns? How much time does she spend in bed and how much of this time is she actually sleeping? Is the problem initiating sleep or maintaining sleep? Does she sleep during the day? Does she have a history of insomnia that is life long and predates her medical problems?

   Does she consume alcohol, caffeine, over-the-counter pills, or eye drops that can disrupt sleep? Does she experience pain at night from her arthritis? Is she eating or drinking late in the evening? Although she denies orthopnea, it would be important to inquire whether she is awakened by the need to urinate, a common problem in late life which can be worsened in CHF, other edematous states, or diuretic use.

   It is also important to rule out primary sleep disorders such as restless leg syndrome or nocturnal myoclonus. This history may be obtained from the live-in aid or other reliable informant. Although snoring is believed to predict obstructive sleep apnea, this association may be unreliable among elderly patients (Young *et al.*, 2002).

   It is also important to ask about daily and evening activities. This patient, like many of her age cohort, retired to bed early. She went to bed at 7 p.m. and woke up at 2 a.m. She stated that she went to bed so early because she had nothing else to do and, when recommendations were made regarding evening activities, she said her friends were all dead, it was difficult to go out at night, her arthritis prevented her from doing needlework, and her vision was poor, so she could not read and did not enjoy the television. One could argue that this litany of complaints masked depression, or was an "excuse," but they are real problems that afflict many elderly and, even if they do not themselves lead to depression, they impose important, practical obstacles to solving her problem.

3. Benzodiazepines exert their effect by enhancing receptors for gamma-aminobutyric acid (GABA), the primary inhibitory neurotransmitter in the central nervous system. With daily use of temazepam, or other benzodiazepines, tolerance will develop over time. Any help the patient is getting from temazepam at this point is likely to be a placebo effect. As with certain other classes of medications, patients who use benzodiazepines daily and for long periods are subject to physiologic dependence. Because of this, abrupt discontinuation may result in rebound insomnia and possibly more severe withdrawal symptoms. Typically, withdrawal symptoms occur in those patients who have been on standing benzodiazepines for more than a few

months. All hypnotics should be tapered slowly over several weeks. An additional problem is that patients who have been taking sleeping pills for a long time are very reluctant to stop. Prior attempts to discontinue medications may have produced rebound insomnia, encouraging prompt resumption of medications.

4. Other pharmacologic agents exist, but all have some disadvantages. Unlike temazepam, which is conjugated in the liver to inactive metabolites, flurazepam (similar to nitrazepam, which is widely used outside of the United States), diazepam, and certain other benzodiazepines are oxidized in the liver to renally excreted metabolites with long half-lives. Because hepatic oxidation and renal function decline with age, the terminal half-lives of these agents may be longer than 1 week and repeated dosing leads to drug accumulation. They often produce morning-after and daytime sedation. Side effects sometimes become apparent only 7 or more days after the medication was instituted. "Short- or intermediate-acting" benzodiazepines, such as triazolam and lorazepam, have inactive metabolites, but have no specific advantages other than more rapid onset of action, or, in the case of triazolam, a low likelihood of morning sedation.

Although the patient has tolerated temazepam well, all benzodiazepines increase the risk of falls and confusion in susceptible elderly. Patients who refuse to discontinue benzodiazepines should use the lowest effective dose and limit use to three times weekly. Use of benzodiazepines as sleep aids should be strictly avoided in patients with dementia, and should be used with the utmost caution in patients with gait abnormalities.

Chloral hydrate has a favorable pharmacokinetic profile, but, like barbiturates (which are now rarely used in the treatment of insomnia), induces cytochrome P450 enzymes and can participate in drug interactions. Chloral hydrate, moreover, has a narrow therapeutic-to-toxic ratio and deaths have been reported from overdose.

Sedating antihistamines, like diphenhydramine (Benadryl, Tylenol PM) are often used as hypnotics because they are considered "mild" and are nonaddicting. The problem is that tolerance to the sedative effects develops fairly soon, but tolerance may not develop to the anticholinergic effects. These agents are available without prescription and patients may self-administer increasing doses to obtain sleep. Elderly patients often develop anticholinergic side effects such as constipation, confusion, blurred vision, urinary retention, and dry mouth. Likewise, melatonin is available without prescription. A hormone secreted by the pineal gland, melatonin plays a role in regulating circadian rhythms. It has been used as a clock-resetting agent and has been demonstrated to have some clinical utility in jet lag and night-shift work. There is a decrease in nocturnal serum levels of melatonin with age, so it is tempting to consider melatonin an "ideal" sleep agent for the elderly. Although there is some evidence that it may reduce the latency to sleep onset in the elderly, no data currently exist to guide optimal dosing or to ascertain safety of melatonin in long-term treatment in older adults. Furthermore, although it is a hormone, melatonin is classified as a dietary supplement and is exempt from federal regulations governing purity, safety, and efficacy of pharmaceuticals (see Case 21).

Zolpidem (Ambien) has recently been marketed as a safe alternative in the elderly when given in lower doses (5 mg). However, caution is called for: the mechanism of action is similar to benzodiazepines in their modulation of GABA receptors. Zolpidem is more selective for specific GABA receptors and is less likely to produce rebound insomnia, tolerance, or withdrawal symptoms. However, although zolpidem has favorable kinetics in the elderly, it may impair memory and has been reported to produce acute confusional states. Like benzodiazepines and certain other centrally acting agents, zolpidem has been associated with a risk of falls and hip fractures in the elderly. Adverse effects include agitation, headaches, gastrointestinal upset, and dizziness.

Although the patient has most likely developed tolerance to temazepam, she may continue to insist on taking a sleeping pill, despite being counseled that long-term use of hypnotics is associated with reduced efficacy. A possible solution to this dilemma is to withdraw the benzodiazepine slowly while instituting a more appropriate agent, such as trazodone, a mild antidepressant with sedating properties. This antidepressant has a relatively short onset of action (30 min) and a half-life of 5–10 hours. It has a low potential for anticholinergic effects and a good safety profile in the elderly, although it rarely causes supine or orthostatic hypotension. If an antidepressant is indicated, the sedating agents such as mirtazepine (Remeron) may be effective for both depression and insomnia. As with trazodone, dependence is unlikely to develop, rebound insomnia is minimal, and abrupt discontinuation is generally associated with mild symptoms.

5. Generally, the approach to treating insomnia depends on the type. According to the International Classification of Sleep Disorders (Diagnostic Classification Steering Committee, 1990), insomnia is classified as transient, short term or long term (chronic). Transient insomnia is the most common, lasts only for a few days, and is usually due to hospitalization, acute illness, or jet lag. Short-term insomnia is defined as lasting less than 3 weeks and is usually related to stressful events. In transient and short-term insomnia, pharmacologic therapy may be appropriate adjunctive treatment to nonpharmacologic therapy. Chronic insomnia, lasting more than 3 weeks, is usually due to medical, psychiatric, or behavioral disorders. Our patient's complaint is chronic, although it may not be true insomnia. Both pharmacologic and nonpharmacologic treatment may be appropriate in transient and short-term insomnia, but nonpharmacologic therapies are the mainstay of chronic insomnia.

Nonpharmacologic approaches in this patient are paramount and should begin with optimizing treatment of her CHF, arthritis, and other medical conditions that interfere with her sleep. Counseling regarding the nature of her problem is key, although this might not overcome her problem or her desire to be treated for "insomnia." In general, nonpharmacologic therapy includes daily exercise, avoiding daytime naps, using the bed for sleep only, and avoiding lying in bed too long without falling asleep. It is most important to address sleep efficiency – the amount of time the patient spends sleeping should be at least 85% of the time spent in bed. This can be addressed with sleep-restriction therapy, a method that has been demonstrated to be effective in the elderly (see Morin *et al.*, 1999). In sleep-restriction therapy, in-bed time is permitted only for the number of hours the patient actually sleeps. For example, if a patient sleeps only 5 of the 8 hours in bed, she is instructed to go to bed 5 hours before her usual waking time, and to be sure to get up at the same time each morning. This slight "sleep debt" promotes the patient's ability to sleep. Every week, the patient adds approximately 15 minutes to initial time in bed and continues to increase this amount as long as the ratio of sleep time to in-bed time remains 85% or greater. Although it is uncertain that this particular patient would comply with the above method, nonpharmacologic therapy should always be attempted either first or in conjunction with pharmacologic sleeping aids. If patients with chronic insomnia cannot adhere to the demand of sleep-restriction therapy or simply do not achieve the desired effect, a trial of a hypnotic agent is sometimes warranted. Other nonpharmacologic approaches to sleep therapy are reviewed in the references (see Kupfer and Reynolds, 1997).

6. A sleep study may be useful in patients with severe daytime somnolence. Sleep-disordered breathing increases in incidence with age, especially in men. There is no consensus as to why a higher prevalence exists in the elderly, but it may be partly due to an age-related increase in hypotonia of the upper airway muscles during sleep, combined with alterations in the neural regulation of breathing and the neuromuscular apparatus.

The absence of snoring does not rule out obstructive sleep apnea, and is a particularly unreliable sign in older patients (see Young *et al.*, 2002). Continuous Positive Airway Pressure (CPAP) is a useful treatment, although many patients have difficulty tolerating the tight-fitting mask.

REFERENCES

Diagnostic Classification Steering Committee (1990). *The International Classification of Sleep Disorders: Diagnostic and Coding Manual.* Rochester, MN: American Sleep Disorders Association.

Kupfer, D. J. and Reynolds, C. F. (1997). Management of insomnia. *New England Journal of Medicine*, **336**, 341–5.

Morin, C. M., Colecchi, C., Stone, J. *et al.* (1999). Behavioral and pharmacological therapies for late-life insomnia. *Journal of the American Medical Association*, **281**, 991–9.

Young, T., Shahar, E., Nieto, F. J. *et al.* (2002). Predictors of sleep-disordered breathing in community dwelling adults. The Sleep Heart Health Study. *Archives of Internal Medicine*, **162**, 892–900.

BIBLIOGRAPHY

Asplund, R. (1999). Sleep disorders in the elderly. *Drugs and Aging*, **14**, 91–103.

Brodeur, M. R. and Stirling, A. L. (2001). Delirium associated with zolpidem. *Annals of Pharmacotherapy*, **35**, 1562–4.

Brzezinski, A. (1997). Melatonin in humans. *New England Journal of Medicine*, **336**, 186–95.

Haria, M., Fitton, A., McTavish, D. *et al.* (1994). Trazodone. A review of its pharmacology, therapeutic use in depression and therapeutic potential in other disorders. *Drugs and Aging*, **4**, 331–55.

Ingbir, M., Freimark, D., Motro, M. *et al.* (2002). The incidence, pathophysiology, treatment and prognosis of Cheyne Stokes breathing disorder in patients with congestive heart failure. *Herz*, **27**, 107–12.

Kirkwood, C. K. (1999). Management of insomnia. *Journal of the American Pharmacists Association*, **39**, 688–96.

Leipzig, R. M., Cumming, R. G., and Tinetti M.E. (1999). Drugs and falls in older people: a systematic review and meta analysis: psychotropic Drugs. *Journal of the American Geriatrics Society*, **47**, 30–9.

McDowell, J. A., Mion, L. C., Lydon, T. J. *et al.* (1998). A nonpharmacologic sleep protocol for hospitalized older patients. *Journal of the American Geriatrics Society*, **46**, 700–5.

National Institute of Health Consensus Development Conference (1984). Drugs and insomnia: the use of medications to promote sleep. *Journal of the American Medical Association*, **251**, 2410–14.

Obermeyer, W. H. and Benca, R. M. (1996). Effects of Drugs on Sleep. *Neurology Clinics* **14**, 827–40.

Pressman, M. R. and Fry, J. M. (1988). What is normal sleep in the elderly? *Clinics in Geriatric Medicine*, **4**, 71–81.

Prinz, P., Vitiello, M., Raskind, M. *et al.* (1990). Geriatrics: sleep Disorders and Aging. *New England Journal of Medicine*, **323**, 520–5.

Salzman, C., for Task Force on Benzodiazepine Dependency, American Psychiatric Association (1990). *Benzodiazepine Dependence, Toxicity, and Abuse: A Task Force Report of the American Psychiatric Association.* Washington, DC: American Psychiatric Association.

Spielman, A. J., Saskin, P., and Thorpy, M. J. (1987). Sleep restriction therapy. *Sleep*, **10**, 45–56.

Wang, P. S., Bohn, R. L., and Glynn, R. J. (2001). Zolpidem use and hip fractures in older people. *Journal of the American Geriatrics Society*, **49**, 1685–90.

White, D. P., Lombard, R. M., Cadieux, R. J. *et al.* (1985). Pharyngeal resistance in normal humans: influence of gender, age and obesity. *Journal of Applied Physiology*, **58**, 365–71.

Case 23

▶▶ Low vision

Mr. L is an 85-year-old Caucasian man who lives with his daughter in a three-story home. He complains that he has had increasing difficulty with his vision over the past year. He has trouble reading and seeing faces when people are speaking to him. His daughter pays his bills and pre-pours his medication, as he can no longer reliably read small print. He denies eye pain, headache, and sudden vision loss. He gave up driving 6 months ago because he couldn't see the road signs.

Mr. L underwent successful bilateral cataract surgeries several years ago. He has been treated for chronic glaucoma with eye drops, but intraocular pressure has been normal, as measured by the ophthalmologist 6 months ago. He has no history of diabetes mellitus, but is being treated for "bladder problems" and hypertension. His medications include oxybutynin and losartan. He also takes eye drops, which he cannot name, and a regimen of antioxidant vitamins prescribed by his ophthalmologist. Mr. L has fallen several times at home, often while trying to get to the bathroom at night. His daughter is quite concerned because her father insists on walking outside unaccompanied and without using his cane. She is afraid that Mr. L may have a serious fall and injure himself.

Questions

1. What eye diseases could be causing this patient's poor vision?
2. How can his condition be managed?
3. How might his medications be affecting his vision? His physical function?
4. What can be done to help Mr. L to manage his activities of daily living and improve his quality of life?

Case Studies in Geriatric Medicine, Judith C. Ahronheim *et al.* Published by Cambridge University Press.
© J. C. Ahronheim, Z.-B. Huang, V. Yen, C. M. Davitt, and D. Barile

5. What environmental changes in the home might decrease the likelihood of falls?
6. What social and psychologic problems can accompany with vision loss?

Answers

1. Low vision is defined as bilateral vision impairment, which significantly impairs the patient's ability to function and is not amenable to correction with medication, surgery, corrective lenses, or contacts. In the elderly, common disorders that cause gradual, painless vision loss include open angle glaucoma, cataracts, diabetic retinopathy, and age-related macular degeneration (ARMD). Diabetic retinopathy is seen in longstanding diabetes; however, undiagnosed diabetes can present with blurred vision due to hyperglycemia and influx of glucose into the lens. This reversible problem occurs when glucose is converted in the lens to sorbitol, leading to hypertonicity, influx of water, and swelling of the lens. Cataract extraction occasionally is accompanied by complications, including macular edema, retinal detachment, and displacement or fracture of the lens implant. Glaucoma can produce visual loss, but peripheral vision is generally lost while central vision is maintained. Because this patient has had "successful" cataract extractions, and has no history of diabetes mellitus, he most likely has ARMD, which presents with loss of central vision. In Mr. L's case, fundoscopic examination by his ophthalmologist demonstrated early macular degeneration a few years ago, but symptoms have now progressed.

   In elderly patients like Mr. L, more than one eye disease can coexist, and many systemic factors can further affect vision.

   ARMD increases in incidence with age and is more often severe in late life. It is more prevalent in nonHispanic whites than in Hispanic or African Americans (in contrast, glaucoma is more common among African Americans). It is caused by degeneration of the macula, the area of the retina responsible for central vision. The hallmarks of ARMD are blurred central vision, image distortion, central scotoma, and difficulty reading, with patients noting that they rely more heavily on increased light or a magnifier to see small print. Mr. L has difficulty with bill paying and reading medication labels, both of which require sharp central vision. Because peripheral vision is spared, patients can often ambulate without assistance and can participate in many activities. Unfortunately, elderly patients may have more than one eye disorder, and physical comorbidities can further impair function.

ARMD is classified as either "wet" (exudative) or "dry" (nonexudative). Wet ARMD often involves dramatic, sudden loss of vision due to acute macular hemorrhage associated with the growth of abnormal vessels ("neovasculature") from the choroidal circulation to the subretinal space. When these friable vessels leak blood or serum in the macula, blurred or distorted central vision results. The exudative form accounts for about 10% of ARMD cases, but for 80–90% of cases with severe vision loss. Dry ARMD is associated with Drusen ("stones") – yellowish-white accumulations of extracellular debris in the macula that distort and lift the retinal pigment epithelium. Visual loss occurs slowly and patients often can accommodate to this by using good lighting and other strategies. Patients with large or multiple Drusen have an increased risk of developing neovasculature and leaking.

2. There is no treatment that restores vision loss, and treatment options are directed at preventing further vision loss in patients with exudative ARMD. Laser photocoagulation is used to ablate new vessels to prevent hemorrhage in patients with neovasculature. New leakage may occur over time, necessitating regular follow up examinations, including fluorescein angiography to identify neovascularization that may respond to additional treatment. In between periodic examination, patients should be instructed to use an Amsler grid, a symmetrical pattern of squares with a central dot, to monitor their vision for any changes (see Figure 8). The Amsler grid is useful as a screening tool in the primary care office and patients can use it at home to monitor their vision for any changes. Any new findings should prompt an immediate visit to the ophthalmologist.

Ablation of new vessels can also be accomplished by photodynamic therapy, which reduces the likelihood of blind spots caused by thermal laser. Other promising options are reviewed in the references (see Fine *et al.*, 2000).

Mr. L's vitamins are probably antioxidants. These are widely prescribed to retard the progression of ARMD based on the theory that they prevent cellular damage by reacting with free radicals produced during light absorption. A large, randomized, placebo-controlled trial of vitamins C and E, beta-carotene, and zinc modestly reduced progression of ARMD to the advanced stages (Age-Related Eye Disease Study Research Group, 2001), but, to date, there is no evidence that antioxidants prevent the development of this disease.

Because people with light-colored irises have an increased risk of developing ARMD, protective sunglasses have been recommended, but they have not been definitively shown to prevent the disease or its progression. However, their use is prudent because this may decrease development of lens opacities. Likewise, smoking cessation is universally recommended and may reduce the risk of ARMD.

3. Anticholinergic medications such as oxybutynin can precipitate acute angle closure glaucoma, thereby causing rapid vision loss. Although these medications are less

Amsler's grid

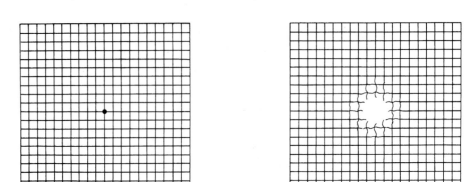

Normal image   Patient's view

Figure 8   Schematic representation of a distortion that might be visualized by a patient with macular degeneration (right) compared with someone with normal vision (left), when utilizing an Amsler grid.

likely to increase intraocular pressure in open angle glaucoma, which Mr. L has, oxybutinin or other bladder antispasmodics could reversibly worsen his vision by reducing pupillary activity and impairing his ability to accommodate vision for near objects. Older, topical antiglaucoma medications, such as pilocarpine, have parasympathomimetic action and cause pupillary constriction, reducing the visual field and impairing visual acuity. This can be a serious problem in patients with ARMD, who already have impaired central vision. Fortunately, more recently introduced topical agents, such as beta-blockers (timolol and others) and prostaglandin analogs (latanoprost and others), lack this problem. Other systemic medications that can affect the eye include systemic corticosteroids, which can increase intraocular pressure, and long-term use can cause cataracts.

Topical antiglaucoma medications can produce systemic effects. These agents are absorbed through conjunctival vessels, and this absorption can be enhanced in conjunctivitis or blepharitis, where vessels are prominent. Ocular agents also enter the nasolacrimal duct through the puncta of the eye, gaining access to the nasal mucosa where they are easily absorbed. Unabsorbed drug reaches the nasopharynx and can be swallowed, but small amounts of swallowed drug are likely to be metabolized, leaving only trivial amounts of active agent available. In contrast, direct mucosal or conjunctival absorption avoids first-pass hepatic metabolism, increasing systemic potency so that, even though small amounts are absorbed, symptoms can result. Systemic absorption can be reduced if the eye is closed and the punctum occluded during installation and for at least 15 seconds afterwards.

Ocular beta-blockers have been reported to produce all the systemic effects seen with systemic agents, including hypotension, bradycardia, bronchospasm, and others. In someone like Mr. L, who is falling, it is important to make sure these agents are not affecting blood pressure or heart rate in any significant way. Parasympathomimetic agents such as pilocarpine are generally well tolerated in doses used in chronic glaucoma but in high doses, as used in acute angle closure, they can produce gastrointestinal symptoms, bradyarrhythmias, and other cholinergic effects. The incidence of these effects is difficult to gauge because they are not frequently considered in differential diagnosis. Oral carbonic anhydrase inhibitors such as acetazolamide (Diamox) can produce systemic acidosis or weakness and, when given together with potassium-losing diuretics, can produce severe hypokalemia; today, these agents are generally instilled topically but drug interactions are theoretically possible, as they have been reported with other ophthalmic agents. Systemic effects of ophthalmic agents are reviewed in the references (see Novack *et al.*, 2002).

Antioxidants are widely used for ARMD and are generally well tolerated, but caution is advised. High doses of zinc can produce copper deficiency and anemia (thus, copper was added to regimens that contained zinc in the Age-Related Eye Disease Study Research Group, 2001), carotenoids produce yellowing of the skin, which is not believed harmful but can look peculiar, and high doses of vitamin E may impair coagulation in certain circumstances (see Case 21).

4. Medications can be pre-poured in dated pill dispensers (boxes) or bottles should be marked with large print labels. Other low vision assistive devices are prism glasses for near work, high-powered magnifying lenses for reading small print, a hand-held monocular telescope for near vision, hand magnifiers with or without illumination, and a signature guide for check writing and form signing. Community agencies offer low- or no cost courses to the visually impaired to help them acquire skills and use assistive devices to maintain independent living. Local libraries may offer large print books or magazines, or books on tape, and some deliver these items to the home. Resources in some communities include courses in the arts, such as ceramics and sculpture. Web-based resources can assist in finding agencies in many countries, as noted in the references (see Lighthouse International, 2004).

Mr. L should be strongly encouraged to accept assistance and to use his cane, especially when walking outside. If he feels stigmatized by this, he may feel more at ease with alternative devices, such as a specially constructed wheeled grocery cart designed for use as a walker or with a strong umbrella fitted with a rubber walking tip.

5. The primary care provider must have an accurate picture of the patient's living arrangements and functional capacity in order to make recommendations. A home visit is an excellent method for assessing the home for environmental hazards and seeing how the patient maneuvers in his environment.

   Many simple home adaptations can be made to increase the safety of someone with impaired vision. There should be good lighting with minimal glare. A bedside commode and a night light can help prevent falls at night. Doorbells should be sufficiently loud, and pathways to the door kept free of clutter. Stove and oven dials should be marked in contrasting colors. Household utensils can be marked with contrasting color tape for easier identification in a kitchen drawer. Keys can be marked with color labels. Emergency telephone numbers should be posted in large contrasting lettering near the telephone. The telephone itself can be a one-touch model with large buttons preprogrammed for emergency numbers and family contacts. Furniture and objects should be kept in the same positions and doors not left half-way open. When possible, the ground floor of a house should be adapted for 24-hour living to decrease the need for going up and down stairs, especially at night; otherwise, the edges of stairs can be painted or marked with contrasting colors or tape. In apartment buildings, entrances and exits should be clearly marked and special attention paid to the adequacy of the lighting.

   In the health care settings, there should be a clear line of sight from the door to the receptionist, good lighting with minimal glare, and forms printed in large contrasting type that patients may take home to review carefully. The staff should use the sighted guide technique to assist patients when they are walking in an unfamiliar environment. The patient walks slightly behind the guide and holds lightly onto the guide's bent elbow. The guide should walk slightly ahead of the patient and announce the presence of steps, doors, and other hazards.

6. Social and psychologic effects of vision loss can be devastating to an elderly patient. The fear of blindness ranks fourth among Americans after the fear of developing AIDS, cancer, and Alzheimer's disease (Faye and Stuen, 1992). Low vision that occurs late in life increases the risk of decreased mobility, social isolation, and loss of independence. This can lead to depression, loss of self-esteem, anxiety, and sometimes dependence on antianxiety agents and alcohol. These problems, often compounded by other chronic physical impairments, need to be addressed with counseling, use of community resources, and even pharmacotherapy for depression if needed. After a period of reluctance, many patients adapt well to alternative living arrangements such as assisted living facilities, where new social contacts and services can improve quality of life.

Caveats

1. Prior to the introduction of intraocular lens implants, aphakic spectacles were needed following cataract extraction, which results in aphakia (absence of a lens). Some patients still use these thick, goggle-like spectacles. While providing useful central vision, they do not provide peripheral vision, which can be problematic. A patient who then develops macular degeneration lacks the additional coping mechanism of useful peripheral vision. Another drawback of aphakic spectacles is that they do not correct unilateral cataract extraction, because they produce magnification and distortion in the corrected eye, and unilateral correction would result in double vision.
2. In some instances, the patient must be declared "legally blind" to obtain community services for the visually impaired. The criteria for legal blindness is generally central visual acuity of 20/200 or less in the better eye, even with corrective lenses, or better than 20/200 but with a peripheral field restricted to a diameter of 20 degrees or less. Clinically, the legally blind cannot read the biggest letter on the Snellen eye chart with or without corrective lenses.

REFERENCES

Age-Related Eye Disease Study Research Group (2001). A randomized, placebo-controlled clinical trial of high dose supplementation with vitamins C and E, beta carotene, and zinc for age-related macular degeneration and vision loss. *Archives of Ophthalmology*, **119**, 1417–36.

Fine, S. L., Berger, J. W., Maguire, M. G. *et al.* (2000). Age-related macular degeneration. *New England Journal of Medicine*, **342**, 483–92.

Lighthouse International. www.visionconnections.org; accessed February 21, 2005.

Novack, G. D., O'Donnell, M. J., and Molloy, D. W. (2002). New glaucoma medications in the geriatric population. Efficacy and safety. *Journal of the American Geriatrics Society*, **50**, 956–62.

BIBLIOGRAPHY

Elner, S. G. (1999). Gradual painless vision loss: retinal causes. *Clinics in Geriatric Medicine*, **15**, 25–46.

Evans, J. R. (2002). Antioxidant vitamins and mineral supplements for age-related macular degeneration. *Cochrane Database of Systematic Reviews*, **2**, CD000254.

Faye, E. E. and Stuen, C. S. (1992). *The Aging Eye – A Study Guide for Physicians*. New York: The Lighthouse Inc.

Fong, D. S. (2000). Age-related macular degeneration, update for primary care. *American Family Physician*, **61**, 3035–42.

Frock, T. (2002). Gaining insight into age-related macular degeneration. *Journal of the American Academy of Nurse Practitioners*, **14**, 207–13.

Klein, R., Klein, B. E., and Jensen, S. C. (1997). The five-year incidence and progression of age-related maculopathy: the Beaver Dam Eye Study. *Ophthalmology*, **104**, 7–21.

Klein, R., Rowland, M. L., and Harris, M. I. (1995). Racial/ethnic differences in age-related maculopathy. Third National Health and Nutrition Examination Survey. *Ophthalmology*, **102**, 371–81.

Quillen, D. A. (1999). Common causes of vision loss in elderly patients. *American Family Physician*, **60**, 99–108.

Shields, S. R. (2000). Managing eye disease in primary care. Part 1. How to screen for occult disease. *Postgraduate Medicine*, **108**, 69–72, 75–6, 78.

Smith, W., Mitchell, P., Webb, K. *et al.* (1999). Dietary antioxidants and age-related maculopathy. The Blue Mountains Eye Study. *Ophthalmology*, **106**, 761–7.

Watson, G. R. (2001). Low vision in the geriatric population: rehabilitation and management. *Journal of the American Geriatrics Society*, **49**, 317–30.

Wormald, R., Evans, J., Smeeth, L. *et al.* (2003). Photodynamic therapy for neovascular age-related macular degeneration. *Cochrane Database of Systematic Reviews*, **2**, CD002030.

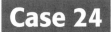

▸▸ Recurrent falls

Mrs. E, an 86-year-old woman, is recovering from a wrist fracture. She has lived alone since her husband died 15 years ago, but has been in relatively good health. Currently, she is being treated for hypertension, constipation, and insomnia. She has fallen three times in the past year but, until the most recent fall, has not sustained an injury. She admits to an occasional feeling of light-headedness, but when you question her closely about the circumstances surrounding the fall, she says, "Oh, I just fell. Maybe I tripped on something." Her medications include ibuprofen as needed for pain, hydrochlorothiazide 25 mg daily, lisinopril 20 mg daily, and temazepam 15 mg for sleep.

Two years ago, Mrs. E was noted to have a heart rate in the 50s. At that time, she had been taking diltiazem for hypertension and, although she denied dizziness or other symptoms, diltiazem was discontinued and lisinopril was instituted.

On physical examination, the patient is alert and oriented but appears somewhat depressed. She has a bruise on her left temple and she says that she hit her head on the table when she fell. She walks slowly but steadily with a cane and her gait appears hesitant. Her blood pressure is 140/70 without postural hypotension. She has cataracts but her corrected near vision is 20/25. She has no jugular venous distension. Her lungs are clear. The heart rate is regular at 56 beats per minute; there is a grade 3/6 systolic murmur most prominent in the upper right sternal border. Her right arm is in a cast. There is no tremor or rigidity of her extremities. The Romberg test is negative, but she is unable to perform tandem gait. An electrocardiogram reveals sinus bradycardia, with a rate of 52 beats per minute.

Case Studies in Geriatric Medicine, Judith C. Ahronheim *et al.* Published by Cambridge University Press.
© J. C. Ahronheim, Z.-B. Huang, V. Yen, C. M. Davitt, and D. Barile

Questions

1. How should you approach this patient's recurrent falls?
2. What is the differential diagnosis?
3. What are the common causes of falls in elderly persons?
4. What modifiable risk factors for falls does Mrs. E have?

Answers

1. Falling in an 86-year-old woman who lives alone needs to be taken very seriously and evaluated carefully: falls account for 70% of accidental deaths in those 70 years and older. One study showed that up to 50% of those who have fallen avoid activities because of fear of falling again (Nevitt, 1989). In addition to injury, falling and loss of confidence result in decreased activity, social isolation, decreasing mobility, and loss of independence. At her age, Mrs. E already has diminished physiologic reserves from loss of muscle mass and diminished aerobic capacity, and decreased physical activity may rapidly diminish her muscle strength and aerobic capacity. This "deconditioning" further increases the risk of falling.

   Although the differential diagnosis of falling in the elderly is very broad, the most fruitful evaluation is one that consists of a careful history and examination with a directed evaluation guided by these findings. Mrs. E, who lives alone, requires a cane for ambulation, and has cataracts and evidence of impaired balance, has many risk factors for falling. The history given by the patient herself is key, but is not always reliable. Some older people fail to report falls or to give precise details because of embarrassment or fear of nursing home placement, or because they are forgetful. In those with poor memory, additional information might be obtained from family or others who have spent time with the patient. In other cases, a home visit to assess for environmental hazards may be very revealing. In this case, the patient cannot remember if she lost consciousness, but the history of recurrent falls as well as hitting her head suggest that loss of consciousness should not be ruled out. There is evidence that many people who deny loss of consciousness during a fall may have actually lost consciousness (Richardson *et al.*, 2002).

2. The history, the finding of bradycardia, and the cardiac murmur raise the suspicion of syncope – a sudden, transient loss of consciousness with loss of postural control. The underlying mechanism of syncope is transient cerebral hypoperfusion. Syncope can present as a fall, but it is important to distinguish syncope from other causes of falling.

Medication review is essential when evaluating falls and syncope, and should give attention to prescribed and nonprescribed (including illicit) drugs and alcohol (see Case 27). Her prescribed medications include a benzodiazepine, a diuretic, and an antihypertensive medication, all of which can contribute to falling. Two years ago, the diltiazem would have been a likely suspect, but, at that time, she was not falling.

The patient's age and physical findings raise the suspicion of a cardiac etiology, such as symptomatic arrhythmia or high-grade aortic stenosis. Neurocardiogenic syncope can occur in patients without underlying cardiovascular disease. Signals from mechanoreceptors and chemoreceptors in the heart, carotid body, and viscera are conducted by afferent neural pathways to the central nervous system. Efferent neural signals can be so strong in some patients that they result in peripheral vasodilatation and bradycardia, leading to hypotension or syncope. This mechanism is involved when patients develop orthostatic hypotension or syncope associated with micturition, defecation, or coughing.

Noncardiac causes of syncope are, likewise, common in the elderly. Orthostatic hypotension – a drop in systolic blood pressure of 20 mm Hg or greater within 3 minutes of standing – is most commonly caused by decreased intravascular volume and medications in the elderly. Older adults are at higher risk of orthostatic hypotension because of impaired baroreceptor responses, including venous insufficiency. The medications most commonly implicated include antihypertensives, tricyclic antidepressants and other agents with anticholinergic activity, and antiangina drugs. Patients who have been lying in the bed for prolonged periods may experience orthostatic hypotension when they need to get up. Chronic orthostatic hypotension without obvious explanation is sometimes due to primary autonomic dysreflexia (see Case 8). A comprehensive discussion of syncope in the elderly is given in the references (see Kapoor, 1994).

The patient is referred for a 48-hour ambulatory electrocardiogram recording (Holter moniter) which identifies occasional sinus pauses of more than 2 seconds, associated with a feeling of lightheadedness. Echocardiogram shows normal left ventricular function, aortic sclerosis with normal aortic valve diameter, mild aortic insufficiency, and mild mitral regurgitation. Blood tests were normal, and specifically ruled out anemia and electrolyte abnormality. A permanent pacemaker was placed and the patient did well.

3. Among community-dwelling older persons, the most common reported cause of falling (30–50%) is an "accident" involving an environmental hazard, such as poor lighting, clutter, unsafe stairs, slippery floors, throw rugs, or poor condition of road or sidewalk surfaces. Often, multiple causes are present. Disease, or age-related change in vision and balance, may predispose older persons to falling in these hazardous conditions, and gait disorders, impaired vision or hearing, decreased reaction time, and dementia may prevent regaining of balance after tripping. Acute

medical illness, as seen in Case 15, or exacerbation of chronic disease can cause weakness or confusion and lead to a fall. Among nursing home residents, the most cited causes are gait or balance disorder, deconditioning due to immobility or a sedentary life, arthritis, neurologic disease, heart failure, and chronic lung disease.

Medications are an important cause of falling. In addition to benzodiazepines and antihypertensive agents, other hypnotics and anxiolytics, major tranquilizers, antidepressants, and anticholinergic medications can produce falls. Selective serotonin reuptake inhibitors (SSRIs) have been as strongly associated with falling as tricyclic antidepressants (TCAs), despite their lack of psychomotor and autonomic effects. It is uncertain if the risk of falls is due to an effect of the antidepressant, to depression itself, or to changes in health that are associated with depression and antidepressant use.

Other common causes of falling in both community and nursing home elders are dizziness or vertigo, confusion and cognitive impairment, visual disorders, and syncope. Frequently, multiple impairments, risk factors, and environmental hazards work together to cause the fall.

4. Mrs. E has some modifiable risk factors for falling, such as medication use and cataracts. Diuretics occasionally cause syncope by acutely decreasing intravascular volume; more commonly, they exacerbate existing urinary frequency and urgency, prompting the patient to dash to the bathroom, a risky practice for someone with other risks for falling (see Case 33). If these issues are of concern, it may be appropriate to replace the diuretic with a different antihypertensive medication, following the patient carefully for any new symptoms.

The patient also takes temazepam, which, like other benzodiazepines, can increase the risk of falls by impairing cognitive function or producing muscle weakness, and should be discontinued if possible. Her cataracts may not be severe enough yet to impair her vision in good lighting, but in poor lighting and at night she may have difficulty seeing things clearly. Thus, it would be important to maintain appropriate lighting in her bedroom and the pathway to the bathroom at night, and it would be very important to remove any environmental hazards in her home. These might include: securing carpet edges, removal of throw rugs, cords, or wires; reducing clutter; and placing grab bars in the bathtub and by the toilet, and placing rubber mats in the bathtub. Mrs. E's gait should be observed carefully to see if her cane is sufficient or if she is using it properly (see Case 18).

Finally, risk of falling due to age-related balance impairment can be reduced by strengthening exercises and appropriate balance exercises. Tai Chi, a form of balance training that has gained popularity among older adults, appears to be a promising intervention. In falls prevention, rehabilitation with gait training, balance and strength exercises, and training in the use of assistive devices is as important as treating the medical problem and modifying the risk factor. Outpatient rehabilitation services exist in hospital settings or office-based rehabilitation facilities, some senior centers and senior day-care programs, and can be provided at home in appropriate circumstances.

For patients at risk for recurrent falls, those like Mrs. E who are cognitively able can employ alerting devices to summon help if needed. Apartments specifically designed for seniors, such as those in assisted living facilities, have installed devices such as pull cords in the bathroom and the bedroom to summon assistance in case of emergency. Because not all falls will happen in arm's reach of a pull cord, a specially designed alerting button can be worn on the wrist or as a pendant that the patient can use to summon help. The system is tied through the telephone to a central monitoring station and the preset-up instructions will alert the service to call the patient's family, health care provider, or emergency services. Some systems can be set so the patient gets a daily call at a predetermined time and, if there is no answer, then the emergency plan goes into effect.

Guidelines for falls prevention in the elderly have been adopted by several professional organizations (see American Geriatrics Society et al., 2001). Strategies for people with low vision are discussed in Case 23.

Caveat

Many patients who require a cane are embarrassed to use one because it makes them "look old," or because they fear that using a cane will make them appear vulnerable and a prey to muggers. For such people, a large umbrella with a heavy rubber tip can be substituted, or a specially constructed wheeled grocery cart designed for use as a walker can be employed. This confers very good stability and may be more acceptable.

REFERENCES

American Geriatrics Society, British Geriatrics Society, and American Academy of Orthopaedic Surgeons Panel on Falls Prevention (2001). Guideline for the prevention of falls in older persons. *Journal of the American Geriatrics Society*, **49**, 664–72.

Kapoor, W. N. (1994). Syncope in older persons. *Journal of American Geriatrics Society*, **42**, 426–36.

Nevitt, M. C. (1989). Risk factors for recurrent nonsyncopal falls. A prospective study. *Journal of the American Medical Association*, **261**, 2663–8.

Richardson, D. A., Shaw, F. E., Bexton, R. *et al.* (2002). Presence of a carotid bruit in adults with unexplained or recurrent falls, implications for carotid sinus massage. *Age and Ageing*, **31**, 379–84.

BIBLIOGRAPHY

Fuller, G. E. (2000). Falls in the elderly. *American Family Physician*, **61**, 2159–68.

Lipsitz, L. A., Wei, J. Y., and Rowe, J. W. (1985). Syncope in an elderly, institutionalised population: prevalence, incidence, and associated risk. *Quarterly Journal of Medicine*, **55**, 45–55.

Thapa, P. B., Gideon, P., and Cost, T. W. (1998). Antidepressants and the risk of falls among nursing home residents. *New England Journal of Medicine*, **339**, 875–82.

Tinetti, M. E. (2003). Preventing falls in elderly persons. *New England Journal of Medicine*, **348**, 42–9.

Van Doorn, C., Gruber-Baldini, A. L., Zimmerman, S. *et al.*, for the Epidemiology of Dementia in Nursing Homes Research Group (2003). Dementia as a risk factor for falls and fall injuries among nursing home residents. *Journal of the American Geriatrics Society*, **51**, 1213–18.

Wolf, S. L., Barnhart, H. X., Kutner, N. G. *et al.* (1996). Reducing frailty and falls in older persons: an investigation of Tai Chi and computerized balance training. Atlanta FICSIT Group: Frailty and injuries – Cooperative Studies of Intervention Techniques. *Journal of the American Geriatrics Society*, **44**, 489–97.

Wu, G. (2000). Evaluation of the effectiveness of Tai Chi for improving balance and preventing falls in the older population – a review. *Journal of the American Geriatrics Society*, **50**, 746–54.

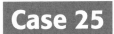

▸▸ Four patients in an osteoporosis clinic

Ms. A

Ms. A is a healthy 53-year-old Caucasian woman who seeks evaluation because of a family history of osteoporosis. Her mother had severe kyphosis as well as a hip fracture at age 80. Ms. A has just finished her menstrual periods, and has hot flushes that awaken her from sleep. She is mildly obese, although as a teenager she was extremely thin and amenorrheic for 2 years, from a possible eating disorder. She leads a sedentary lifestyle. She does not smoke or drink alcohol. She tried calcium supplements because she rarely eats dairy products, but discontinued them because of constipation.

Questions

1. What are her risk factors for osteoporosis?
2. How can her risk be confirmed?
3. Should she receive hormone replacement therapy (HRT) to prevent fractures?
4. What other approaches are available for this early postmenopausal woman?

Answers

1. This patient's most important risk factors are female sex, postmenopausal state, and family history. Much of the variance in peak bone mass and sensitivity to environmental stimuli or insults appears to be genetic, making her family history

Case Studies in Geriatric Medicine, Judith C. Ahronheim *et al.* Published by Cambridge University Press.
© J. C. Ahronheim, Z.-B. Huang, V. Yen, C. M. Davitt, and D. Barile

important. Age-related bone loss, which begins at approximately age 30, accelerates in women for approximately 7 years following menopause. Ms. A's low calcium intake is also a risk factor, as epidemiologic studies have repeatedly shown that this dietary factor is associated with a higher rate of fractures.

She is mildly obese and, although obesity reduces fracture risk (see below), her history of low body mass in her youth, associated with a possible eating disorder, might be an additional risk factor. Eating disorders leading to extreme low weight in adolescence may lead to amenorrhea; because 60% of bone is acquired during the pubertal growth spurt, amenorrhea during this time may interrupt bone acquisition, resulting in suboptimal peak bone mass and low bone mineral density (BMD). In contrast to the postmenopausal state, in which osteoporosis is related to excess bone loss, amenorrhea during adolescence or early adulthood leads to deficits in achieving peak bone mass. This mechanism also contributes to low bone mass that develops in some "super athletes," in whom excessive exercise is associated to low body weight and amenorrhea.

2. Measurement of BMD by dual electron X-ray absorptiometry (DEXA) would help to establish her current risk of developing osteoporosis. Measurements are generally performed at the spine or midforearm (trabecular or spongy bone) and the hip (primarily cortical or "dense" bone). BMD is reported as standardized scores, which compare the patient's bone density with reference populations of adults and express the result in standard deviations above or below the mean. The "T score" reflects comparison with young adults (those at lowest risk), and the "Z score" with one's same-age peers. According to current World Health Organization (WHO) criteria, a T score less than -2.5 indicates osteoporosis, and a score between -1 and -2.5 indicates "osteopenia," a less advanced stage of bone loss. There is no true "fracture threshold;" rather, the risk is continuous, each standard deviation below the mean conferring approximately twice the relative risk of subsequent fracture. Ms. A's T score was -1.7 at the spine and -1.2 at the hip, putting her at high risk for future fractures.

Another popular method of measuring BMD is heel ultrasound but this method may miss approximately 5% of cases that would otherwise be diagnosed by DEXA measurements of the axial skeleton. Methods of measuring BMD are reviewed in the references (see Nelson *et al.*, 2002).

Biochemical markers of bone resorption and formation, such as urinary N-telopeptide or osteocalcin, respectively, can yield useful information in selected patients who are undergoing treatment but do not in and of themselves predict fracture risk because they are nonspecific, varying with factors such as the degree of the patient's mobility.

3. This patient in her early postmenopausal years already has evidence of bone loss and a program of prevention is needed. Because estrogen is the most effective treatment

for menopausal hot flushes, it would seem to be a logical choice for short-term treatment. However, long-term use of HRT for the prevention of fractures has become increasingly controversial.

In bone, estrogen appears to act by blocking cytokine-mediated stimulation of osteoclastic bone resorption. Most evidence indicates that estrogen retards bone loss and reduces fracture risk, even when treatment is initiated as late as age 70, but, when estrogen is discontinued, a period of accelerated rate of bone loss ensues, mimicking postmenopausal bone loss. Thus, initiation of treatment at this time implies long-term exposure to hormones, subjecting her to the risk of side effects, including deep vein thrombosis, gallstones, and breast and endometrial cancer. The risk of endometrial cancer can be minimized with concurrent use of progestin, but progestin has not been ruled out as the cause of the slightly increased risk of breast cancer attributed to HRT. Finally, recent evidence suggests that combination HRT may increase rather than decrease the risk of coronary heart disease.

In addition to dramatic peri- and postmenopausal changes in estrogen status, there is a gradual decline in androgen levels in women with age. The place of androgen replacement in women is highly controversial (see Morley *et al.*, 2003).

4. Given her risk factors for osteoporosis, a program to prevent fractures should include calcium supplementation, vitamin D to promote intestinal calcium absorption and to prevent vitamin D deficiency, and exercise. Weight-bearing exercise is generally recommended, but nonweight bearing, resistive exercise may also increase bone density of the underlying muscle groups, and may have the additional benefit of improving balance.

Although there is sufficient reason to attribute her low BMD to osteoporosis alone, at her relatively young age it would be useful to rule out common "secondary causes" such as hyperthyroidism, hyperparathyroidism, and vitamin D deficiency. Screening for these tests can be done using simple laboratory tests, as discussed below.

Management of osteoporosis is geared to addressing the mechanism of bone fragility. In osteoporosis, there is both a reduction in the amount of bone and an abnormal architecture, which results from an accumulation of the remodeling deficits that occur with each cycle of bone turnover, wherein osteoclastic bone resorption is not completely balanced by osteoblastic bone formation. "Antiresorptive" agents, including calcium, bisphosphonates, calcitonin, and estrogen, reestablish the balance between bone resorption and formation, and retard further bone loss, although these agents do not appear to increase bone mass in a sustained fashion.

Calcium supplementation slows the rate of bone loss, although it only modestly reduces fracture rate. Intestinal calcium absorption declines with age, and in women this begins around menopause. In order to maintain "zero calcium balance," such patients must ingest 1500 mg of elemental calcium per day – the equivalent of more than a quart of skim milk – which is difficult for most people to achieve through diet alone. As this patient has noticed, supplements can cause constipation, but she might be able to tolerate small doses of calcium tablets, supplemented by nondairy sources of calcium, such as greens, sardines, and fortified cereals or orange juice.

Raloxifene, a selective estrogen receptor modulator (SERM), has the bone protective effects of estrogen, although to a lesser degree. The agonist/antagonist effects of the SERMs are not the same in every tissue. Thus, raloxifene, unlike estrogen, may not be acceptable to this patient because it can cause hot flushes (vasomotor symptoms). Raloxifene does not appear to cause endometrial changes and may reduce rather than increase the risk of breast cancer. However, there is concern that SERMs may, in fact, prove to be pro-oncogenic if given on the long term, as has been shown with tamoxifen. Like estrogen, raloxifene may increase the risk of deep vein thrombosis.

Bisphosphonates would be an acceptable option for Ms. A, but would need to be given with the admonition that few long-term data exist regarding the quality of bone that results when turnover/replacement has been shut down. Bisphosphonates have a prolonged half-life in bone and an earlier bisphosphonate – etidronate – was found to impair bone mineralization. Antiresorptive effects of newer bisphosphonates – alendronate (Fosamax) and residronate (Actonel) – occur at dosages that do not cause mineralization defects.

Given the possibility that this patient's low BMD might be partly related to failure to attain peak bone mass during adolescence, it is possible that she has a degree of "low turnover" osteoporosis (see below). Such patients might benefit from parathyroid hormone injections (see Neer *et al.*, 2001).

Mrs. B

Mrs. B, an 82-year-old woman with multiple compression fractures of the spine, is brought to the clinic by her daughter because of back pain. Mrs. B has dementia and lives with her daughter on the fourth floor of an apartment building that has no elevator.

The patient experienced a right wrist fracture 15 years ago when she slipped in her apartment. She has not fallen recently, although the daughter worries about her balance. She has some memory loss but otherwise has been healthy and takes no medications.

Mrs. B is able to walk with a cane, but appears to be in pain, especially when she transfers to the examining table. She has severe kyphoscoliosis, and percussion tenderness along the spine. X-ray of the spine reveals about 50%

reduction in height in one thoracic and three lumbar vertebrae. There are no flattened vertebrae and the pedicles are intact.

Serum total calcium is 7.9 mg/dl ($n = 8.5{-}10.5$), phosphate is 2.4 mg/dl ($n = 2.5{-}4.5$), and alkaline phosphatase 220 U/l ($n = 35{-}100$). Complete blood count (CBC) and other blood chemistries are normal.

Questions

1. In addition to her advanced age, what might be causing her bone fragility? How can this be confirmed?
2. What is the best initial treatment?
3. What is the utility of bone mineral density measurements in this case?
4. The patient's daughter has found a local radiologist through a vertebroplasty website. Should this treatment be recommended for this patient?

Answers

1. This elderly patient is home bound and has limited mobility. Immobility and lack of exercise promote bone resorption and osteoporosis. In addition, she lacks sunlight exposure and, unless she has a very good dietary source of vitamin D, such as the equivalent of one quart of vitamin D-fortified milk per day, she is likely to have vitamin D deficiency, the most common cause of adult osteomalacia. Her low serum calcium and phosphate levels also suggest vitamin D deficiency. Osteomalacia frequently coexists with osteoporosis in the elderly.

   Age-associated factors also increase the risk for vitamin D deficiency. With aging, the skin thins and contains less vitamin D substrate 7-dehydrocholesterol (provitamin D), which is converted to previtamin D by ultraviolet light, and then isomerized to cholecalciferol (vitamin D). Provitamin production requires only approximately 20 minutes of exposure to ultraviolet beta rays, but persons with deeply pigmented skin require 3–6 times longer to produce the same amount of vitamin. An additional problem is a seasonal variation in levels of 25-hydroxy (25-OH) vitamin D, which decline as much as 25% in the winter. The rate of hip fractures peaks in the early spring, as most fractures occur indoors. Vitamin D deficiency and fracture can be prevented by adequate vitamin D intake. When intake is less than 220 IU per day, parathyroid hormone level rises to compensate. The recommended daily allowance (RDA) of 400 IU prevents this "secondary hyperparathyroidism," but adults 70 years of age and older require 600 IU daily, and 800 IU in the winter months.

Osteomalacia in the elderly is generally clinically indistinguishable from, and usually occurs in conjunction with, osteoporosis, although patients with osteomalacia sometimes have bone tenderness even in the absence of apparent fracture, and may also have muscle weakness due to accompanying hypophosphatemia. Technically, confirmation of osteomalacia requires bone biopsy, with measurement of the mineralization rate after tetracycline labeling, which binds to the sites of active mineralization. Clinically, vitamin D-deficient osteomalacia is diagnosed by measuring serum levels of 25-OH vitamin D.

2. Initial management should consist of analgesia to reduce pain and encourage ambulation. Bone density will increase as mechanical load increases.

This patient's serum 25-OH D level was only 8 ng/ml ($n = 20-50$ ng/ml). In addition to vitamin D, calcium supplementation should be given. Although calcium intake alone does not improve osteomalacia, in this age group, calcium supplementation improves both BMD and fracture risk.

A bisphosphonate should be considered, if Mrs. B can take the medication as prescribed. Bisphosphonates should be taken with water and away from other medications in order to avoid drug–nutrient or drug–drug interactions. The patient must then avoid reclining for 30 minutes after taking the medication because of the risk of esophageal ulcer due to direct mucosal contact with the medication. Patients with limited ability to cooperate with their care or who have a history of esophageal or gastroduodenal disease, are unable to sit up, or have swallowing difficulties are at greater risk of complications. For patients with contraindictions to oral bisphosphonates, periodic intravenous infusions of bisphosphonates such as pamidronate or zolodronate may be effective.

Another option is nasal or subcutaneous injectable calcitonin. This antiresorptive agent may have analgesic effects, perhaps related to calcitonin receptors in the central nervous system. The antiresorptive effect is weaker than that of bisphosphonates or estrogen, and, although calcitonin increases BMD, fracture reduction data are limited.

Ultimately, the patient's risk of fractures depends on falls prevention, as discussed in Case 24. External hip protectors may be useful if acceptable to the patient (see Kannus *et al.*, 2000).

3. The value of DEXA in this patient is questionable. Given her age, and her history of wrist and multiple vertebral fractures, it would be extremely unlikely that she would *not* have poor BMD, and demonstrating it would not change decisions about treatment. Although there is growing evidence that identifying and treating symptomatic women with low BMD reduces fracture risk, there is no current agreement regarding who should be tested and when. A baseline DEXA would also have to be interpreted with caution, given her existing spinal pathology, and one must question

the rationale for the common practice of intermittent follow up examinations (see Miss. D, below).

4. Percutaneous vertebroplasty, using an injection of polymethylacrylate cement into the marrow of osteoporotic vertebral bodies that have collapsed to one-third of their height, may relieve pain. There is a paucity of data in the very elderly, and there have been cases of death due to inadvertent injection of cement into cerebrospinal fluid. In experienced hands, this treatment may be very useful in selected patients with acute fracture, but more study is needed to determine its efficacy in patients with multiple fractures.

Mr. C

Mr. C, a 70-year-old man, develops severe back pain after lifting a box. X-ray reveals a severely compressed L-4 vertebral body and poor mineralization of other vertebrae. He describes generalized fatigue but no paralysis. He has a 40-pack-year history of smoking but stopped 2 years ago on the advice of his physician when he was admitted for a severe exacerbation of chronic obstructive pulmonary disease (COPD). He has been following a strict medication regimen since then.

On examination, he is thin and chronically ill appearing. Pertinent laboratory values include hemoglobin 11 g/dl, serum albumin 3.0 g/dl ($n = 3.5–5.0$), total calcium 10.5 mg/dl, and phosphate 2.5 mg/dl.

Questions

1. What factors have contributed to his bone fragility?
2. How will a bone mineral density study contribute to his assessment?
3. How does the approach to osteoporosis in an older man differ from that in an older woman?
4. What treatment should he receive?

Answers

1. Osteoporotic vertebral fractures are uncommon in men, even at the age of 70, so secondary causes should be considered. Among young and middle-aged men, approximately 30–60% are found to have a "secondary cause." Although a 70-year-old man would be expected to have some age-related bone loss, patients being treated for COPD have generally been exposed to systemic corticosteroids, which

produce a severe form of osteoporosis. Even inhaled corticosteroids can lead to a dose-dependent decrease in BMD. Glucocorticoids act by directly inhibiting renal tubular calcium reabsorption and intestinal calcium absorption, with apparent increased expression of parathyroid hormone action in the bone and kidney. In addition, glucocorticoids inhibit osteoblastic maturation and activity and promote osteoblastic death by apoptosis. The overall effect is to accentuate the remodeling deficit that occurs in age-related osteoporosis. Chronic pharmacologic doses of glucocorticoids also suppress the hypothalamic–pituitary–gonadal axis, decreasing androgen production. Osteoporosis may also result from endogenous Cushing's syndrome, which has many causes, including ectopic adrenocorticotropic hormone production by tumors, such as small cell lung cancer, for which this long-time smoker would be at risk. Cigarette smoking itself is an important risk factor for osteoporosis (see Miss. D, below). Osteoporosis in COPD may also be related to chronic acidosis.

2. In men, BMD measurement has specific limitations. DEXA reports bone density as standardized scores in comparison with reference populations, generally young or postmenopausal white women, and these reference populations are generally not specified in radiology reports. Men of all races have greater peak bone mass than women, and black individuals have greater peak bone mass than other groups. Overall, individuals with greater peak bone mass develop fractures significantly later than others. However, men and other populations, such as blacks, Asians, and young people, may fracture at different levels of BMD than white women. Moreover, it cannot be assumed that their fracture risk correlates with BMD in the typical way. For example, a large study of multiple ethnic groups revealed that Asian American women have a lower BMD than Caucasians, but they also have a lower rate of hip fracture (see Siris *et al.*, 2001). It is not known if this is related to anatomic differences, such as height or pelvic configuration, or to criteria used to assess BMD. In short, it is important to determine the reference population when ordering DEXA and, if possible, to compute a T score based on ideal BMD for the patient in question.

   Despite these problems, the patient's history and clinical presentation make it apparent that his BMD would be far less than in a young, healthy male. A more productive use of DEXA in a male (or a female) might be to assist in the diagnosis of a patient with no apparent risk of osteoporosis who fractures bone after minimal trauma.

3. The approach should first be to suspect osteoporosis in any man in late life because it is underdiagnosed. Among people aged 65 and older, women have two to three times the incidence of hip fracture than men, but, by age 85, the incidence of hip fracture is equal in men and women. This probably reflects the clinical appearance of age-related "senile" osteoporosis, which occurs in both sexes as a result of steady decline in bone mass following its peak in the third and fourth decades of life, but which,

in women, is superimposed on postmenopausal bone loss. "Senile" osteoporosis involves cortical bone of the femur (hip) and humerus (shoulder), whereas postmenopausal osteoporosis is manifested largely as loss of trabecular bone (spine), and accounts for the elevated female-to-male ratio of vertebral fractures.

An important secondary cause in men is hypogonadism. Hypogonadism in men is due to androgen deficiency, and estrogen deficiency may also play a role, as a male's lifetime exposure to estrogens may actually exceed a female's. Younger men with genetic aromatase deficiency and low estrogen levels develop severe osteoporosis. Testosterone status declines with age, as discussed in detail in Case 35, but the clinical significance of this age-related change has not been fully determined, and the degree to which it contributes to age-related bone loss is not known.

Mr. C had mild hypercalcemia, suggesting primary hyperparathyroidism. Intact parathyroid hormone (PTH) should be determined to distinguish between hyperparathyroidism and malignancy caused by a nonparathyroid tumor, such as squamous cell tumors of the head and neck and lung, which would have to be considered in a smoker. These and other solid tumors sometimes secrete PTH-related peptide, which is not detected by intact PTH assays. Hypercalcemia and osteoporosis can also be caused by hematologic malignancies that are associated with secretion of osteoclast-activating cytokines, such as interleukin (IL)-1, IL-6, and tumor necrosis factor. This patient's PTH level was 45 pg/ml, which is technically in the normal range, but "inappropriately high" for an elevated serum calcium level, suggesting mild primary hyperparathyroidism; if the PTH level were suppressed, ectopic production would have to be considered.

Mr. C should receive a bisphosphonate because these agents are effective in corticosteroid-induced osteoporosis, even though corticosteroids do not increase bone resorption. Bisphosphonates and other antiresorptive agents exert their effect by reducing the "normal" background bone resorption that ultimately produces age-related bone loss. Bisphosphonates may also have some effect in lowering serum calcium in primary hyperparathyroidism.

Miss. D

Miss. D is a 72-year-old woman of Irish descent with a history of three compression fractures of the spine. She states that she has lost 3 inches in height and has occasional pain in her back. Her mother had a history of breast cancer, kyphosis, and dementia. Miss. D's last menstrual period was at about age 45 years. She has a history of hypothyroidism, hypertension, and noninsulin-dependent diabetes mellitus managed on diet alone. She smokes ten cigarettes a day and drinks two cocktails every evening. Her medications include atenolol 50 mg, aspirin 81 mg, levothyroxine 175 μg daily, and occasional diazepam for anxiety.

On physical examination, she is 5 feet 5 inches tall, and weighs 110 pounds. Blood pressure is 160/70, and pulse is 96 and regular. She has kyphoscoliosis without spinal tenderness, and a grade III/VI systolic murmur. She has no goiter or breast masses. Her uterus is intact. Her gait is slightly unstable.

Bone mineral density by DEXA, 6 months ago, reveal a T score of −1.5 at the lumbar spine and −3.0 at the total hip. CBC and comprehensive metabolic panel were normal. Hemoglobin A1c was 6.9%.

Questions

1. What are the patient's risk factors for bone fragility?
2. How should the DEXA study be interpreted?
3. What treatment should be given?
4. What studies should be used to follow the course of her treatment?

Answers

1. In addition to being an elderly, thin, Caucasian, postmenopausal female, this patient's main risk factor is her prior history of fracture. Fracture in an osteoporotic site, such as the spine, hip, or wrist, confers a 4–5-fold risk of subsequent fracture. Her risk is further increased by her risk factors for falling, including her unsteady gait and her use of alcohol, a benzodiazepine, and an antihypertensive, all of which have been associated with a risk of falls and fractures in older individuals (see Cases 24 and 27).

   This patient's cigarette smoking confers additional risk. Tobacco has an antiosteoblastic effect as well as an antiestrogen effect and inhibits production of nonovarian estrogen. She underwent menopause over 25 years ago and her age at menopause was somewhat earlier than average, like many women who smoke. Diabetes is associated with an increased risk of osteoporosis, perhaps due to advanced glycosylation end products interfering with bone microarchitecture.

   An additional risk factor in this patient is her thin body habitus. Patients with higher weights and increased body fat have higher estrogen levels than thin patients, owing to nonovarian production of estrogen in adipose tissue. Nonovarian androgens are converted to estrogen under the direction of aromatase enzymes that exist in adipose tissue, and estrone is converted to the more potent estradiol, and thin patients lack this advantage.

Finally, her thyroxine dose is somewhat higher than average and it would be important to ascertain that the dose is correct, as excessive thyroid hormone replacement – as well as hyperthyroidism – increase bone turnover and accelerate osteoporosis.

2. Miss. D's T score of −3.0 convers a risk of hip fracture about six times that of a young adult. This score seems disproportionately worse than her score of −1.5 at the lumbar spine, and her history of three spinal compression fractures suggests this score is misleading. Measurements of BMD can be misleadingly high in the presence of spinal compression fractures, degenerative joint disease, and scoliosis, so it is likely that the patient has significant osteoporosis in the spine as well as the hip.

3. In addition to calcium and vitamin D, a bisphosphonate would be a reasonable choice for someone in her age group. These powerful antiresorptive agents have long-lasting antiosteoclastic effects. They reduce hip and spine fracture incidence by up to 50%, and can be used both for the treatment and prevention of osteoporosis. In contrast to estrogen, discontinuation of bisphosphonates is not followed by accelerated bone loss or decreased BMD. However, bisphosphonates remain in bone for many years and their long-term effect is not known.

   An additional option includes adding a thiazide diuretic to her blood pressure regimen. Thiazides decrease calciuria and have been shown to increase bone density and decrease fracture risk. Blood glucose should be followed closely and antidiabetic medications used if indicated.

   Unlike Ms. A, who suffered from hot flushes, there is no compelling reason to give estrogen to Miss. D, and there may be additional risks, given the history of breast cancer in the first-degree relative and her atherosclerotic risk factors, including diabetes and cigarette smoking.

4. Although it is tempting to repeat the DEXA on a regular basis, the utility of this practice is not known. Increases in BMD on repeated measurements may be due to random error, or the statistical principle of "regression to the mean;" for example, a patient taking an antiresorptive agent who appears to lose (or gain) more than would be expected from the mean response might, on repeat measurement, demonstrate a more "normal" response (closer to the mean) or even an exaggerated one (see Cummings *et al.*, 2000).

   Biochemical markers of bone resorption are sometimes suggested to evaluate the level of resorption at baseline or to monitor effectiveness of therapy. Urinary N-telopeptide (NTP) and pyridinoline crosslinks, which are fragments of type 1 collagen, if high, indicate a state of high bone turnover (such as early postmenopause, hyperparathyroidism, or hyperthyroidism) and, if low, indicate low turnover (as in Cushing's syndrome). A reduction in urinary NTP following treatment (generally less than 30 BCE/mmol creatinine) indicates suppression of bone resorption, but currently no data exist regarding whether this suppression is reflected in a reduced fracture rate. These tests are expensive and not routinely used in the primary care setting, where, in most cases, they would not lead to a change in therapy. Use of biochemical markers is discussed in the references (see Garnero *et al.*, 2000; Reginster *et al.*, 2001).

Caveats

1. Anticonvulsants, especially phenytoin and phenobarbital, are an important cause of vitamin D deficiency and osteomalacia. These drugs induce hepatic enzymes and may preferentially lead to inactive vitamin D metabolites.

2. The commonly used supplement calcium carbonate (Os-Cal and others), which has the highest calcium content per gram weight of supplement (400 mg/g), requires gastric acidity in order to be absorbed; thus, patients who have low gastric acid secretion on the basis of age or medication use may fail to absorb calcium adequately in this form. Absorption tends to be improved if calcium carbonate is taken with, or right after, meals, which stimulate gastric acid secretion. Calcium citrate, which does not depend on gastric acid for absorption, has only 210 mg calcium per gram of supplement, so more pills need to be taken to achieve zero calcium balance.

3. Plant sources of estrogen (phytoestrogens), which are popularly perceived as safe, contain plant sterols such as isoflavones derived from soy that have estrogen-like properties. Although these can improve bone mineral density, phytoestrogens have diverse estrogen-binding properties, and, like approved selective estrogen receptor modulators, their beneficial and potentially harmful effects on various organs and tissues remain to be elucidated.

REFERENCES

Cummings, S. R., Palermo, L., Browner, W. *et al.* (2000). Monitoring osteoporosis therapy with bone densitometry: misleading changes and regression to the mean. *Journal of the American Medical Association*, **283**, 1318–21.

Garnero, P., Sornay-Rendu, E., Claustrat, B. *et al.* (2000). Biochemical markers of bone turnover, endogenous hormones, and the risk of fractures in postmenopausal women: the OFELY study. *Journal of Bone and Mineral Research*, **15**, 1526–36.

Kannus, P., Palvanen, M., Kaprio, J. *et al.* (1999). Genetic factors and osteoporotic fractures in elderly people: prospective 25 year follow up of a nationwide cohort of elderly Finnish twins. *British Medical Journal*, **319**, 1334–7.

Morley, J. E. and Perry, H. M. (2003). Androgens and women at the menopause and beyond. *Journals of Gerontology Series A: Biological Sciences and Medical Sciences*, **58**, M409–16.

Neer, R. M., Arnaud, C. D., Zanchetta, J. R. *et al.* (2001). Effect of parathyroid hormone (1–34) on fractures and bone mineral density in postmenopausal women with osteoporosis. *New England Journal of Medicine*, **344**, 1434–41.

Nelson, H. D., Rizzo, J., Harris, E. *et al.* (2002). Osteoporosis and fractures in postmenopausal women using estrogen. *Archives of Internal Medicine*, **162**, 2278–84.

Reginster, J. Y., Henrotin, Y., Christiansen, C. *et al.* (2001). Bone resorption in postmenopausal women with normal and low bone mineral density assessed with biochemical markers specific for telopeptide derived degradation products of collagen type I. *Calcified Tissue International*, **69**, 130–7.

Siris, E. S., Miller, P. D., Barrett-Connor, E. *et al.* (2001). Identification and fracture outcomes of undiagnosed low bone mineral density in postmenopausal women: results from the National Osteoporosis Risk Assessment. *Journal of the American Medical Association*, **286**, 2815–22.

BIBLIOGRAPHY

Adachi, J. D., Saag, K. G., Delmas, P. D. *et al.* (2001). Two year effects of alendronate on bone mineral density and vertebral fractures in patients receiving glucocorticoids. *Arthritis and Rheumatism*, **44**, 202–11.

Amin, S., Zhang, Y., Sawin, C. T. *et al.* (2000). Association of hypogonadism and estradiol levels with bone mineral density in elderly men from the Framingham study. *Annals of Internal Medicine*, **133**, 951–63.

Bai, J. C., Gonzalez, D., Mautalen, C. *et al.* (1997). Long term effect of gluten restriction on bone mineral density of patients with coeliac disease. *Alimentary Pharamacology and Therapeutics*, **11**, 157–64.

Bauer, D. C., Ettinger, B., Nevitt, M. C. *et al.*, for the Study of Osteoporotic Fractures Research Group (2001). Risk for fracture in women with low serum levels of thyroid-stimulating hormone. *Annals of Internal Medicine*, **134**, 561–8.

Bauer, D. C., Mundy, G. R., Jamal, S. A. *et al.* (2004). Use of statins and fracture: results of 4 prospective studies and cumulative meta-analysis of observational studies and controlled trials. *Archives of Internal Medicine*, **164**, 146–52.

Bone, H. G., Greenspan, S. L., McKeever, C. *et al.* (2000). Alendronate and estrogen effects in postmenopausal women with low bone density. *Journal of Clinical Endocrinology and Metabolism*, **85**, 720–6.

Canalis, E. (2003). Mechanisms of glucocorticoid-induced osteoporosis. *Current Opinions in Rheumatology*, **15**, 454–7.

Cauley, J. A., Robbins, J., Chen, Z. *et al.* (2003). Effects of estrogen plus progestin on risk of fracture and bone mineral density. The Women's Health Initiative Randomized Trial. *Journal of the American Medical Association*, **290**, 1729–38.

Cooper, C., Atkinson, E. J., O'Fallon, W. M. *et al.* (1992). Incidence of clinically diagnosed vertebral fractures: a population-based study in Rochester, Minnesota, 1985–1989. *Journal of Bone and Mineral Research*, **7**, 221–7.

Cummings, S. R., Black, D. M., Thompson, D. E. *et al.* (1998). Effect of alendronate on risk of fracture in women with low bone density but without vertebral fractures: results from the Fracture Intervention Trial. *Journal of the American Medical Association*, **280**, 2077–82.

Dawson-Hughes, B., Harris, S. H., Krall, E. A. *et al.* (1997). Effect of calcium and vitamin D supplementation on bone density in men and women 65 years of age or older. *New England Journal of Medicine*, **337**, 670–6.

Downs, R. W., Bell, N. H., Ettinger, M. P. *et al.* (2000). Comparison of alendronate and intranasal calcitonin for treatment of osteoporosis in postmenopausal women. *Journal of Clinical Endocrinology and Metabolism*, **85**, 1783–8.

Ettinger, B., Black, D. M., Mitlak, B. H. *et al.*, for the Multiple Outcomes of Raloxifene Evaluation (MORE) Investigators (1999). Reduction of vertebral fracture risk in postmenopausal women with osteoporosis treated with raloxifene. Results from a 3-year randomized clinical trial. *Journal of the American Medical Association*, **282**, 637–44.

Ettinger, M. P. (2003). Aging bone and osteoporosis: strategies for preventing fractures in the elderly. *Archives of Internal Medicine*, **163**, 2237–46.

Gregg, E. W., Cauley, J. A., Seeley, D. G. *et al.* (1998). Physical activity and osteoporotic fracture risk in older women. Study of Osteoporotic Fractures Research Group. *Annals of Internal Medicine*, **129**, 81–8.

Hulley, S., Furberg, C., Barrett-Connor, E. *et al.* (2002). Noncardiovascular disease outcomes during 6.8 years of hormone therapy. Heart and Estrogen/Progestin Replacement Study Follow-up (HERS II). *Journal of the American Medical Association*, **288**, 58–66.

Kannus, P., Parkkaru, J., Niemi, S. *et al.* (2000). Prevention of hip fracture in elderly people with the use of a hip protector. *New England Journal of Medicine*, **343**, 1506–13.

Kelepouris, N., Harper, K. D., Gannon, F. *et al.* (1995). Severe osteoporosis in men. *Annals of Internal Medicine*, **123**, 452–60.

Klebzak, G. M., Beinart, G. A., Perser, K. *et al.* (2002). Undertreatment of osteoporosis in men with hip fracture. *Archives of Internal Medicine*, **162**, 2217–22.

Lacroix, A. Z., Ott, S. M., Ichikawa, L. *et al.* (2000). Low-dose hydrochlorthiazide and preservation of bone mineral density in older adults. A randomized, double blind, placebo controlled trial. *Annals of Internal Medicine*, **133**, 516–26.

Lanza, F. L., Hunt, R. H., Thomson, A. B. *et al.* (2000). Endoscopic comparison of esophageal and gastroduodenal effects of risedronate and alendronate in postmenopausal women. *Gastroenterology*, **119**, 631–8.

LeBoff, M. S., Kohlmeier, L., Hurwitz, S. *et al.* (1999). Occult vitamin D deficiency in postmenopausal US women with acute hip fracture. *Journal of the American Medical Association*, **281**, 1505–11.

Liberman, U. A., Weiss, S. R., Broll, J. *et al.* (1995). Effect of oral alendronate on bone mineral density and the incidence of fractures in postmenopausal osteoporosis. *New England Journal of Medicine*, **333**, 1437–43.

MacLaughlin, J. and Holick, M. F. (1985). Aging decreases the capacity of human skin to produce vitamin D3. *Journal of Clinical Investigation*, **76**, 1536–8.

Manolagas, S. C. and Jilka, R. L. (1995). Bone marrow, cytokines, and bone remodeling. *New England Journal of Medicine*, **332**, 305–11.

McClung, M. R., Geusens, P., Miller, P. D. *et al.*, for the Hip Intervention Program Study Group (2001). Effect of risedronate on the risk of hip fracture in elderly women. *New England Journal of Medicine*, **344**, 333–40.

Orwoll, E., Ettinger, M., Weiss, S. *et al.* (2000). Alendronate for the treatment of osteoporosis in men. *New England Journal of Medicine*, **343**, 604–10.

Peh, W. C. G., Gilula, L. A., and Peck, D. D. (2002). Percutaneous vertebroplasty for severe osteoporotic vertebral body compression fractures. *Radiology*, **223**, 121–6.

Reid, I. R., Ames, R. W., Evans, M. C. *et al.* (1993). Effect of calcium supplementation on bone loss in postmenopausal women. *New England Journal of Medicine*, **328**, 460–4.

Standing Committee on the Scientific Evaluation of Dietary Reference Intakes Food and Nutrition Board Institute of Medicine (1997). *Dietary Reference Intakes for Calcium, Phosphorus, Magnesium, Vitamin D, and Fluoride*. Washington, DC: National Academy Press, pp. 274–5.

Tonino, R. P., Meunier, P. J., Emkey, R. *et al.* (2000). Skeletal benefits of alendronate: 7-year treatment of postmenopausal osteoporotic women. Phase III Osteoporosis Treatment Study Group. *Journal of Clinical Endocrinology and Metabolism*, **85**, 3109–15.

U.S. Preventive Services Task Force (2002). Screening for osteoporosis in postmenopausal women: recommendations and rationale. *Annals of Internal Medicine*, **137**, 526–8.

Van Staa, T. P., Leufkens, H. G. M., and Cooper, C. (2001). Use of inhaled corticosteroids and risk of fractures. *Journal of Bone and Mineral Research*, **15**, 993–1000.

Vogel, J. M., Davis, J. W., Nomura, A. *et al.* (1997). The effect of smoking on bone mass and the rates of bone loss among elderly Japanese-American men. *Journal of Bone and Mineral Research*, **12**, 1495–501.

Wasnich, R. D. and Miller, P. D. (2000). Antifracture efficacy of antiresorptive agents are related to changes in bone density. *Journal of Clinical Endocrinology and Metabolism*, **85**, 231–6.

Writing Group for the Women's Health Initiative Investigators (2002). Risks and benefits of estrogen plus progestin in healthy postmenopausal women. Principle results from the Women's Health Initiative Randomized Controlled Trial. *Journal of the American Medical Association*, **288**, 321–33.

Case 26

►► Hip fracture

Miss. D, whom we met in Case 25, was standing uncomfortably for 20 minutes while waiting for a taxi when she developed severe pain in her right hip and fell to the ground. She was unable to bear weight on her affected leg and, when she finally got a taxi, she took it directly to her doctor's office where an X-ray of the hip was done. The X-ray was said to be normal, but her symptoms persisted. Three days later, she went to a local hospital emergency room where a repeat hip X-ray revealed a subcapital hip fracture. Hemiarthroplasty is planned.

Questions

1. When did the hip fracture occur?
2. Why was the first X-ray read as normal?
3. What sort of perioperative issues need to be considered?

Answers

1. Hip fractures sometimes occur after apparently nontraumatic stress if the femoral neck is severely osteopenic. A patient may report struggling to break a fall and applying torsion to the hip, or may report no obvious trauma at all, so the fall sometimes is caused by the fracture, and not the other way around. Miss. D probably had such a "stress" or "insufficiency" fracture after standing uncomfortably for a prolonged period of time.
2. Severe osteopenia and a "paper-thin" cortex are common radiographic features in the bones of elderly patients, making small fractures hard to detect. Early healing may make fractures more apparent on X-ray several days later. Lateral and oblique

Case Studies in Geriatric Medicine, Judith C. Ahronheim *et al.* Published by Cambridge University Press.
© J. C. Ahronheim, Z.-B. Huang, V. Yen, C. M. Davitt, and D. Barile

views may be needed to confirm a fracture. Positional rotation may obscure radiographic signs of fractures.

It is important to maintain a high index of suspicion when there is clinical evidence of hip fracture in a patient at risk. Although stress fractures such as this patient describes probably comprise a small minority, any high-risk patient with even minor trauma who develops hip pain or difficulty ambulating must be considered to have a hip fracture until proven otherwise. Surgical repair is the treatment of choice in elderly patients, who cannot tolerate prolonged bed rest. Morbidity and mortality increase when surgery is delayed for more than 48–72 hours. It is likely that prompt surgery improves outcome in patients who are otherwise relatively healthy, although delay may be necessary in patients with comorbidities that require medical attention prior to surgery.

A negative X-ray in an elderly patient with probable osteoporosis, who has clinical symptoms or signs suggestive of hip fracture, should prompt further investivation. Magnetic resonance imaging (MRI) is the most sensitive test and has been shown to detect fractures in patients with negative X-rays; in one study of 70 patients with clinically suspected hip fractures undetected by X-ray, 27 had MRI evidence of hip fracture and an additional 11 had a pelvic fracture (Bogost et al., 1995). MRI immediately reveals the bone marrow disruption that occurs at the time of fracture. Bone scan is less expensive and is a reasonable alternative if MRI is unavailable, contraindicated, or cannot be tolerated by a patient. However, bone scan is slightly less sensitive than MRI; it depends on osteoblastic activity, which is impaired in late life, and, although generally helpful and usually positive within the first 24 hours after fracture, bone scans occasionally may not become positive for several days in elderly patients. Computed tomography scan is another alternative, although false negative results sometimes occur.

3. The patient is at low operative risk, given her overall high function (see Case 12). However, certain perioperative issues are particularly important to consider in the setting of hip fracture.

Elderly patients with acute hip fracture are at extremely high risk for deep vein thrombosis (DVT), having virtually the highest incidence of any risk group, as high as 80% detected by venography (Geerts et al., 1994). This risk is likely to be due to trauma-related activation of the coagulation system, compounded by tissue disruption near the femoral vein. Because DVT associated with hip fracture is often in the proximal venous system, the risk of pulmonary embolism is also elevated. The DVT is often established at the time of surgery, and unanticipated surgical delay is common, so anticoagulation should be initiated prior to surgery if practical and not contraindicated. Methods of prophylaxis and their rationale are discussed in the references (see Morrison et al., 1998; Geerts et al., 2001). Increasingly, the low molecular weight heparin, enoxaparin (Lovenox), has been used for DVT prophylaxis in various settings, because of its greater pharmacologic predictability and safety compared with heparin, and its lack of pharmacokinetic drug interactions also makes it preferable to warfarin. Caution is required in elderly patients, however. Enoxaparin is eliminated by the kidney, and, although major bleeding is unusual, it occurs primarily in patients with renal insufficiency and the elderly if "usual" doses are used. Because normal serum creatinine often masks impaired creatinine clearance in the elderly, and because routine laboratory monitoring of factor Xa activity is not generally available, lower doses should be given to elderly patients and those with known renal insufficiency. Unfortunately, no specific dosing guidelines exist for these high-risk groups.

Prophylactic antibiotics are routinely given to prevent wound infection. Other perioperative infections are common in the elderly hip fracture patient, including pneumonia and urinary tract infection (UTI). The risk of UTI could possibly be reduced by early removal of indwelling catheters, which are routinely placed pre-operatively and often unnecessarily left in place when there is no clear indication. This may be because of the assumption that certain elderly patients are unable to assist in care or are incontinent. An indication for bladder catheterization in the immediate postoperative period is urinary retention, which is generally related to a delayed effect of anesthetic agents or opioid analgesia. In general, the indwelling catheter should be removed promptly and intermittent catheterization performed if needed. This will help to avoid the problem of the neglected indwelling catheter and its elevated risk of UTI, and may have the added benefit of promoting more rapid patient mobilization.

Delirium occurs commonly in elderly hip fracture patients, especially in the postoperative period. This is likely to be due to delayed effects of anesthesia, analgesic agents, and infection, but multiple factors may exist in frail elderly with comorbidities. Careful attention to risk factors can reduce the risk and severity of postoperative delirium. Early mobilization, reorientation, hearing and vision aids when necessary, optimization of hydration status, and using nonpharmacologic methods for sleep and agitation while avoiding sedation medications are some of the methods found to be successful by geriatric consultants (see Inouye *et al.*, 1999; Marcantonio *et al.*, 2001). Postoperative analgesia with opioids is generally required but dosing must be cautious. Initial doses in the opioid-naive patient over 80 years of age should generally be one-half of that given to younger adults. Although around-the-clock analgesia is helpful, patients must be re-evaluated often because opioids and their renally eliminated active metabolites may accumulate over a few hours.

Hip surgery was performed 12 hours later and hemiprosthesis was inserted. Within a week, Miss. D was able to ambulate with a walker and, within a few weeks, she was walking with a cane, although with somewhat more difficulty than before the hip fracture.

Two years later, she began to notice pain in her right hip, and, disillusioned with her original physician because of the misdiagnosis, she comes to you for help. Her overall medical condition has been stable except for extraction of two "infected molars" 1 month ago.

On physical examination, she is alert and interactive. Blood pressure, pulse, and temperature are normal. Her right leg is 1 inch shorter than her left. There is no erythema, swelling, or tenderness at the surgical site. She walks with a stooped posture and limps slightly "because of the pain."

Questions

1. Why did her orthopedic surgeon insert a hemiprosthesis and not perform the simpler repair consisting of transcutaneous pinning?
2. What might be causing her *new* hip pain?

Answers

1. Subcapital fractures may cut off the major arterial blood supply to the femoral head since the artery of the round ligament provides adequate supply in only 5% of individuals (see Figure 9), and avascular necrosis may occur. Avascular necrosis of the femoral head occurs as a late complication in over 30% of subcapital fractures that have been nailed or pinned at surgery, but is extremely rare after trochanteric fracture since blood supply is not interrupted. Hemiarthroplasty circumvents the problem of avascular necrosis because the femoral head is removed and replaced by the prosthesis. Moreover, the hemiprosthesis allows early weight bearing, speeding rehabilitation and lowering the likelihood of complications that occur as a result of prolonged bed rest. Intertrochanteric fractures, in contrast, are repaired by approximating the ends of the fracture and internally fixing the fracture with a sliding screw and plate.
2. The prosthesis may have loosened in the femoral shaft, or might have been the wrong "fit" for the patient's acetabulum. Both factors could result in acetabular erosion and secondary osteoarthritis. Latent infection around the prosthesis can present with pain in the absence of classic signs of infection. Such infection can be introduced at the time of surgery or can be caused by bacteremia from an invasive procedure, including dental work, but the incidence of this problem is not known and routine prophylaxis in patients with orthopedic appliances is controversial.

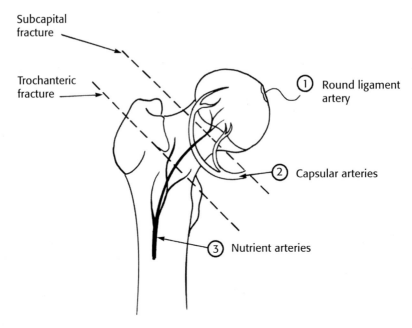

Subcapital
fracture

Trochanteric
fracture

① Round ligament
artery

② Capsular arteries

③ Nutrient arteries

Figure 9   Vascular supply to the femoral head. A trochanteric fracture could disrupt blood supply from arteries that course through the femoral shaft, leaving the capsular supply intact. A subcapital fracture could, in addition, disrupt the capsular blood supply; the artery of the ligament is insufficient to compensate.

Although Miss. D had recent dental work, an X-ray revealed early acetabular erosion, a condition which is clinically comparable to arthritis of the hip. She was treated with analgesia and other conservative measures, and was informed that total hip replacement could be offered in the future if her symptoms demanded.

Diagnostic imaging of pain in hip arthroplasty is reviewed in the references (see Keogh *et al.*, 2003).

REFERENCES

Bogost, G. A., Lizerbram, E. K., and Crues, J. V. (1995). MR imaging in evaluation of suspected hip fracture: frequency of unsuspected bone and soft-tissue injury. *Radiology*, **197**, 263–7.

Geerts, W. H., Code, K. I., Jay, R. M. *et al.* (1994). A prospective study of venous thromboembolism after major trauma. *New England Journal of Medicine*, **331**, 1601–6.

Geerts, W. H., Heit, J. A., Clagett, G. P. *et al.* (2001). Prevention of venous thromboembolism. *Chest*, **119**, S132–75.

Inouye, S. K., Bogardus, S. T., Charpentier, P. A. *et al.* (1999). A multicomponent intervention to prevent delirium in hospitalized older patients. *New England Journal of Medicine*, **340**, 669–76.

Keogh, C. F., Munk, P. L., Gee, R. *et al.* (2003). Imaging of the painful hip arthroplasty. *American Journal of Roentgenology*, **180**, 115–20.

Marcantonio, E. R., Flacker, J. M., Wright, R. J. *et al.* (2001). Reducing delirium after hip fracture: a randomized trial. *Journal of the American Geriatrics Society*, **49**, 516–22.

Morrison, R. S., Chassin, M. R., and Siu, A. L. (1998). The medical consultant's role in caring for patients with hip fracture. *Annals of Internal Medicine*, **128**, 1010–20.

BIBLIOGRAPHY

American Dental Association and American Academy of Orthopedic Surgeons Advisory Statement (1997). Antibiotic prophylaxis for dental patients with total joint replacement. *Journal of the American Dental Association*, **128**, 1004–8.

Ching, D. W., Gould, I. M., Rennie, J. A. *et al.* (1989). Prevention of late haematogenous infection in major prosthetic joints. *Journal of Antimicrobial Chemotherapy*, **23**, 676–80.

Curry, S. and Phillips, H. (2002). Joint arthroplasty, dental treatment, and antibiotics: a review. *Journal of Arthroplasty*, **17**, 111–13.

Grimes, J. P., Gregory, P. M., Noveck, H. *et al.* (2002). The effects of time-to-surgery on mortality and morbidity in patients following hip fracture. *American Journal of Medicine*, **112**, 702–9.

Perron, A. D., Miller, M. D., and Brady, W. J. (2002). Orthopedic pitfalls in the ED: radiographically occult hip fracture. *American Journal of Emergency Medicine*, **20**, 234–7.

Sanderink, G. J., Guimart, C. G., Ozoux, M. L. *et al.* (2002). Pharmacokinetics and pharmacodynamics of the prophylactic dose of enoxaparin once daily over 4 days with renal impairment. *Thrombosis Research*, **105**, 225–31.

Vaya, A. Mira, Y., Azner, J. *et al.* (2003). Enoxaparin-related fatal spontaneous retroperitoneal hematoma in the elderly. *Thrombosis Research*, **110**, 69–71.

Zuckerman, J. D. (1996). Hip fracture. *New England Journal of Medicine*, **334**, 1519–25.

Zuckerman, J. D., Skovron, M. L., Koval, K. J. *et al.* (1995). Postoperative complications and mortality associated with operative delay in older patients who have a fracture of the hip. *Journal of Bone and Joint Surgery, American volume*, **77**, 1551–6.

▸▸ Headache

Ms. J is a 75-year-old woman who first came to your office 1 year ago after a hospital admission for new-onset atrial fibrillation with a ventricular rate of 138 beats per minute. Sinus rhythm was restored following intravenous diltiazem and digoxin, and warfarin was begun. She was referred for visiting nurse services for medication supervision, and monitoring of her cardiac status and international normalized ratio (INR). The nurse found a bottle of ranitidine in the home, which had been prescribed by the patient's previous physician, and a medication review in the office 1 week after hospital discharge revealed that the patient had been taking generic levothyroxine as well as Synthroid.

Ms. J is seen in the office today for a follow up visit. She is a well-dressed, slim white woman whose shoes and bag perfectly match her outfit. Her make-up is expertly applied. She steadies her tremulous right hand on the top of an elegantly decorated cane. She is accompanied by a young woman who is a student at the local university whom she privately pays for 2 hours twice a week to help with the shopping and laundry and "little things around the house." A medication review reveals that the patient is taking oxy-codone/acetaminophen and she states that she suffers from headaches. They occur upon awakening and last throughout the day, and are relieved only with these tablets and a glass of champagne. The headaches are not associated with nausea, vomiting, or aura. They are usually on the top of her head and sometimes behind her eyes. She has no history of migraine, but says she has had these headaches for years. When you ask her about alcohol use, she states that she has an occasional "social" drink when friends stop by to see her, but denies that's she's ever been a "drinker." Besides, she has heard that alcohol is "good for the heart."

Her other medical problems include difficulty sleeping. She has taken flurazepam in the past and currently takes either temazepam or zolpidem, saying she "can't sleep without a little help." The temazepam helps a little,

Case Studies in Geriatric Medicine, Judith C. Ahronheim *et al*. Published by Cambridge University Press.
© J. C. Ahronheim, Z.-B. Huang, V. Yen, C. M. Davitt, and D. Barile

but she still lies awake until 2.30 a.m. when she looks for "something to take." She has tried over-the-counter diphenhydramine/acetaminophen (Tylenol PM) as well. You would like her to stop taking sleeping pills, and, thinking she might be a little depressed, you prescribe mirtazapine 15 mg, but the patient stopped it after 1 week because "it wasn't strong enough."

On questioning, the patient reports that she broke her shoulder in a "nasty fall" last winter.

Questions

1. What is causing her headaches?
2. What changes of aging compound her problem?
3. What medical problems could be due to her problem?
4. What drug interactions should you be concerned about?
5. How can this problem be better recognized and diagnosed in the elderly?
6. What treatment options might you offer this patient?

Answers

1. Tension, cluster, and migraine headaches decrease in prevalence with aging. Headaches that first present late in life suggest a secondary cause, sometimes serious, such as a neoplasm or temporal arteritis, but the course of Ms. J's headache does not suggest either etiology. Subdural hematoma can present with headaches, but, in the elderly, altered mental status and other neurologic signs usually predominate. Sleep apnea can produce headaches and are usually associated with daytime somnolence; if Ms. J reported daytime somnolence, however, it would be difficult to determine its origin, given her use of opioids and alcohol during the day.

Alcohol use can be a contributing factor to Ms. J's headaches, although it may not be the only cause. Two-thirds of persons with an alcohol hangover suffer from a morning-after headache. The mechanism of this headache, though once believed to represent a form of alcohol withdrawal, is complex (see Wiese *et al.*, 2000). The features of hangover ("veisalgia") vary from episode to episode and it is unknown if a daily headache can be attributed exclusively to alcohol use. The patient's report that the headache is relieved by alcohol would suggest this etiology, but it is also possible that her complaint of headache is partly a rationale for her use of alcohol, as well as opioids.

Ms. J eventually revealed that her alcohol consumption was higher than she first reported. She admitted to one to two glasses of champagne daily at lunch, a drink before dinner, a glass of red wine with dinner, and, most nights, a "night cap" to fall asleep. The visiting nurse also reported that there were multiple empty liquor bottles in the apartment, raising the concern that her intake is even higher. Ms. J may be caught in the vicious cycle of headache related to a hangover, drinking more to relieve the headache and tremor (perceived as anxiety), daytime sleeping, and using the alcohol to try and induce sleep at night. The tremulousness, which the patient experiences as anxiety, is also part of the veisalgia syndrome.

2. Aging is associated with a diminished tolerance to alcohol. With age, there is a decrease in lean body mass and total body water; alcohol distributes in body water, so there is a decreased volume of distribution with age, and an increase in blood alcohol level for any given dose. There is also an age-related decrease in gastric alcohol dehydrogenase, which metabolizes alcohol prior to systemic absorption; this leads to an increase in the amount of ingested alcohol that is systemically absorbed. Probably less than 10% of alcohol is metabolized by the liver (alcohol dehydrogenase [ADH] and oxidation by cytochrome P450 isoenzymes), but hepatic oxidation declines with age, although the contribution of this phenomenon to alcohol's effect in late life is not known. Young women have twice as much gastric ADH activity than men but this difference disappears after midlife. Alcohol ingestion impairs cognitive function (perception and attention), in proportion to the blood alcohol content, and at all levels the elderly do worse than the young. This effect is magnified in the presence of dementia.

One drink per day is generally considered the maximum amount for "moderate" drinking for men and women aged 65 and older (see National Institute on Alcohol Abuse, 2004), compared with two drinks for younger adults, although some guidelines recommend one-half the amount for women. One drink is generally considered equivalent to 12 ounces of beer, 5 ounces of wine, or 1.5 ounce of 80-proof spirits.

3. Although atrial fibrillation occurs commonly in late life, the risk of atrial fibrillation and other cardiac arrhythmias can be further increased by alcohol. "Holiday Heart" is a syndrome of increased atrial and ventricular arrhythmias related to binge drinking. Although moderate drinking may reduce the risk of coronary artery disease, alcohol and its metabolite acetaldehyde are toxic to the myocardium. Chronic (six drinks a day for 5–10 years in nonelderly adults), as well as binge drinking, can produce myocardial depression and chronic abuse can cause permanent myocardial damage and cardiomyopathy. Any mortality benefit achieved from moderate drinking is small, and is most pronounced in persons at risk for coronary artery disease. Despite the popular perception that people should drink because "it's good for their heart," only light consumption has potential health benefit, and a physician's

prescription could be interpreted as a stamp of approval for potentially harmful behavior.

Hyperthyroidism also increases the risk of developing atrial fibrillation. Ms. J was unintentionally taking twice her prescribed dose of thyroxine, which could have acted in concert with excessive alcohol use to precipitate her arrhythmia. It is uncertain if her alcohol abuse impaired comprehension of the prescribed regimen.

Another problem associated with alcohol use is falling. This risk is also increased by the use of sedating medications. Ms. J has a history of falling and a shoulder fracture, a typical fracture seen in osteoporosis. In addition to advanced age, chronic heavy use of alcohol may increase bone fragility.

Alcohol can disrupt sleep. Although alcohol shortens sleep latency (the time it takes to fall asleep), it stimulates the reticular-activating system, and reduces REM sleep, resulting in a decrease in total time of restful sleep. Time spent in REM sleep declines with age, and alcohol would make this worse. Age is associated with "phase advance," in which sleep onset and awakening occur earlier, and this pattern can be mimicked and worsened by alcohol. The patient may also experience increased early morning awakening and night-time restlessness, leading to daytime lethargy and sleepiness. Among recovering alcoholics, insomnia is a known risk factor for relapse, presumably because they use alcohol to induce sleep.

Heavy alcohol use and binge drinking increase the risk of stroke, possibly hemorrhagic more so than ischemic stroke. Alcohol can furthermore acutely elevate blood pressure, another risk factor for stroke. Other potential consequences in the elderly include decreased mental function, falls, accidents, depression, lack of self-care, decreased immune function and increased susceptibility to infections, and social isolation.

Recent epidemiologic studies suggest an association between alcohol use and breast cancer in postmenopausal women, possibly because of elevated levels of estrone sulfate concentration and dehydroepiandrosterone (DHEA) with the consumption of 15 or 30 g of alcohol daily, or concurrent dietary deficiencies such as low folate intake. Alcohol consumption also increases estrogen levels in post-menopausal women taking estrogen replacement therapy.

4. Alcohol participates in many pharmacokinetic and pharmacodynamic interactions with medications. Pharmacokinetic interactions are difficult to predict because alcohol's effect on metabolic enzymes is complex and absorption and rapidity of alcohol's entry into the circulation varies depending on a number of factors. Potential drug interactions in Ms. J's regimen include ranitidine, a histamine-2 blocker which can inhibit alcohol dehydrogenase, and warfarin, whose metabolism can be inhibited by alcohol. Heavy alcohol use causes induction of certain hepatic microsomal enzymes; when the drinker is intoxicated, the enzymes are being employed to metabolize alcohol and less enzyme is available to metabolize other drugs, such

as warfarin. When the chronic heavy drinker is sober, the induced enzymes can accelerate drug metabolism. Like many drinkers, Ms. J has either failed to adhere to her prescribed regimen or has made medication errors. Acute alcohol intake decreases warfarin metabolism, increasing the risk of bleeding, a particularly worrisome problem in someone who falls. Ms. J did, in fact, present several times to the office and the emergency department with significant hematomas, sometimes with a therapeutic or subtherapeutic INR, indicating the complexity of her situation.

Alcohol participates in pharmacodynamic interactions as well, mostly by enhancing the effects of sedating medications, such as opioids and hypnotic agents, which this patient was taking. Benzodiazepines which undergo hepatic oxidation, such as flurazepam, chlordiazepoxide, and alprazolam, may also interact pharmacokinetically with alcohol. Interactions with sedating medications are responsible for falls, fractures, and head trauma, and Ms. J was at very high risk of developing a subdural hematoma on account of her warfarin use. On one occasion, she presented with multiple hematomas and it was discovered that she had been taking Aleve (naproxen) along with her warfarin. By impairing platelet function, nonsteroidal anti-inflammatory agents can increase the risk of bleeding in patients taking warfarin. Interactions of alcohol with prescription and nonprescription medications are reviewed in detail in the references (see Weathermon *et al.*, 1999).

5. It is often difficult to recognize elderly alcoholics, especially when they are women. The elderly alcoholic may be misdiagnosed with dementia, malnutrition, "failure to thrive," or other chronic illness, and medication nonadherence can be attributed to numerous other causes. Family members may cover for their relative out of embarrassment at the discovery of the alcoholism.

In general, elderly alcoholics fall into three groups: those who have survived a long history of heavy drinking and present with chronic medical problems, those who binge infrequently and otherwise abstain or drink moderately, and those who take up drinking late in life as a response to a significant stressor such as retirement, loss of a spouse, or out of loneliness or boredom (O'Connor and Schottenfeld, 1998). Ms. J may fall into the first group. An articulate, well-dressed woman complaining of headaches, she exemplifies the alcoholic who does not fit the "stereotype," and points out the importance of vigilance on the part of the primary care provider. This patient's denial of the seriousness of the problem led to a delay in diagnosis.

Blood alcohol content (BAC) is sometimes used to confirm the diagnosis of alcoholism. With a blood alcohol content (BAC) of 100 mg/100 ml, the average nonalcohol-abusing patient will exhibit signs of intoxication. A BAC of 150 mg/100 ml or higher without signs or symptoms of intoxication indicates tolerance to alcohol, supporting the diagnosis. However, these levels should be adjusted downward in elderly individuals because, for any given amount of alcohol ingestion, the

BAC of a 60-year-old person is 20% higher, and that of a 90-year-old person 50% higher, than that of a 20-year-old person.

Serum liver function tests may provide clues in suspected alcohol abusers. Early diagnostic clues at any age also include insomnia, easy bruising, anxiety, tachycardia, hypertension, and reluctance to discuss the issue of drinking. Elderly patients should be queried regarding social isolation, falls, accidents, and family problems. They should also be asked about quantity and frequency of drinking as well as binges. Memory impairment may affect the history so it is important to corroborate answers with a reliable informant.

Several screening tools to detect alcohol use disorders have been studied in the geriatric population. The 10-item Short Michigan Alcohol Screening Test (SMAST-G) is a geriatric version of the Michigan Alcohol Screening Test (MAST). Although sensitive and specific in elderly American patients, the SMAST-G may not have universal applicability because of cultural differences. The Alcohol Use Disorders Identification Test (AUDIT), developed by the World Health Organization, was developed specifically to identify patients with current drinking problems but its sensitivity among the elderly population is limited. The CAGE questionnaire is a four-item screen that is widely used. Each item answered positively is given a score of one point, with a score of two or greater suggesting alcohol problems and the need for further evaluation. This score may be too conservative for elderly patients, and reducing the cut-off score to one positive answer increases the sensitivity of the screen. Applicability of screening methods to the elderly is reviewed in the references (see Conigliaro *et al.*, 2000).

6. Only a small minority of alcoholics are referred for treatment. If patients are reluctant to enter a formal program, simple advice or brief counseling by the primary care provider have been shown to reduce significantly the number of drinks per week. Counseling can include a contract with the patient to limit or eliminate drinking, providing alternatives to drinking, and stress management techniques. Patients should also be informed about high concentrations of alcohol in consumer products such as mouthwash – Geritol (12% alcohol), Nyquil (25% alcohol) – and some liquid multivitamin preparations. A referral for outpatient treatment may be necessary. Self-help groups such as Alcoholics Anonymous are among the most effective tools to help a patient toward recovery. Although specific 12-step groups for the elderly exist, information on their effectiveness is limited.

Older persons undergoing detoxification should be closely supervised, preferably in a hospital setting due to the risk of seizures, falls, delirium, and decreased ability to care for themselves. Inpatient treatment could be an option for this patient, if she were to acknowledge her problem.

Medications approved for the treatment of alcohol use disorders to prevent relapse include disulfiram and naltrexone. Disulfiram is mediated by acetaldehyde dehydrogenase and causes the unpleasant side effects of nausea, vomiting, and diarrhea if the patient drinks alcohol. It is not recommended for use in the elderly due to the risk of hepatotoxicity and neuropathy. Naltrexone is an opioid antagonist that decreases the craving for alcohol. It is used as an adjunct for patients enrolled in supportive psychotherapy programs, but its specific role in the treatment of the elderly alcoholic has not been established.

Despite much effort and extensive counseling, Ms. J was unwilling to admit that many of her problems were related to chronic alcohol abuse and was unwilling to consider outpatient or inpatient treatment. She had no actively interested family to help her to seek treatment. Further research is needed to quantify the most effective means of identifying and successfully treating alcohol use disorders in late life.

REFERENCES

Conigliaro, J., Kraemer, K., and McNeil, M. (2000). Screening and identification of older adults with alcohol problems in primary care. *Journal of Geriatric Psychiatry and Neurology*, **13**, 106–14.

National Institute on Alcohol Abuse. http://www.niaaa.nih.gov/; accessed February 27, 2005.

O'Connor, P. G. and Schottenfeld, R. S. (1998). Patients with alcohol problems. *New England Journal of Medicine*, **338**, 592–602.

Weathermon, R. and Crabb, D. W. (1999). Alcohol and medication interactions. *Alcohol Research and Health*, **23**, 40–54.

Wiese, J. G., Shlipak, M. G., and Browmer, W. (2000). The alcohol hangover. *Annals of Internal Medicine*, **132**, 897–902.

BIBLIOGRAPHY

Blow, F. C., Gillespie, B. W., Barry, K. L. *et al.* (1992). Brief screening for alcohol problems in elderly populations using the Short Michigan Alcoholism Screening Test-Geriatric Version (SMAST-G): a new elderly-specific screening instrument. *Alcoholism: Clinical and Experimental Research*, **22** (Suppl), 131A.

Brower, K. J., Aldrich, M. S., Robinson, E. A. *et al.* (2001). Insomnia, self-medication and relapse to alcoholism. *American Journal of Psychiatry*, **158**, 399–404.

Edmeads, J. (1997). Headaches in older people: how are they different in this age group? *Postgraduate Medicine*, **105**, 91–100.

Fingerhood, M. (2000). Substance abuse in older people. *Journal of the American Geriatrics Society*, **48**, 985–95.

Fink, A., Hays, R. D., Moore, A. A. *et al.* (1996). Alcohol-related problems in older persons: determinants, consequences and screening. *Archives of Internal Medicine*, **156**, 1150–6.

Mayfield, D., McLeod, G., and Hall, P. (1974). The CAGE questionnaire: validation of a new alcoholism screening instrument. *American Journal of Psychiatry*, **131**, 238–46.

Mazzaglia, G., Britton, A. R., Altman D. R. *et al.* (2001). Exploring the relationship between alcohol consumption and non-fatal or fatal stroke: a systematic review. *Addiction*, **96**, 1743–56.

Moore, A. A., Seeman, T., Morgenstern, H. *et al.* (2002). Are there differences between older persons who screen positive on the CAGE Questionnaire and the Short Michigan Alcoholism Screening Test-Geriatric version? *Journal of the American Geriatrics Society*, **50**, 858–62.

Reinert, D. F. and Allen, J. P. (2002). The Alcohol Use Disorders Identification Test (AUDIT). *Alcoholism: Clinical and Experimental Research*, **26**, 272–9.

Saper, J. R. (1999). Headache disorders. *Medical Clinics of North America*, **83**, 663–90.

Singletary, K. W. and Gapstur, S. M. (2001). Alcohol and breast cancer: review of epidemiologic and experimental evidence and potential mechanisms. *Journal of the American Medical Association*, **286**, 2143–51.

Case 28

▶▶ Pain

A 78-year-old woman complains of pain in the left lower back. The pain is burning in nature and has increased in severity over a period of 2 days. On physical examination, there is mild local tenderness but normal range of motion and no pain on straight leg raising. Lumbosacral spine films and urinalysis are ordered, and acetaminophen is prescribed.

A week later, the patient returns, complaining of a rash and disabling pain in her left side and back. The rash appeared 5 days before. Medication is given and the rash subsides after 10 days, but the pain diminishes only slightly. For the next few months, the patient is plagued by burning and lancinating pain and hyperaesthesia of the affected area. The symptoms are unrelieved by maximum doses of analgesics, including acetaminophen, ibuprofen, and acetaminophen–codeine combination (Tylenol #3).

On her latest visit to you, the patient is accompanied by her son, who worries that his mother is getting Alzheimer's disease because she has been very "mixed up" the past few days. The son explains apologetically that he had read about a "pain clinic" in the local newspaper and took his mother there "out of desperation." At the pain clinic, the patient received doxepin, which she has taken nightly for the past week.

Questions

1. How could this patient's current pain have been prevented?
2. What could be contributing to her change in mental status?
3. What treatment alternatives exist at this point?
4. What has predisposed her to the rash and the pain that followed?

Case Studies in Geriatric Medicine, Judith C. Ahronheim *et al.* Published by Cambridge University Press.
© J. C. Ahronheim, Z.-B. Huang, V. Yen, C. M. Davitt, and D. Barile

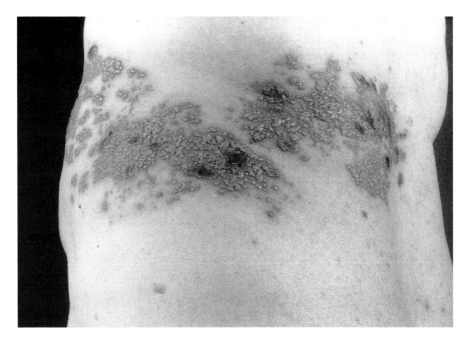

Figure 10   Vesicular rash of acute herpes zoster ("Shingles").

Answers

1. The patient has recovered from shingles – acute cutaneous herpes zoster (see Figure 10) and now has postherpetic neuralgia (PHN), which is generally defined as pain persisting for more than 1 month after the disappearance of the rash. PHN may persist for months, and is much more common in the elderly than in younger adults. Antiviral agents taken during the acute episode reduce the likelihood of PHN, and randomized controlled study has shown valacyclovir and famciclovir to be superior to acyclovir in reducing the risk and duration of PHN (see Beutner *et al.*, 1995). This is likely to be due to the increased oral bioavailability of these drugs over acyclovir. In addition, valacyclovir and famciclovir have longer half-lives than acyclovir and require less frequent dosing than acyclovir, improving adherence to the regimen.

    The benefits of antiviral therapy in promoting rapid healing and reducing the likelihood of PHN appear to require that therapy be started within 72 hours after the onset of the rash. Antiviral agents are beneficial as long as new lesions are actively being formed, but they are unlikely to help if lesions are crusted. Treatment with corticosteroids may speed healing of lesions when added to antiviral therapy, and may reduce the duration of acute pain (that lasting less than 1 month), but does not reduce the likelihood of PHN.

2. Tricyclic antidepressants (TCAs), including doxepin, are often effective in treating neuropathic pain, including PHN. However, their strong anticholinergic properties make them problematic in the elderly, and probably contributed to this patient's change in mental status. As discussed elsewhere in this volume, elderly patients are predisposed to reversible cognitive impairment when given medications with anticholinergic properties. This may be due to an age-related decrease in acetylcholine reserve, an existing mild cognitive impairment, or preclinical Alzheimer's disease, now unmasked with an anticholinergic agent.

3. Opioids, anticonvulsants, and some topical agents may be effective in the management of PHN, although head-to-head comparisons of various agents are lacking. Anticonvulsant medication such as gabapentin may be effective in reducing various forms of neuropathic pain through actions on the axon or synapse, and may be used alone or in combination with a TCA. Among the anticonvulsants, gabapentin has often been recommended because of an improved side effect profile, but it too can cause mental status changes and even urinary retention in the elderly. Moreover, gabapentin also is eliminated by the kidney and dose adjustments often need to be made.

Because nortriptyline and desipramine are less anticholinergic than other TCAs, they may be an option if a TCA is needed, but have the potential to cause the same array of side effects as other TCAs. The analgesic action of TCAs is thought to be at least partly independent of the antidepressant action, and may be related to their ability to inhibit the enzymatic degradation of enkephalin and to enhance serotonin at the synaptic cleft. These drugs may also block the sodium channels that are upregulated at the site of neuronal injury, thereby blocking the pain message as it travels to the central nervous system. Although some evidence exists to support the use of selective serotonin reuptake inhibitors (SSRIs) in other neuropathies, they are less effective than TCAs and anticonvulsants. Thus far, no studies exist evaluating their use in PHN.

Topical treatment may be a good alternative for this patient. Capsaicin topical analgesic cream provides some pain relief in patients with PHN. It is used after herpetic lesions have healed and is thought to act by depleting substance P, a mediator of pain impulses, from peripheral neurons. Topical lidocaine patches may also provide short-term pain relief without systemic absorption or adverse systemic effects.

Although not studied in controlled trials, nonpharmacologic treatment includes transcutaneous electrical nerve stimulation ("TENS"), ethyl chloride coolant spray followed by rubbing of the affected area, or injection of local anesthetics. Acupuncture and ultrasound have not been found to be effective. In intractable and prolonged cases, nerve block may be helpful.

4. The greatest risk factor for acute zoster, as well as PHN, is advanced age. It is believed that the risk of acute zoster is due to age-related declines in cell-mediated immunity, including specific cell-mediated immunity to varicella zoster virus (VZV). It has been postulated that this results in persistently elevated viral burden, producing chronic neural inflammation and damage.

Certain malignancies and other immunosuppressive states may also predispose to acute zoster, but underlying malignancies are found no more often in older adults who develop this condition than their same-age peers, making a malignancy workup unwarranted in most circumstances. Likewise, HIV infection predisposes to herpes zoster; although HIV testing might be warranted in a younger patient, it is not warranted in an elderly person without other HIV risk factors.

Risk factors for PHN are discussed in detail in the references (see Dworkin and Portenoy, 1996).

Caveat

In ophthalmic zoster, serious eye complications are a threat. An ophthalmologic consultation should be obtained immediately to diagnose and manage potentially serious manifestations such as keratitis and iridocyclitis. Long-term ophthalmologic follow up is essential, since possible late effects include glaucoma, cataracts, and blindness. One hint that suggests ophthalmic involvement is a lesion at the tip of the nose. This indicates involvement of the nasociliary nerve which also supplies the cornea.

A rare complication of ophthalmic zoster is cerebral angiitis with delayed contralateral hemiplegia. This is thought to be due to viral invasion of cerebral vessels from the contiguous cranial nerve. Despite its rarity, this complication is of interest in geriatric practice because it can be confused with thromboembolic stroke. Other neurologic complications of shingles are rare, especially in nonimmunocompromised hosts. Reported syndromes include encephalitis, myelitis, or motor neuropathy with segmental paralysis in the dermatome of the rash.

REFERENCES

Beutner, K. R., Friedman, D. J., and Forszpaniak, C. (1995). Valacyclovir compared with acyclovir for improved therapy for herpes zoster in immunocompetent adults. *Antimicrobial Agents and Chemotherapy*, **39**, 1546–53.

Dworkin, R. H. and Portenoy, R. K. (1996). Pain and its persistence in herpes zoster. *Pain*, **67**, 241–51.

BIBLIOGRAPHY

Dworkin, R. H. and Schmader, K. E. (2003). Treatment and prevention of postherpetic neuralgia. *Clinical Infectious Diseases*, **36**, 877–82.

Francis, P. T., Palmer, A. M., Snape, M. *et al.* (1999). The cholinergic hypothesis of Alzheimer's disease: a review of progress. *Journal of Neurology, Neurosurgery, and Psychiatry*, **66**, 137–47.

Freedman, G. M. and Pervemba, R. (2000). Geriatric pain. *Anesthesiology Clinics of North America*, **18**, 123–41.

Galer, B. S., Rowbotham, M. C., Perander, J. *et al.* (1999). Topical lidocaine patch relieves postherpetic neuralgia more effectively than a vehicle topical patch: results of an enriched enrollment study. *Pain*, **80**, 533–8.

Gnann, J. W. and Whitley, R. J. (2002). Herpes zoster. *New England Journal of Medicine*, **347**, 340–6.

Raja, S. N., Haythornthwaite, J. A., Pappagallo, M. *et al.* (2002). Opioid versus antidepressants in postherpetic neuralgia. *Neurology*, **59**, 1015–21.

Rowbotham, M. C., Davies, P. S., Verkempinck, C. *et al.* (1996). Lidocaine patch, double-blind controlled study of a new treatment method for postherpetic neuralgia. *Pain*, **65**, 39–44.

Watson, C. P., Tyler, K. L., and Bickers, D. R. (1993). A randomized vehicle-controlled trial of topical capsaicin in the treatment of postherpetic neuralgia. *Clinical Therapeutics*, **15**, 510–26.

Whitley, R. J., Weiss, H., and Ghann, J. W. (1996). Acyclovir with and without prednisone for the treatment of herpes zoster. *Annals of Internal Medicine*, **125**, 376–83.

Case 29

▶▶ Leg ulcer

Mr. W, an 85-year-old man with chronic venous stasis, develops a leg ulcer. He has congestive heart failure, history of a stroke with residual weakness in his left hand and leg, and history of a fractured right hand. Topical treatment and leg elevations are prescribed, but 1 month later, his ulcer is larger and there is abundant necrotic tissue, purulent discharge, and surrounding erythema. On the involved leg, and to a lesser extent the other leg, there is scaling of the skin, mild to moderate erythema, and areas of brownish discoloration. Both legs are edematous.

The patient, who lives in a single room occupancy hotel (SRO), cannot care for his ulcer adequately because of poor manual dexterity and his reluctance to transfer between chair and bed. He refuses to hire someone to give him daily care because he says he cannot afford it. You advise temporary hospitalization, noting that his insurance, Medicare, would pay most of the cost, but he refuses, fearing that his television, his most prized possession, would be stolen.

The patient has never married and has no known living relatives. However, he has lived independently for many years, shops for himself, and has not had trouble managing his finances. He does not appear depressed and answers questions appropriately.

Questions

1. Does this elderly stroke patient have the mental capacity to refuse hospitalization for this serious condition?
2. How can his ulcer be managed at home?
3. What types of dressing would be appropriate for this patient?
4. What additional management should be provided for his skin rash?
5. What adjunctive treatment should be recommended, if any?

Case Studies in Geriatric Medicine, Judith C. Ahronheim *et al.* Published by Cambridge University Press. © J. C. Ahronheim, Z.-B. Huang, V. Yen, C. M. Davitt, and D. Barile

Answers

1. Mental capacity (or, more specifically, decisional capacity) relates to a patient's general decisional abilities, such as understanding treatment information, reasoning, and appreciating consequences. Capacity is specific to the decision at hand, and to the particular patient, not to his diagnosis, and not according to a predetermined score on mental status testing. Capacity can be assessed during a discussion between the physician and the patient. If a coexisting psychiatric disorder exists that may be affecting judgment, than a consultation by an experienced psychiatrist may be necessary. Otherwise, capacity should be assessed by the physician treating the patient. This discussion should be in language the patient can readily understand, and not complicated by medical jargon.

   In determining the patient's ability to refuse hospitalization (or his ability to accept or refuse any medical intervention), the physician needs to make sure the patient understands the purpose, the risks and benefits of any treatments he would receive, the alternatives, and the outcome of his decision. Mr. W's position was that loss of his television was more important than care of his leg, a seemingly unreasonable decision to the physician. However, a patient has the right to refuse medical treatment for any reason, however "quirky" that decision may seem, as long as the decision is a "reasoned" one. If Mr. W were subject to "command hallucinations" and refused hospitalization because voices were telling him not to go, this would not be a reasoned decision.

   Patients with limited capacity (such as those with early dementia) may be able to make straightforward decisions, such as permitting (or refusing) phlebotomy or even more invasive procedures such as surgery, but may be unable to make more complex decisions, such as agreeing to or avoiding hemodialysis. In this case, the patient is refusing hospitalization. Although his decision was based on what may seem a peculiar reason to the physician, it may be entirely valid to Mr. W, and consistent with his limited resources, lifestyle, and personal value system. It may, furthermore, be based on real concerns that have grown out of his prior experiences. If the patient refused hospitalization because he was sufficiently depressed or had another psychiatric illness that impaired his judgment, it would be essential to obtain consultation from an experienced psychiatrist to assess his capacity carefully, and to treat any reversible cause of cognitive impairment that would present an obstacle to appropriate treatment of his medical condition.

   Determination of capacity, a clinical judgment, differs from a competency determination, which is a legal decision made in a court of law, albeit with medical or psychiatric testimony. Legally, Mr. W is presumed to be competent, and, if he also has the capacity to decide about hospitalization, no one other than himself is legally authorized to make this decision.

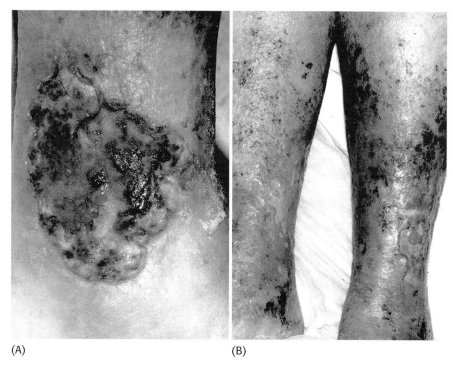

(A)   (B)

Figure 11   A. A typical venous stasis ulcer over the medial malleolus. B. The patient's legs showing chronic stasis changes and stasis dermatitis.

Even if Mr. W were found to lack decisional capacity and could not give informed *consent* to hospitalization – e.g. if he had significant dementia – it would still be important to obtain his *assent* – that is, willingness to undergo treatment – because use of physical force would be inappropriate. Thus, as a practical matter, his refusal to go to the hospital requires a humane and pragmatic approach rather than a legalistic one, such as a court hearing. Health care decisions made by others ("surrogates") are discussed in Case 7.

2. Innovative approaches will be needed to augment whatever home-based care would be available to him through government entitlements or any available personal funds. A visiting nurse will be essential for assisting with dressing changes and monitoring disease, which will be partly paid for by Medicare (see Case 5), as would home visits by the physician.

Although numerous causes of leg ulcers exist (see Sarkar and Ballantyne, 2000), this patient has a typical venous stasis ulcer (see Figure 11A). Strict attention must be given to reducing edema. Diuretics are needed and medications that can worsen edema (such as calcium channel blockers) should be avoided. Leg elevation and compression stockings are first-line treatment for edema of venous insufficiency, if the patient can adhere to these measures. Compression stockings are highly effective but, very difficult to put on. Assistive appliances are available, but given the patient's poor manual dexterity, would not be sufficient. Mr. W is unlikely to stand for prolonged periods, but when sitting or recumbent should rest the feet high enough to ensure venous return – namely, at a level above the right atrium. At other times, he should exercise the leg muscles to stimulate the venous pump. Although the value of exercise in reducing venous pressure in venous insufficiency is uncertain, activity should be encouraged for its potential ability to prevent venous thrombosis, especially in a high-risk patient like Mr. W.

Mr. W's ulcer has pierced the dermal layer and penetrated into subcutaneous fat (stage III). The wound should be carefully examined for lateral tunneling below intact skin. Necrotic tissue, if present, should be debrided with a scalpel to rule out pockets of purulent tissue or extension of the ulcer through the fascia to muscle or bone (stage IV). Mr. W might agree to visit a physician's office for this. Wet-to-dry dressings are effective in debriding small areas of necrotic tissue and can help to prevent development of new necrotic areas. Chemical or enzymatic debriding agents are not as efficient as sharp debridement, but are useful for patients who refuse or cannot tolerate sharp debridement.

Mr. W finally agreed to hospitalization where he received intravenous antibiotics, treatment of heart failure, and mechanical debridement of his ulcer. Unfortunately, when he returned home, he found that his television had been stolen.

3. Many types of dressings exist. Although nonadherent gauze (Telfa and others) may be effective for stage II ulcers, which involve epidermal disruption, moist or occlusive dressings are preferred for deeper ulcers because they prevent drying of the wound. Wound fluid has intrinsic healing capabilities, containing enzymes produced by white blood cells and bacteria, which digest necrotic tissue and fight infection. Occlusive dressings, like the roof of a blister, keep the wound moist. Commercially available hydrocolloid dressings (DuoDerm and others) form a gel as the wound heals, allow granulation to occur, and, when removed, do not damage new epithelium. Unless there is significant infection or excessive oozing, the dressing can be kept on for days, reducing nursing time, and are ideal for patients who cannot perform wound care themselves. In the early stages of treating an ulcer in an edematous leg, oozing may require more frequent dressing changes. Alginate dressings (complex polysaccharides) have high absorbency properties and may circumvent this problem to a certain extent. A wet-to-wet dressing composed of gauze that has been soaked in saline is also effective, but this approach would require diligent care and manual dexterity.

An external compression dressing should be applied over the primary dressing if possible because this pressure facilitates healing of venous stasis ulcers. However, high compression dressings require adequate arterial circulation, which should be assessed if arterial as well as venous insufficiency is suspected.

A useful alternative for patients like Mr. W, who cannot perform self-care, is an Unna boot, which is a roll bandage impregnated with zinc oxide, calamine lotion, glycerine, and gelatine. It is molded to the leg and kept on for a week. This method keeps the wound clean and promotes drying, and has an added advantage of external compression, which can reduce edema if applied correctly.

Dressings and other approaches to ulcer management are reviewed in detail in the references (see Thomas, 2001; DeAraujo *et al.*, 2003).

4. The patient's skin rash suggest chronic stasis dermatitis (see Figure 11B). Venous stasis alone produces extravasation of blood with petechiae. In longstanding cases, fibrosis, nonpitting edema, and hyperpigmentation from hemosiderin deposition occur. Stasis dermatitis with erythema, scaling, and edema can be superimposed, and can resemble or be complicated by cellulitis. In the absence of cellulitis, this can be treated with topical corticosteroids. Caution should be used when applying corticosteroids in the vicinity of the ulcer because direct application would impair wound healing.

Cellulitis frequently accompanies skin ulcers, especially those that have been neglected. Cellulitis should be treated with systemic antibiotics that cover *Streptococcus* or *Staphylococcus* species. Swabbing the wound for culture is generally not revealing, since skin ulcers are "dirty wounds" that are colonized by many species of bacteria.

5. Although nutrition is an important factor in wound healing and specific vitamins, amino acids, and protein promoted as supplements, no evidence exists that routine supplementation speeds healing. Vitamin C deficiency may impair wound healing, but research has not proven that vitamin C accelerates healing in patients who do not have deficiency of that vitamin. Likewise, zinc is commonly prescribed; pharmacologic doses of zinc improve immune function in vitro, but, in the absence of deficiency, this does not speed healing of skin ulcers. Furthermore, zinc supplementation can cause gastrointestinal symptoms and copper deficiency. It is difficult to diagnose zinc deficiency accurately because is a trace element; however, Mr. W is theoretically at risk because of his use of potassium-losing diuretics, which can increase renal loss of zinc. The recommended daily allowance of zinc is no more than 8 mg per day, but zinc sulfate supplements typically contain approximately 100 mg of elemental zinc and are probably not needed.

Topical use of zinc oxide has been shown to inhibit bacterial growth and is a frequent ingredient in protective skin moisture barriers. Topical zinc is unlikely to cause systemic problems.

Topical antibiotics, such as neomycin and bacitracin, may sensitize the skin and lead to contact dermatitis; this is especially common in patients with stasis dermatitis. Skin sensitization is less common with other agents, such as silver sulfasalazine. Overall, however, debate exists over whether topical antibiotics accelerate wound healing, and concerns have been raised about the development of antimicrobial-resistant strains of bacteria, especially with agents such as neomycin and bacitracin. Antiseptic agents may be more effective than topical antibiotics but they are also more irritating and can damage normal skin.

Systemic antibiotics should be reserved for wounds complicated by cellulitis or systemic infection.

Caveat

A feature that distinguishes a venous stasis ulcer from an arterial ulcer is the location. Venous ulcers occur in the malleolar area, usually on the medial aspect, but not involving the malleolus itself. Arterial ulcers tend to occur more distally, on the heel, the toes, or on bony prominences, such as the malleolus. Venous ulcers are usually accompanied by other signs of chronic stasis. However, arterial insufficiency commonly coexists in elderly patients with venous insufficiency and should be suspected in patients with a history of atherosclerotic disease, diabetes, or cigarette smoking, as this may modify management.

REFERENCES

DeAraujo, T., Valencia, I., Federman, D. G. *et al.* (2003). Managing the patient with venous ulcers. *Annals of Internal Medicine*, **138**, 326–34.

Sarkar, P. K. and Ballantyne, S. (2000). Management of leg ulcers. *Postgraduate Medical Journal*, **76**, 674–82.

Thomas, D. R. (2001). Issues and dilemmas in the prevention and treatment of pressure ulcers: a review. *Journal of Gerontology, Medical Sciences*, **56A**, M328–40.

BIBLIOGRAPHY

Ahronheim, J. C., Moreno, J. D., and Zuckerman, C. (2000). *Ethics in Clinical Practice*, 2nd edn. Gaithersburg, MD: Aspen Publishers, Inc., pp. 17–50.

Clark, J. J. (2002). Wound repair and factors influencing healing. *Critical Care Nursing Quarterly*, **25**, 1–12.

Cullum, N. and Fletcher, A. W. (1999). Compression bandages and stockings in the treatment of venous leg ulcers. *Cochrane Library*, **1**, 1–10.

Houston, S., Haggard, J., Williford, J. *et al.* (2001). Adverse effects of large-dose zinc supplementation in an institutionalized older population with pressure ulcers. *Journal of the American Geriatrics Society*, **49**, 1130.

Kim, S., Karlawish, J. H. T., and Caine, E. D. (2002). Current state of research on decision-making competence of cognitively impaired elderly persons. *American Journal of Geriatric Psychiatry*, **10**, 151–65.

Spann, C. T., Tutrone, W. D., Weinberg, J. M. *et al.* (2000). Topic antibacterial agents for wound care: a primer. *Dermatologic Surgery*, **29**, 620–6.

Sugarman, J., McCrory, D. C., and Hubal, R. C. (1998). Getting meaningful informed consent from older adults: a structured review of the literature. *Journal of the American Geriatric Society*, **46**, 517–24.

Thomas, D. R. (1997). Specific nutritional factors in wound healing. *Advances in Wound Care*, **10**, 40–3.

Werteim, D., Melhuish, J., and Williams, R. (1999). Measurement of forces associated with compression therapy. *Medical and Biological Engineering and Computing*, **37**, 31–4.

Wilkinson, E. A. and Hawke, C. I. (1998). Does oral zinc aid the healing of chronic leg ulcers? A systematic literature review. *Archives of Dermatology*, **134**, 1556–60.

Case 30

▸▸ Chronic cough

An 87-year-old widower, who was living alone in a studio apartment of a senior housing development, complained of a cough productive of scant amounts of grayish sputum for several weeks. He had no fevers, sweats, or other constitutional symptoms. On physical examination, he appeared vigorous and was not coughing. Temperature was 98 °F. Auscultation of the lungs revealed scattered rhonchi, which cleared on coughing. He was a nonsmoker and denied a history of lung disease or exposure to tuberculosis.

Chest X-ray was done and an infiltrate was seen. Sputum culture was sent and a 10-day course of clarithromycin was instituted. The cultures were negative and the patient went about his normal business. Six months later, he reappeared at the doctor's office complaining of persistent coughing, again without constitutional symptoms. Physical examination was unchanged and the infiltrate was again demonstrated on chest X-ray. The patient now revealed that, "after thinking about it," he remembered that 70 years before his college roommate had been forced to leave school because of "consumption."

Except for excision of a melanoma 2 years ago, and a remote history of duodenal ulcer, the patient has been otherwise well. He was widowed over 1 year before the onset of his cough, but has been socially active and in relatively good spirits.

Questions

1. What further tests are required?
2. Of what diagnostic significance is the chest X-ray?
3. What risk factors have contributed to the patient's problem?
4. What preventive measure should be implemented within the patient's housing complex?

Case Studies in Geriatric Medicine, Judith C. Ahronheim *et al.* Published by Cambridge University Press.
© J. C. Ahronheim, Z.-B. Huang, V. Yen, C. M. Davitt, and D. Barile

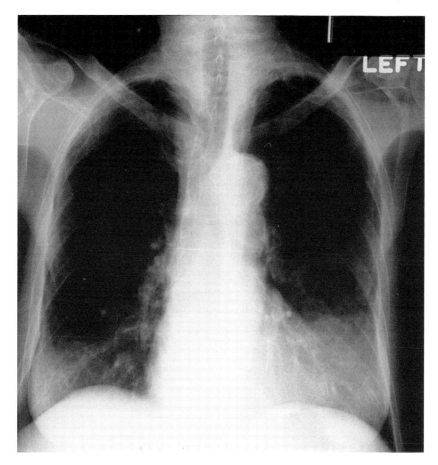

Figure 12   The patient's chest X-ray showing an infiltrate in the lingula.

Answers

1. This patient has an unresolving infiltrate of the lingula (see Figure 12) and a chronic cough, making tuberculosis (TB) a strong consideration. Expectorated sputum should be sent for cytologic and microbiologic evaluation for bacteria, fungi, and acid-fast bacillus (AFB). Although the patient does not have constitutional symptoms or weight loss, and is a nonsmoker, a lung malignancy should also be considered, as lung cancer increases with age, cancer and other serious comorbidities increase risk of TB, and this patient has a history of melanoma. Flexible bronchoscopy, which is tolerated in the elderly, should be strongly considered if expectorated sputum stain does not reveal AFB. AFB cultures obtained by fiberoptic bronchoscopy are more likely to be positive than expectorated sputum. Fiberoptic bronchoscopy also has a high yield for identifying endobronchial

obstructing lesions and would be appropriate – perhaps in addition to a chest computed tomography scan – to assist in ruling out carcinoma.

Although safe and simple, and useful in TB surveillance, skin testing to diagnose TB is controversial, especially when there is strong clinical suspicion of active TB. The negative predictive value of the test (the likelihood that a negative test indicates no infection) is very low in this setting and may divert attention from definitive microbiologic testing. Moreover, because skin test anergy is common in late life, the likelihood of negative skin test in active TB rises with age. An additional problem is that the disease itself can cause anergy, and even specific anergy to tuberculin, perhaps because of saturation of T-cell receptors by disease-associated antigen, or because of T-cell sequestration. Skin testing would be more useful in this case if it were known to be negative at baseline. The booster phenomenon (skin test positivity upon retesting 1–3 weeks after a negative test) is more common in the elderly than the young, possibly because of a higher incidence of remote TB infection or exposure, or remote exposure to nonpathogenic atypical mycobacteria. Skin test positivity wanes with time after exposure to *Mycobacterium tuberculosis*, as the population of memory CD4 T cells declines. This population can be augmented with exposure to tuberculin during skin testing, and subsequent exposure by repeated skin testing will "boost" the response. Elderly patients undergoing skin testing whose initial test is negative should be retested after 2–3 weeks. Skin test positivity is sometimes delayed for as long as 1 week after the first skin test is placed. This phenomenon is also more common in older as compared with younger adults.

In this patient, the smear obtained from expectorated sputum was positive for AFB.

2. The patient's isolated lingular infiltrate is a "classic" finding in primary TB. This, at first, seems surprising because his history of remote exposure suggests reactivation TB, and because of the belief that the majority of elderly with TB have reactivation disease, in which the lingular infiltrate would be seen as an extension of upper lobe disease. However, primary as well as postprimary pulmonary TB may present without these classic radiographic features, especially in the elderly, who are less likely to have cavitary or apical lesions and more likely to have mid and basal zone lesions (see Morris, 1989). These findings are similar to those seen in patients with profoundly decreased cell-mediated immunity, such as patients with HIV infection.

The differentiation of primary from postprimary TB, if reliable, could help to guide TB surveillance in the housing complex, but would not change the patient's therapy, nor would it eliminate the need for careful surveillance.

The breast shadows seen on the patient's X-ray represent gynecomastia. This had been noted on his physical examination, and is a finding that increases in incidence with age in men. It is unrelated to his present disease.

3. Among all ethnic groups and both sexes, TB is much more common in the elderly population as a whole than in younger age groups. However, there is no evidence

that age alone is an independent risk factor for TB. This age-associated risk might be related to comorbidities impacting on immunologic function, such as diabetes, chronic obstructive pulmonary disease, cardiovascular disease, renal insufficiency, cancer, or even gastrectomy, which was a more common treatment for peptic ulcer in the past than today. The mechanism is speculative and may be related to a "dumping syndrome," which would result in malnutrition and impaired immune function. Additionally, age itself brings with it a decline in T-cell function and perhaps other defects in cellular immunity that would otherwise sequester the organism after TB exposure. In this way, the present patient would be theoretically at risk of either primary or reactivation disease. Our patient has a history of melanoma excision, and it would be important to consider recurrent tumor, especially if no other recent exposure history were found. He denied a history of surgery for peptic ulcer.

The incidence of TB is particularly high in nursing homes. Although there are no specific data about senior housing, the patient's likelihood of exposure in a closed senior community might be higher than in the community at large.

The issue of emotional stress has been raised as a precipitant of a variety of diseases. In late life, stress often comes as a result of losses, such as death of a spouse or loss of employment. There is evidence that the hypothalamic–pituitary–adrenal axis and the sympathetic nervous system play a role in the depression of T-helper cells, which are important in controlling infection. Bereavement has been associated with excess mortality from a number of diseases, including TB, alcoholism, heart disease, and others. Men are at greater risk of mortality following loss and bereavement than are women.

4. Regardless of whether the patient had primary or postprimary disease, interviews, skin testing, and chest X-rays of the patient's contacts should be conducted. If TB skin testing had been required of new residents and employees in the housing complex, retesting at this time would facilitate discovery of the index case if the patient had primary TB, and would identify his contacts at risk for primary disease if he had reactivation TB.

Caveat

TB often presents "atypically" in the elderly, either as "failure to thrive" or as an apparently mild disease without fever or other constitutional symptoms. TB is more likely to be missed in late life when its "protean manifestations" (such as mental status changes, weight loss, or respiratory symptoms) are mistaken for comorbidities of late life. TB is often not diagnosed until autopsy. In one study, the proportion of TB cases diagnosed at death increased with age from 2% in adults 25–34 years of age to 18.6% in people aged 85 years of age and older; 60.3% of cases not diagnosed until death were in people aged 65 years and older (Reider *et al.*, 1991).

REFERENCES

Morris, C. D. W. (1989). The radiography, hematology and biochemistry of pulmonary tuberculosis in the aged. *Quarterly Journal of Medicine*, **71**, 529–35.

Reider, H. L., Kelly, G. D., Block, A. B. *et al.* (1991). Tuberculosis diagnosed at death in the United States. *Chest*, **100**, 678–81.

BIBLIOGRAPHY

American Thoracic Society (1981). The tuberculin skin test. *American Review of Respiratory Diseases*, **124**, 356–63.

(2000). Diagnostic standards and classification of tuberculosis in adults and children. *American Journal of Respiratory and Critical Care Medicine*, **161**, 1376–95.

Biondi, M. and Picardi, A. (1996). The clinical and biological aspects of bereavement and loss-induced depression: a reappraisal. *Psychotherapy and Psychosomatics*, **64**, 229–45.

Bobrowitz, I. D. (1982). Active tuberculosis undiagnosed until autopsy. *American Journal of Medicine*, **72**, 650–8.

Delafuente, J. C., Mueleman, J. R., and Nelson, R. C. (1988). Anergy testing in nursing home residents. *Journal of the American Geriatrics Society*, **36**, 733–5.

Knox, A. J., Mascie-Taylor, B. H., and Page, R. L. (1988). Fiberoptic bronchoscopy in the elderly: four years' experience. *British Journal of Diseases of the Chest*, **82**, 290–3.

Liaw, Y. S., Yang, P. C., Yu, C. J. *et al.* (1995). Clinical spectrum of tuberculosis in older patients. *Journal of the American Geriatrics Society*, **43**, 256–60.

Marrie, T. J., Johnson, S., and Durant, H. (1988). Cell-mediated immunity of healthy adult Nova Scotians in various age groups compared with nursing home and hospitalized senior citizens. *Journal of Allergy and Clinical Immunology*, **81**, 836–43.

Patel, Y. R., Mehta, J. B., and Harvill, L. (1993). Flexible bronchoscopy as a diagnostic tool in the evaluation of pulmonary tuberculosis in an elderly population. *Journal of the American Geriatrics Society*, **41**, 629–32.

Perez-Guzman, C., Vargas, M. H., and Torres-Cruz, A. (1999). Does aging modify pulmonary tuberculosis? *Chest*, **116**, 961–7.

Pitchenik, A. E. and Robinson, H. A. (1985). The radiographic appearance of tuberculosis in patients with AIDS and pre-AIDS. *American Review of Respiratory Disease*, **131**, 393–6.

Slovis, B. S., Plitman, J. D., and Haas, D. W. (2002). The case against anergy testing as a routine adjunct to tuberculin skin testing. *Journal of the American Medical Association*, **283**, 2003–7.

Slutkin, G., Perez-Stable, E. J., and Hopewell, P. C. (1986). Time course and boosting of tuberculin reactions in nursing home residents. *American Review of Respiratory Disease*, **134**, 1048–51.

Snider, D. E. (1995). Tuberculosis and gastrectomy. *Chest*, **87**, 414–15.

Stead, W. W., Lofgren, J. P., Warren, E. *et al.* (1985). Tuberculosis as an endemic and nosocomial infection among the elderly in nursing homes. *New England Journal of Medicine*, **312**, 1483–7.

Case 31

▸▸ Diarrhea

An 84-year-old woman has resided in a nursing home for 2 years. She has a history of thrombotic stroke, myocardial infarction, and memory loss, and is wheelchair bound. She develops watery diarrhea and you are called to evaluate her. She has no complaint of nausea, vomiting, or abdominal pain; there are no other cases of diarrhea on her floor. The patient had been briefly admitted to a nearby hospital a few week ago, where she was treated for fecal impaction. She now has "PRN" orders for a stool softener, senna, milk of magnesia, and acetaminophen.

On physical examination, the patient is lying in bed and slightly lethargic, but, when you ask her how she feels, she says, "Oh, not so bad." Her blood pressure is 100/60, heart rate 102 and regular, and temperature is 98 °F. Examination of her lungs reveals coarse crepitations at both bases, which were present on admission 2 years ago. The abdomen is somewhat distended and there is mild, nonlocalized tenderness without rebound. Bowel sounds are decreased. There are no surgical scars. Rectal examination reveals no masses. Stool is brown and positive for occult blood. The remainder of the physical examination is normal. According to the chart, her usual systolic blood pressure has been 110–130, and the lung findings have been present since her admission 1 year ago.

You send blood and stool samples to the laboratory and start intravenous fluid.

Question

What is the differential diagnosis?

Case Studies in Geriatric Medicine, Judith C. Ahronheim *et al.* Published by Cambridge University Press.
© J. C. Ahronheim, Z.-B. Huang, V. Yen, C. M. Davitt, and D. Barile

Answer

New-onset diarrhea in this frail, elderly nursing home patient could be due to many things. Overtreatment with laxatives commonly causes diarrhea, and should be considered in this patient. Fecal impaction sometimes presents with diarrhea as loose stool is expelled around the impaction, and is frequently misdiagnosed and treated incorrectly with antidiarrheal agents, worsening the problem. Failure to detect stool in the rectum does not rule out a high impaction. Fecal impaction is an important consideration in bed-bound or wheelchair-bound patients, especially one with a known history of this problem. However, the presence of occult blood in the stool raises the suspicion of more invasive causes, such as infectious diarrhea, diverticulitis, inflammatory bowel disease, or ischemic colitis. It is also possible that more than one disease exists in an old, frail patient, and there could be coincidental pathology, such as colorectal cancer.

The absence of fever does not rule out an infectious etiology, and the patient's physician originally considered viral gastroenteritis. Infection with *Clostridium difficile* should also be considered, however. *C. difficile* can be transmitted through environmental contamination, is the most common cause of hospital-acquired diarrhea, and should always be considered in a nursing home patient, especially one who was recently hospitalized, because a history of antibiotic treatment is frequently not communicated in cursory notes that accompany patients when they are transferred back to the nursing home. Other toxigenic bacteria, such as *Escherichia coli, Staphylococcus aureus,* and *Salmonella* are usually related to contaminated food. *E. coli* 0157:H7 can cause particularly severe illness and is associated with high morbidity and mortality among frail elderly. These agents, as well as viral etiologies, are less likely in this patient because no other residents are ill. However, there is evidence that *S. aureus* can cause antibiotic-associated colitis, and, although a cause and effect relationship has not been proved, there is a strong association of this organism among elderly patients with antibiotic-associated diarrhea (see Gravet, 1999).

Inflammatory bowel disease is another consideration. Although generally considered a disease that presents in younger adults, late-onset disease does occur and a bimodal distribution has been described in some, though not all, series (see Robertson *et al.,* 2001). Because of the patient's advanced age and atherosclerotic disease affecting other systems, ischemic colitis should be considered. Diverticulitis, likewise, is a possibility and is very common in elderly patients.

After 3 hours, the laboratory calls to report that the white blood cell count (WBC) was 35 800 with 91% neutrophils.

Questions

1. What should marked leukocytosis prompt you to do?
2. Explain the patient's early presentation.
3. What is the relationship between the diarrhea and her current problem?

Answers

1. The marked increase in WBC in an occult blood-positive diarrhea requires an immediate re-evaluation. On re-examination, she is more lethargic. Her abdomen is firm but not markedly tender; there is no rebound, but bowel sounds are markedly diminished. In addition to worsening infection from extrinsic infection or diverticulitis, intestinal ischemia with bowel infarction become strong possibilities. The patient should be sent to the hospital for appropriate investigations.

   In the emergency room, the patient was found to have board-like rigidity of the abdomen and absent bowel sounds. She underwent emergency laparotomy and was found to have extensive infarction of the small intestine with gangrene and the diseased portion was excised. A few hours later, her abdominal signs again deteriorated and repeat laparotomy was performed, but bowel infarction had extended and the patient expired.

   Although intestinal ischemia is often reversible or runs an indolent course, this patient's course was fulminant and there was little time for investigation. Earlier, given the broad differential diagnosis, the choice of imaging studies would have depended on practical considerations, such as the ready availability of specific studies for a nursing home patient and her ability to tolerate certain procedures or a series of them. Plain abdominal films and abdominal computed tomography (CT) scans are often nonspecific but may be helpful in ruling out other causes of acute abdominal pain. CT scans are often normal in early colonic ischemia as well as in established ischemic colitis. The most common findings are nonspecific, and include circumferential wall thickening in the involved segments secondary to edema or hemorrhage. However, CT scanning is a useful method of detecting mesenteric vein thrombosis, which can produce ischemic syndromes of the gut. Colonoscopy can help to establish the diagnosis of ischemic colitis, grade its severity, and follow the course, and can help to distinguish it from other diseases of the colon. Barium enema, which is rarely used today for this purpose, commonly reveals "thumbprinting" due to submucosal edema and hemorrhage.

Colonoscopy or barium enema, which might have detected this patient's condition early on, would have been risky as she deteriorated because distension can further diminish intestinal blood flow. Angiography, which is a useful diagnostic test in mesenteric ischemia, cannot be justified when surgical delay would be disastrous. This patient's outcome reflects the high mortality rate of bowel infarction, which ranges from 59% to 93% in published series (see Brandt *et al.*, 2000). This is likely to be related not only to the seriousness of the disease, but to patient-associated factors including atherosclerotic disease in other organs, advanced age, comorbidities, and factors leading to the bowel infarction.

2. Minimal symptoms in the face of serious, acute abdominal pathology are not unusual in elderly patients, particularly those who are neurologically impaired. This nonspecific presentation initially led the physician to consider uncomplicated gastroenteritis, although it was also consistent with mild, reversible colonic ischemia, a diagnosis which is frequently not considered. Her mild tachycardia and slightly reduced blood pressure could have been explained by dehydration, but occult blood-positive stool and lethargy suggested a more serious etiology. Leukocytosis with left shift and deteriorating abdominal signs denoted a possible abdominal catastrophe, triggering an immediate intensive workup. A high index of suspicion is critical for an early diagnosis, which helps to improve outcome significantly.

   Subtle presentations of serious illness in the elderly have been attributed to an inability to express pain and impaired perceptions of pain, but the latter mechanism has never been confirmed (see Cases 15 and 39). Likewise, absence of fever is not unusual, even in the setting of leukocytosis and serious infection. Alterations in immune response decrease the production of endogenous pyrogens, and abnormalities in thermoregulation have also been proposed as causes of attenuated fever in the elderly (see Case 41). In addition, oral temperature measurement may be particularly unreliable in impaired or debilitated elderly if they fail to cooperate, or in the presence of mouth breathing.

3. It is possible that this patient's diarrhea represented an acute, early manifestation of a fulminant process. The mesenteric circulation is complex, but, most frequently, the superior mesenteric artery (SMA) supplies the small intestine and the proximal colon. This patient, who had evidence of atherosclerosis in other organs, may have had ischemic colitis due to arterial narrowing or ruptured plaque of the SMA, followed by in situ thrombosis, which extended and led to extensive bowel infarction. Likewise, she may have had nonocclusive disease due to a "low-flow" state seen in severe congestive heart failure or hypotensive states. However, intestinal ischemia comprises numerous syndromes, and some are often not recognized, including chronic ischemic colitis, which may be remitting and relapsing. Chronic

mesenteric ischemia may be asymptomatic, may present with postprandial pain and constipation, or symptoms might be unrecognized in a patient who cannot communicate. Ischemic colitis could have been missed in this patient who has previously had bowel problems. Syndromes of intestinal ischemia are discussed in the references (see Greenwald *et al.*, 2001).

Caveats

1. Although a bimodal distribution of inflammatory colitis (notably, inflammatory bowel disease and Crohn's colitis) has been disputed, two atypical forms – collagenous colitis and lymphocytic colitis – almost always present at midlife or later. The onset is usually insidious and diarrhea is watery rather than bloody; the course is generally benign, but can be prolonged or chronic.
2. Mesenteric vein thrombosis can cause intestinal ischemic syndromes. Although an unusual cause, it should be considered, especially if there is a reason to suspect hypercoagulable syndromes. Despite its low sensitivity in diagnosing intestinal ischemia per se, CT scanning is a sensitive method of detecting mesenteric venous thrombosis.

REFERENCES

Brandt, L. J. and Boley, S. J. (2000). AGA technical review on intestinal ischemia. *Gastroenterology*, **118**, 954–68.

Gravet, A. (1999). Predominant *Staphylococcus aureus* isolated from antibiotic-associated diarrhea is clinically relevant and produces enterotoxin A and biocomponent toxin LukE-lukD. *Journal of Clinical Microbiology*, **37**, 4012–19.

Greenwald, D. A., Brandt, L. J., and Reinus, J. F. (2001). Ischemic bowel disease in the elderly. *Gastroenterology Clinics*, **30**, 445–73.

Robertson, D. J. and Grimm, I. S. (2001). Inflammatory bowel disease in the elderly. *Gastroenterology Clinics*, **30**, 409–26.

BIBLIOGRAPHY

Barbut, F. and Petit, J. C. (2001). Epidemiology of *Clostridium difficile*-associated infections. *Clinical Microbiology and Infection*, **7**, 405–10.

Carter, A. O., Borczyk, A. A., Carlson, J. A. *et al.* (1987). A severe outbreak of *Escherichia coli* 0157:H7-associated hemorrhagic colitis in a nursing home. *New England Journal of Medicine*, **317**, 1496–500.

Finucane, P. M., Arunachalam, T., O'Dowd, J. *et al.* (1989). Acute mesenteric infarction in elderly patients. *Journal of the American Geriatrics Society*, **37**, 355–8.

Jarvinen, O., Laurikka, J., Sisto, T. *et al.* (1995). Atherosclerosis of the visceral arteries. *Vasa*, **24**, 9–14.

Kumar, S., Sarr, M. G., and Kamath, P. S. (2001). Mesenteric venous thrombosis. *New England Journal of Medicine*, **345**, 1683–8.

Case 32

▶▶ Upper gastrointestinal bleeding

A 78-year-old woman is brought to the hospital by her neighbor because of generalized weakness and inability to walk. She states that she had felt increasing fatigue and was occasionally dizzy for about 1 week. She recently had experienced nausea but no abdominal pain. She denies chest pain, shortness of breath, palpitations, diarrhea, or black stools.

She is a nonsmoker and does not drink alcoholic beverages. She denies the use of aspirin and arthritis pills.

Her physical examination reveals orthostatic hypotension, mild epigastric tenderness, and positive occult stool test. Her hemoglobin is 8 gm/dl and hematocrit 25%. Other routine admission labs are within normal limits. Esophogastric endoscopy reveals erosive hemorrhagic gastritis. A biopsy is performed.

Questions

1. What factors have led to this patient's bleeding?
2. Why did this patient not have pain?
3. How should the gastritis be managed?
4. How should her medical problems be managed in the future?

Answers

1. Although it is possible that the patient has *Helicobacter pylori*-associated disease, the most common cause of hemorrhagic gastritis in the elderly is medication, notably aspirin and antiarthritis preparations. Thus, a more probing history of medication

Case Studies in Geriatric Medicine, Judith C. Ahronheim *et al.* Published by Cambridge University Press.
© J. C. Ahronheim, Z.-B. Huang, V. Yen, C. M. Davitt, and D. Barile

use is called for. A review of systems indicated that the patient suffered from knee arthritis for which she took medications which she could not name, but, she indicated, 2 months ago she saw her doctor, who wrote a prescription for "new arthritis medication." She never filled the prescription because it was "too expensive." The patient's daughter was asked to bring in the patient's medications, which included acetaminophen, acetaminophen with codeine, and the unfilled prescription for Celebrex (celocoxib). When asked about over-the-counter medications, it was revealed that the daughter, who suffers from low back pain, takes a nonprescription preparation of naproxen (Aleve) and recommended this to her mother, who has been taking it for several weeks. When asked how it made her feel, she admitted it made her "sick at the stomach," so she took Alka-Seltzer, which contains not only antacid but also 325 mg aspirin per tablet. This made her feel worse, so she purchased Alka-Seltzer Extra Strength, which contains 500 mg aspirin per tablet.

This case, like Cases 19, 21, and others, illustrates the importance of a detailed medication history. Many patients do not consider over-the-counter agents to be medications, since they are available without prescription. Likewise, patients may not be aware that aspirin or other potentially problematic agents are ingredients in their favorite brand-name remedies. In addition to asking specifically about any active agent, it is important to ask about topical and transdermal agents, injectables, vitamins, and herbal supplements (see Case 21). Naproxen is one of the nonsteroidal anti-inflammatory agents (NSAIDs) available without prescription. As weak organic acids, NSAIDs can diffuse into epithelial cells in the low pH environment of the stomach, causing ionization and rapid destruction of the epithelium. More importantly, NSAIDs systemically inhibit production of cyclooxygenase and eventually of prostaglandin E2 (PGE2). Depletion of PGE2 compromises the barrier function of mucosa and thus facilitates the penetration of acid and pepsin to the submucosa, resulting in injury. The variety of gastric pathology, which includes mucosal erythema, erosive or diffuse gastritis, and gastric ulcer, has been termed "NSAID gastropathy." NSAIDs produce gastric more often than duodenal lesions, but NSAID users have a 2–4-fold greater risk of duodenal ulcer than the general population. Other gastrointestinal lesions produced by NSAIDs include pill esophagitis, esophageal or small bowel ulceration, and exacerbation of inflammatory bowel disease.

Prostaglandins also play an important role in the inhibition of gastric acid secretion. By reducing endogenous prostaglandins, NSAIDs can cause hyperacidity and facilitate NSAID-induced injury. The interference of NSAIDs with platelet aggregation also contributes to the risk of bleeding. This problem is greater with aspirin, which irreversibly inhibits cyclooxygenase and impairs platelet function for its life span. Aspirin can also produce gastric erosions via a direct effect on the mucosa.

The greatest risk factor for NSAID gastropathy is advanced age, probably because of underlying atrophic gastritis, making the gastric mucosa vulnerable to NSAID-induced damage. In addition, age-related pharmacokinetic changes can slow the elimination of many NSAIDs. Casual use of NSAIDs tends to be well tolerated, but regular use is associated with an increased risk of gastropathy and bleeding. This patient was taking over-the-counter naproxen (Aleve) 200 mg three times a day (her daughter's dose). Unlike the widely available over-the-counter ibuprofen (Advil, Motrin, and others), which has a half-life of only 2–3 hours, the average half-life of naproxen is 14 hours, and even longer in older individuals. This long half-life makes infrequent dosing practical, but also increases the likelihood of toxicity. In addition, naproxen is a more potent (though reversible) inhibitor of platelet function than ibuprofen, and, like other nonacetylated NSAIDs, the duration of antiplatelet activity is correlated with presence of drug in the serum. Higher doses of NSAIDs confer additional risk; although this patient was taking a low dose (for a nonelderly person) of naproxen sodium, prolonged half-life may have resulted in accumulation. Likewise, age-associated changes in the gastric mucosa probably enhanced the pharmacodynamic effect of the drug.

Use of aspirin, even in small doses, is associated with an increased risk of NSAID gastropathy, especially ulcer. Other risk factors for bleeding include a past history of ulcer, concurrent use of corticosteroids, anticoagulants, or other NSAIDs, as well as alcohol use, cigarette smoking, and concurrent serious illness.

One recent meta-analysis suggested that *H. pylori* infection and NSAIDs act synergistically in the development of peptic ulcer and ulcer bleeding (Huang *et al.*, 2002). This patient's biopsy for *H. pylori* was negative. However, some evidence suggests that elderly patients are more likely to have a falsely negative biopsy for *H. pylori*, requiring carefully localized and sometimes repeated biopsies, in conjunction with other diagnostic testing for diagnosis (see Pilotto and Malfertheiner, 2002). Thus, even if patients have been taking NSAIDs, it is important carefully to rule out *H. pylori* infection.

2. Elderly patients with NSAID-associated gastric or duodenal damage are often asymptomatic until upper gastrointestinal bleeding or perforation occurs. The uncommon occurrence of dyspeptic symptoms has been attributed to blunted pain perception, analgesic effect of NSAIDs, or both, but these explanations are speculative, and, in fact, younger adults with peptic ulcer also sometimes present with painless bleeding. Bleeding may be gradual, intermittent, and insidious, only detected by chemical testing. Even overt bleeding may not be recognized if the patient is unaware that coffee ground vomitus and black stool contains blood. Visual impairment and functional limitations may affect the ability of older patients to recognize bleeding. The patient, as well as the physician, may attribute nonspecific

symptoms such as dizziness, fatigue, and shortness of breath to aging or common age-associated comorbidities.

3. Gastritis induced by NSAIDs without *H. pylori* infection should be treated with a proton-pump inhibitor (PPI), or a histamine-2 (H-2) blocker, and discontinuation of the NSAID. The best way to prevent NSAID-associated gastrointestinal problems is to avoid NSAIDs entirely. If there is no alternative, the patient needs to avoid the modifiable risk factors noted above. Cotherapy with H-2 blockers, PPIs, or prostaglandin analogs (misoprostol) reduce the risk of NSAID-associated ulcer and can be used in patients at high risk. If NSAIDs are necessary, short-acting agents, such as ibuprofen, in the lowest possible dose, are preferable.

Cyclooxygenase 2 (COX-2) selective inhibitors, such as celocoxib and rofecoxib, have generally been recommended over nonselective cyclooxygenase inhibitors (NSAIDs) because they have a lower risk of gastrointestinal side effects compared with NSAIDs. COX-2 inhibitors virtually lack activity against COX-1 at therapeutic doses and can be given once or twice a day. This improves adherence but also could increase the risk of toxicity, and gastrointestinal bleeding may still occur. Both nonselective and COX-2 selective inhibitors should probably be avoided entirely in patients with previous NSAID-associated gastrointestinal bleeding and should generally be avoided in patients taking platelet inhibitors or warfarin.

In addition, COX-2 inhibitors may be more likely than NSAIDs to cause edema or elevate blood pressure. Recent evidence that COX-2 inhibitors are associated with cardiac morbidity has created considerable concern about their use.

4. There are other ways to manage osteoarthritis besides anti-inflammatory medications. Mild joint pain often responds to acetaminophen, although it stopped helping this patient. Opioid and opioid-like analgesics (such as tramadol) can be helpful in patients who do not respond to or cannot tolerate NSAIDs. Glucosamine sulfate may control symptoms and prevent joint-space narrowing in arthritis, but, pending further study, this agent has not been approved for use in the United States, is currently classified as a dietary supplement, and is not subject to rigorous quality control (see Case 21). Topical agents such as capsaicin, transdermal lidocaine, and over-the-counter creams and liniments (salicylates, or cooling agents such as menthol) may be useful adjunctive therapy in painful joints.

Nonpharmacologic therapies are very important but underused in osteoarthritis. Therapeutic exercises (designed, conducted, and supervised by professionally trained physiotherapists), weight reduction, walking aids, shoe insoles, and braces may reduce pain and improve function in some patients. Therapeutic heat and cold, electrotherapeutics, ultrasound, and acupuncture are widely used, although their benefits are yet to be established. Finally, joint replacement remains an excellent treatment for selected patients in whom medical treatment has failed to provide adequate pain relief and maintenance of function.

Caveats

1. Anemia is a risk factor for acute ischemic cardiac syndromes. Anemia induced by aspirin-associated gastrointestinal bleeding, like other causes of anemia, can induce angina and acute myocardial infarction. In one report, 15 patients (mean age 72) who were on low-dose aspirin for secondary prevention of ischemic heart disease were admitted for unstable angina or myocardial infarction due to gastrointestinal bleeding (Bar-Dayan *et al.*, 1997).
2. Other important side effects of both NSAIDs and COX-2 inhibitors include exacerbation of hypertension, congestive heart failure, and renal toxicity. COX-2 inhibitors may be as likely or possibly even more likely to affect blood pressure and fluid status than nonselective NSAIDs.
3. Although sucralfate is effective against NSAID-induced duodenal disease, it has not been shown to be effective in the prevention or treatment of NSAID-induced gastric ulcers.

REFERENCES

Bar-Dayan, Y., Levy, Y. L., Amital, H. *et al.* (1997). Aspirin for prevention of myocardial infarction. A double-edged sword. *Annales de Medecine Interne (Paris)*, **148**, 430–3.

Huang, J., Sridhar, S., and Hunt, R. H. (2002). Role of *Helicobacter pylori* infection and non-steroidal anti-inflammatory drugs in peptic-ulcer disease: a meta-analysis. *Lancet*, **359**, 14–22.

Pilotto, A. and Malfertheiner, P. (2002). An approach to *Helicobacter pylori* infection in the elderly. *Alimentary Pharmacology and Therapeutics*, **16**, 683–91.

BIBLIOGRAPHY

Johnson, D. L., Hisel, T. M., and Phillips, B. B. (2003). Effect of cyclooxygenase-2 inhibitors on blood pressure. *Annals of Pharmacotherapy*, **37**, 442–6.

Laine, L. (2001). Approaches to nonsteroidal anti-inflammatory drug use in the high-risk patient. *Gastroenterology*, **120**, 594–606.

Lichtenstein, D. R., Syngal, S., and Wolfe, M. M. (1995). Nonsteroidal antiinflammatory drugs and the gastrointestinal tract: the double-edged sword. *Arthritis and Rheumatism*, **38**, 5–18.

Linder, J. D., Monkemuller, K. E., Davis, J. V. *et al.* (2000). Cyclooxygenase-2 inhibitor cele-coxib, a possible cause of gastropathy and hypothrombinemia. *Southern Medical Journal*, **93**, 930–2.

Ling, S. M. and Bathon, J. M. (1998). Osteoarthritis in older adults. *Journal of American Geriatrics Society*, **46**, 216–25.

McAlindon, T. E., Va Valley, M. P., Gulin J. P. *et al.* (2000). Glucosamine and chondroitin for treatment of osteoarthritis: a systematic quality assessment and meta-analysis. *Journal of the American Medical Association*, **283**, 1469–75.

Rains, C. and Bryson, H. M. (1995). Topical capsaicin. A review of its pharmacological properties and therapeutic potential in post-herpetic neuralgia, diabetic neuropathy and osteoarthritis. *Drugs and Aging*, **7**, 317–28.

Reginster, J. Y., Deroisy, R., Rovati, L. C. *et al.* (2001). Long-term effects of glucosamine sulphate on osteoarthritis progression: a randomized, placebo-controlled clinical trial. *Lancet*, **357**, 251–6.

Silverstein, F. E., Faich, G., Goldstein, J. L. *et al.* (2000). Gastrointestinal toxicity with celecoxib vs nonsteroidal anti-inflammatory drugs for osteoarthritis and rheumatoid arthritis: the CLASS study, a randomized controlled trial. Celecoxib Long-term Arthritis Safety Study. *Journal of the American Medical Association*, **284**, 1247–55.

Stiel, D. (2000). Exploring the link between gastrointestinal complications and over-the-counter analgesics: current issues and considerations. *American Journal of Therapeutics*, **7**, 91–8.

Wolfe, M. M., Lichtenstein, D. R., and Singh, G. (1999). Gastrointestinal toxicity of non-steroidal antiinflammatory agents. *New England Journal of Medicine*, **340**, 1888–99.

Case 33

▸▸ Urinary incontinence

Mrs. L, a 75-year-old widow, came to your office after being discharged from the hospital, where she underwent surgery for a fracture of her right shoulder. Mrs. L has been under your care for several years and has been treated for hypertension, osteoarthritis of both knees, and obesity. She had a stroke 4 years ago but the deficit resolved. She has no history of diabetes or glaucoma. Her hypertension had been well controlled with daily hydrochlorothiazide 25 mg and atenonol 50 mg. Because she does not tolerate nonsteroidal anti-inflammatory agents, she takes acetaminophen for her knee pain but still has pain when she walks and sometimes uses a cane. Other medications include enteric-coated aspirin and a multivitamin.

Mrs. L explains that, on the night of the fracture, she woke up to urinate around midnight, and then fell and broke her shoulder. She related her fall to drinking wine that night with a friend, which had made her a little drowsier than usual when she got up at midnight. She drinks alcohol only occasionally, and has not had trouble before. The conversation reminded Mrs. L that she experienced frequent nocturnal urination during the hospitalization and on several occasions was unable to get to the toilet on time and became incontinent. When questioned, she admits that she has had urinary frequency for several years but managed it by avoiding beverages before sleep or before leaving her house. She also avoids going out for long periods during the day, and, whenever she returns from her brief excursions, she develops urinary urgency "as soon as the key goes into the lock." She has occasionally experienced leakage when sneezing, standing, or coughing, but this most commonly occurs when she is trying to hold her urine during one of her "urgent" episodes. Still, she did not view her urinary pattern as a big problem until her recent hospitalization.

Mrs. L last visited her gynecologist 1 year ago. She has no cystocele, rectocele, or uterine prolapse. She denies dysuria, fever, or constipation.

Case Studies in Geriatric Medicine, Judith C. Ahronheim *et al.* Published by Cambridge University Press.
© J. C. Ahronheim, Z.-B. Huang, V. Yen, C. M. Davitt, and D. Barile

Questions

1. What factors contributed to this patient's urinary incontinence?
2. How should her problem be approached?
3. What nonpharmacologic approaches could be of benefit to this patient?
4. What is the place of cystometry in the evaluation of urinary incontinence?

Answers

1. The patient's chronic urinary urgency suggests that she suffers from detrusor instability, but her problem may be multifactorial. She has been taking diuretics, which could be exacerbating her problem. Although she has found her bladder problems annoying, she coped with them until she became incontinent in the hospital.

   Urinary "urge incontinence" is a typical presentation of detrusor instability. The diagnosis of detrusor instability (also referred to as "overactive," "unstable," "hyperreflexic," "spastic," or "uninhibited neurogenic" bladder) is generally apparent from the history alone. Typically, the affected patient reports frequent involuntary contractions or severe urgency at a relatively lower bladder volume.

   Detrusor instability is the most common cause of urinary incontinence in elderly men and women. It can be caused by a neurologic condition, such as dementia or stroke, which releases the brainstem detrusor-reflex from cerebrocortical inhibition. In most cases, however, no specific neurologic illness is identified, and incontinent elderly patients who develop stroke or other brain lesions may previously have had detrusor instability. In the setting of detrusor instability, bladder irritation due to infection, bladder tumor, or stone can worsen existing urgency and frequency. In Mrs. L's case, the long history of bladder symptoms, and the absence of fever and dysuria, make urinary tract infection a less likely cause of acute incontinence.

   Mrs. L also has occasional stress incontinence, which can coexist with detrusor instability in women, and which may present in the perimenopausal years and even earlier. This "true" stress incontinence (in contrast to stress incontinence in the presence of urinary retention) is characterized by leakage of urine in association with sudden increased intra-abdominal pressure during coughing, sneezing, laughing, or, in severe cases, merely standing up. It is due to insufficiency of the internal urethral sphincter or pelvic floor weakness. The syndrome has been attributed to estrogen deficiency and childbirth, but variable clinical response to estrogen replacement, and existence of the problem in nulliparous women, challenge those explanations or suggest that other factors are involved.

Overflow urinary incontinence occurs in the setting of significant urinary retention. Incontinence may be precipitated by increased intra-abdominal pressure, causing a reflex micturition contraction and loss of a small amount of urine. Persistent urinary retention is uncommon in women and, on examination, Mrs. L's bladder was not palpable. Urinary retention, its causes, and management are discussed in detail in Case 34.

Mrs. L's "acute" incontinence was partially functional in nature and was precipitated by circumstances associated with hospitalization. Functional urinary incontinence (also called "pseudoincontinence") occurs when the patient is unable to reach the toilet on time because of physical limitations, environmental barriers, or a pharmacologic effect, such as sedation. In Mrs. L's case, ambulatory problems due to arthritis, now complicated by problems with her right arm and deconditioning during hospitalization, prevented her from toileting quickly enough and she became incontinent. In addition to her ambulatory limitations, detrusor instability, diuretics, and alcohol (with its sedating as well as diuretic properties) were all important factors in her fall.

2. Like many patients, Mrs. L's long-standing urinary frequency did not prompt her to seek medical attention, and her physicians did not inquire. In general, it is important to inquire routinely about bladder problems in older adults. Because Mrs. L recently underwent surgery and probably had an indwelling catheter, urinalysis and culture should now be performed to rule out a hospital-acquired urinary tract infection as a factor in her "acute" incontinence. However, asymptomatic bacteriuria often exists in late life (see Case 34) and treatment of the infection does not reverse the incontinence.

In order to address her ongoing bladder problem, the diuretic could be replaced by an antihypertensive agent that would not exacerbate her bladder problems. It is best to avoid certain antihypertensive agents, such as alpha-blockers, which can relax the urethral sphincter and are, in fact, commonly given to promote voiding in benign prostatic hyperplasia. Calcium channel blockers, though generally well tolerated, have occasionally been reported to cause urinary retention, probably because detrusor contractions are dependent on calcium channels. Other medications that can be problematic are sedatives, which can cause confusion and missed bladder cues.

Medications that relax the detrusor muscle, such as oxybutynin (Ditropan) or tolterodine (Detrol), can sometimes ameliorate detrusor instability but can cause dry mouth, visual blurring, and other anticholinergic effects. Systemic and topical estrogen are frequently given for urinary stress incontinence but clinical trials have not consistently supported their benefit, even in younger women.

Mrs. L was given enalapril instead of hydrochlorothiazide. Her urinalysis was normal, and on follow up 1 week later, and her blood pressure was still under control. Her urinary frequency seemed diminished, but she still had to urinate two to three times per night and continued to have frequency during the day. Oxybutynin was instituted at a very small dose, and she was instructed to take the medication only at specific times, such as prior to a social activity, a physical therapy session, or at bedtime. This reduced her urinary frequency somewhat.

3. Removal of environmental hazards and a good night light can make it easier to get to the bathroom safely and on time. A bedside commode can make night-time toileting easier and can help to prevent functional incontinence. These interventions would be particularly important in this patient who fractured her arm on the way to the bathroom at night.

   Pelvic muscle exercises are helpful for patients with stress incontinence and for some with urge incontinence. The patient first is taught to identify the pelvic muscles that will be exercised, then to try to stop the stream in the middle of urination, let it resume, and then stop the stream again. The exercise consists of 10-second contractions followed by 10-second relaxations, and the exercise is repeated 15 times approximately three times a day. The ideal patient is cognitively intact, ambulatory, and able to perform this exercise correctly, so it is not suitable for many frail older patients. Biofeedback instruments are sometimes used to help the patient learn to identify pelvic muscles and to master the technique of exercising pelvic muscles selectively while keeping abdominal muscle relaxed.

   Bladder training is another approach that could be helpful. This consists of the patient or caregiver observing and recording the patient's micturition needs, and toileting at the longest possible interval (usually 30 minutes to 2 hours) to keep her dry. If continence is maintained for 48 hours, the interval can be lengthened. This method is repeated until a reasonable goal is achieved, such as 4 hours of continence. Patients with urge incontinence are taught to employ "urge strategies," which are adaptive responses to the sensation of urgency. These include distraction, relaxation of the entire body, or contracting pelvic muscles instead of rushing to the toilet. After urgency subsides, the patient proceeds to the toilet at a normal pace. For patients with dementia, who will be unable to use these strategies or for others who cannot toilet on their own, a caregiver observes the patient's voiding patterns and maintains a regular toileting schedule in accordance with the observed pattern. Adult incontinence garments and pads are commercially available or can be improvised in the home or hospital and can be used as a backup for "accidents" to maintain dryness and to give the patient confidence to participate in social activities.

4. Although the history is usually sufficient to distinguish between types of urinary incontinence, cystometry is probably not necessary in most patients like Mrs. L. However, when diagnostic uncertainty exists, certain measurements can be helpful.

   Simple cystometry can be conducted in the office or bedside, and consists of several steps. First, the patient is asked to cough while standing, holding a pad over the

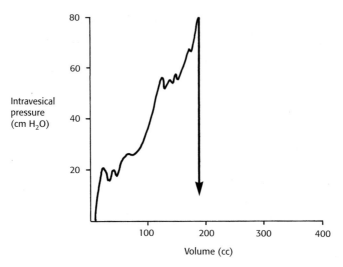

80 —

60 —

Intravesical
pressure
(cm H₂O)   40 —

20 —

100   200   300   400

Volume (cc)

Figure 13   Cystogram depicting volume–pressure relationship in detrusor instability. Micturition contractions are occurring at inappropriately low volumes while the bladder is being filled with water. Descending arrow indicates that the bladder has emptied at a volume of less than 200 cubic centimeters (cc).

urethral area. Ideally, this step is performed when the patient feels the bladder is full. Leakage of urine while coughing confirms stress urinary incontinence. Next, the patient voids privately, collecting the urine for volume measurement, and reports any symptoms of hesitancy, straining, or intermittent stream, which may suggest outlet obstruction or atonic bladder. Immediately after voiding, postvoid residual (PVR) is determined; the patient lies supine and a straight catheter is inserted into the bladder with sterile technique and the volume of remaining urine is measured. Greater than 100 cc suggests urinary retention, and difficulty passing the catheter suggests obstruction. (Alternatively, PVR can be estimated by portable bladder ultrasound, which is reasonably sensitive and very specific for determining PVR greater than 100 cc.) With the catheter in place, a 50 cc syringe without a piston is attached to the catheter, held about 15 cm above the pubic symphysis, and sterile water at room temperature is poured into the syringe 50 cc at a time. When the patient reports the feeling of fullness and urge to void, filling amount is reduced to 25 ml until the patient requires immediate voiding, or an involuntary contraction is observed; this consists of rapid or continuous upward movement of the fluid column, sometimes with leaking around or expulsion of the catheter. Involuntary contraction or severe urgency at a relatively low bladder volume (less than 250–300 ml) suggest detrusor instability. This volume–pressure relationship is depicted in the cystometrogram (see Figure 13), which is generated during formal cystometry in which precise measurements are made.

The stress maneuver can be repeated, as a full bladder increases the sensitivity of detecting stress incontinence. Finally, the patient can void again and PVR calculated by subtracting voided volume from instilled volume. This calculation may more accurately determine PVR if the patient did not have full bladder at the beginning of the test.

Caveats

1. Nocturnal urinary frequency is sometimes related to congestive heart failure or fluid overload from other causes. When supine, blood flow to the kidney increases, increasing urine production. In these cases, diuretics can paradoxically decrease nocturia.
2. Indwelling urethral or suprapubic catheters are not indicated in the treatment of chronic urinary incontinence unless it is associated with intractable urinary retention that can not be managed without intermittent catheterization. Indwelling catheters may be indicated for short-term use in patients with severe pressure ulcers on buttocks or sacrum until healing is established. A potential pitfall of an indwelling catheter in this setting is reduced nursing vigilance; pressure sores require removal of pressure, frequent turning, and avoidance of excessive moisture and soilage caused not only by urine but also by feces and perspiration.
3. Most elderly diabetics with urinary incontinence have detrusor instability, not atonic bladder. The "diabetic cystopathy" of atonic bladder is an autonomic neuropathy that occurs as a result of longstanding uncontrolled diabetes. It involves a disturbance in the afferent limb of the brainstem detrusor reflex, so messages are not sent to the brainstem about bladder filling.

BIBLIOGRAPHY

Burgio, K. L., Locher, J. L., Goode, P. S. *et al.* (1998). Behavioral vs drug treatment for urge urinary incontinence in older women: a randomized controlled trial. *Journal of American Medical Association*, **280**, 1995–2000.

Fantl, J. A., Bump, R. C., Robinson, D. *et al.*, for the Continence Program for Women Research Group (1996). Efficacy of estrogen supplementation in the treatment of urinary incontinence. *Obstetrics and Gynecology*, **88**, 745–9.

Goode, P. S., Locher J. L., Bryant, R. L. *et al.* (2000). Measurement of postvoid residual urine with portable transabdominal bladder ultrasound scanner and urethral catheterization. *International Urogynecology Journal and Pelvic Floor Dysfunction*, **11**, 296–300.

Grady, D., Brown, J. S., Vittinghoff, E. *et al.*, for the HERS Research Group (2001). Postmenopausal hormones and incontinence: the Heart and Estrogen/Progestin Replacement Study. *Obstetrics and Gynecology*, **97**, 116–20.

Ouslander J. G., Greendale, G. A., Uman, G. *et al.* (2001). Effects of oral estrogen and progestin on the lower urinary tract among female nursing home residents. *Journal of the American Geriatrics Society*, **49**, 803–7.

Ouslander, J. G., Leach, G. E., and Staskin, D. R. (1989). Simplified tests of lower urinary tract function in the evaluation of geriatric urinary incontinence. *Journal of the American Geriatrics Society*, **37**, 706–14.

Starer, P. and Libow, L. (1990). Cystometric evaluation of bladder dysfunction in elderly diabetic patients. *Archives of Internal Medicine*, **150**, 810–13.

▶▶ Urinary retention

An 84-year-old retired professor was admitted to the coronary care unit of an acute care hospital with tachycardia and congestive heart failure. He had a history of chronic constipation for which he had taken various senna-containing preparations for many years. His most recent bowel regimen also included psyllium hydrophilic mucilloid (Metamucil) twice daily, docusate sodium (Colace) 300 mg daily, daily prune juice, and milk of magnesia 30 cc as needed. He had no known history of urinary difficulties.

Physical findings included atrial fibrillation with a ventricular rate of 150, and bibasilar rales. Treatment consisted of enalapril and furosemide, diltiazem for rate control, and morphine for dyspnea. A low salt diet was ordered and Colace 100 mg daily was prescribed for constipation. The patient was kept on bed rest.

On the second hospital day, the patient complained that he was "not being given enough laxatives," and his diet orders were modified to include 10 g of bran with his breakfast cereal, and two high-fiber cookies (5 g of fiber each) for dessert at lunch and dinner. At this time, diphenhydramine (Benadryl) was added for insomnia.

By the third hospital day, his cardiac status had improved but he began to complain of an inability to void, whereupon it was noted that he had not passed urine for at least 8 hours, although he had been eating and drinking normally. A Foley catheter was inserted and 550 cc of clear urine was passed. The catheter remained in place while cardiac workup was completed over the next few days.

On the fifth hospital day, the patient developed a temperature of 101 °F (oral) and urinalysis revealed many bacteria and eight to ten white blood cells per high power field. Urine and blood cultures were sent to the laboratory and ciprofloxacin was begun. The patient began to complain that the catheter

Case Studies in Geriatric Medicine, Judith C. Ahronheim *et al.* Published by Cambridge University Press.
© J. C. Ahronheim, Z.-B. Huang, V. Yen, C. M. Davitt, and D. Barile

was "annoying" him and that it was "probably to blame for the infection in the first place." He demanded that it be removed. The catheter was removed but, when the patient was unable to pass urine 8 hours later, it was reinserted.

Questions

1. What factors have contributed to this patient's problem?
2. How should this problem be managed?
3. What factors contributed to the urinary tract infection?
4. What additional factors contributed to this patient's dilemma?

Answers

1. The patient's constipation, imposition of bed rest, medications, and, as an elderly male, his likelihood of underlying benign prostatic hyperplasia (BPH; see Figure 14) have all contributed to acute urinary retention. Rectal examination revealed a hard mass that had resulted in fecal impaction and accumulation of abundant feces in the rectum, compressing the bladder and resulting in urinary retention. Stool impaction is implicated as a cause of urinary retention in up to 10% of older hospitalized patients.

   Morphine, diltiazem, and diphenhydramine are likely to have contributed to this patient's fecal impaction by slowing bowel transit time. The anticholinergic activity of morphine and diphenhydramine also contributed to urinary retention directly, by inhibiting the detrusor muscle of the bladder, which contracts in response to cholinergic stimulation. Common offenders include tricyclic antidepressants, first-generation antihistamines, opioids, and gastrointestinal antispasmodics. Antispasmodics such as oxybutinin (Ditropan) and tamsulosin (Detrol), which are used to treat detrusor instability (see Case 33), may result in unwanted urinary retention.

   The probability that this patient had some degree of BPH increased the likelihood that he would develop acute urinary retention. The prevalence of BPH increases with age and, by age 80, approximately 80% of men have pathologic evidence of BPH. According to a large prospective study, men aged 70–79 years have a one in ten chance of developing acute urinary retention in the next 5 years, and the risk for men in their eighties is almost one in three (see Jacobsen et al., 1997).

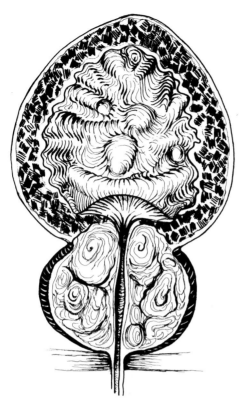

Figure 14   An enlarged prostate gland with adenomatous growth in the periurethral region. The bladder wall is trabeculated, probably as a result of chronically elevated intravesicular pressures.

2. Fecal impaction can be treated with enemas, but, when a hard mass is felt on digital rectal examination, manual disimpaction should be initiated first. This patient was treated with manual disimpaction, after which he expelled soft feces spontaneously. Appropriate treatment would also include discontinuation, when possible, of medications that interfere with bladder and bowel function – in this case, morphine and diphenhydramine. Diltiazem, which is very constipating, should be replaced if possible with a beta-blocker.

   Enemas can be given if necessary, and follow up should include bathroom or commode privileges, physical activity as soon as possible, and removal of the catheter. Antibiotics are not always necessary in catheter-induced urinary tract infections, once the catheter has been removed, as most catheter-induced infections are asymptomatic and bacteriuria may resolve on its own.

   Acute urinary retention is extremely common in older men when they are hospitalized. Bowel function needs to be monitored on a daily basis in patients at risk, and constipation treated right away in order to prevent fecal impaction. Early mobilization, avoidance of dehydration, avoidance of constipating medications, and avoidance of anticholinergic medications are other maneuvers that need to be employed. Male patients should be assisted to get out of bed and stand to urinate if possible, or, if they are unable to use a urinal or urinate effectively with one, a bedside commode may help. Likewise, bowel movements are easier if the patient can be seated on the toilet, in the privacy of the bathroom. Bladder catheters should be discontinued as soon as minute-to-minute measurement of urinary output is no longer necessary, in order to avoid infection.

Patients who have no history of symptomatic urinary retention prior to hospitalization generally are again able to urinate if precipitating factors are rectified. However, it is not unusual for an elderly man to be unaware of a high urine residual volume, and urinary retention sometimes stubbornly persists. In these cases, tamsulosin (Flomax) should be considered. This alpha-blocking agent selectively inhibits alpha-1a adrenergic receptors, reducing smooth muscle contractions, reducing intraurethral pressure, and increasing urine flow. Because tamsulosin has a greater specificity for the receptors in the bladder and prostate, it does not lower systemic blood pressure and is an appropriate first-line treatment for obstructive symptoms in BPH. Alternatively, a nonselective alpha-blocker such as terazosin (Hytrin) can be given in patients requiring treatment for hypertension.

3. The indwelling catheter, acute urinary retention, and likelihood that the patient had underlying BPH probably all contributed to the urinary tract infection. The incidence of catheter-related urinary tract infections increases rapidly with the duration of catheterization at a rate of about 10% per day. In addition, this patient had developed urinary retention prior to catheterization and was already predisposed to infection. With BPH, this patient probably would have had an elevated postvoid residual urine (see Case 33), increasing his risk of stasis and bacteriuria.

Loss of barrier defenses is an additional risk factor for urinary tract infections and bacterial colonization in elderly patients. The uroepithelium appears to be less effective in providing a barrier to infection. Changes in surface glycosaminoglycans and fibronectins contribute to adherence of bacteria. In elderly women, predisposing factors include increased adherence of vaginal uropathogens to uroepithelial cells, cystocele, which can increase postvoid residual volume, and estrogen deficiency, which promotes colonization of the vagina with urinary pathogens.

4. The patient was known to suffer from chronic constipation. Intestinal transit time is prolonged with age, but constipation is not a universal complaint. Chronic use of such laxatives may permanently damage the electrical system of the colon. Irritant laxatives such as senna, and possibly others, may directly affect the myenteric plexus. The result is "cathartic bowel," an overdistended colon with loss of haustrations and poor motility. Other irritant laxatives that may cause cathartic bowel include

castor oil, cascara, aloe, bisacodyl, and phenolphthalein. Prunes and prune juice contain a phenolphthalein derivative but have not been reported to cause cathartic bowel.

This patient's bowel movements occurred to his satisfaction only with a strict bowel regimen. This regimen was not given to him in the hospital, possibly because it was viewed by the staff as an eccentric and excessive use of laxatives. Also, medications are not always part of the hospital formulary and alternatives are not always sought for what might be perceived as a "nonessential" medication. The sudden imposition of bed rest probably reduced his bowel motility further. The diuretic and salt restriction, combined with age-related decline in renal concentrating ability, is likely to have caused a relative dehydration and reduced water content of feces. Although bran has been shown to reduce intestinal transit time in elderly hospitalized patients, bran supplementation can sometimes form a bulky mass and cause fecal impaction, especially when the water content of the diet is not concurrently increased, or if the patient is bedridden. The difficulty of supine defecation and the lack of privacy are also likely to be contributors to this patient's dilemma, but these modifiable risk factors are often overlooked in the hospital setting.

Caveats

1. The incidence of asymptomatic bacteriuria rises dramatically after midlife in men and is ten times more common in men over 80 than in the 65–70-year age group, and in the setting of fever should not be assumed to be the source of infection. In one study of nursing home elderly, fewer than 10% of febrile episodes could be attributed to urinary tract infection, and a high proportion of patients with other infections had coincidental bacteriuria (Orr *et al.*, 1996).

2. The rectal examination is important in determining the cause of urinary obstruction but must be interpreted with caution. The size of the prostate gland on digital examination does not necessarily correlate with the degree of obstructive symptoms since adenomatous growth of tissue begins in the periurethral area. The prostate may feel relatively normal on digital examination in cases where there may be a high degree of obstruction. Likewise, many patients with BPH have a preponderance of fibromuscular stroma, which contributes to spasm and outlet obstruction, but this is not appreciated on digital rectal examination. Conversely, a patient may have a prostate gland that is large in size but nonobstructing. Prostatic carcinoma tends to originate in the periphery of the gland and does not usually cause obstructive symptoms early in the course of the disease.

3. Cystometry is sometimes performed in acute urinary retention. However, it can be misleading in patients who are taking medications that cause pharmacologic

bladder paralysis and can divert attention from the search for reversible causes. Cystometry is discussed in detail in Case 33.

4. The cholinomimetic drug, bethanachol, is sometimes used in the setting of urinary retention but should generally be avoided. This agent can increase detrusor contractions, but is usually clinically ineffective and may cause bradycardia. This would be particularly risky in a patient who is being treated with negative chronotropic agents.

5. Acute urinary retention in elderly women rarely persists, and a secondary cause should always be vigorously sought. Chronic urinary retention in women tends to occur in specific neurologic conditions that can affect both sexes, such as multiple sclerosis or spinal cord transection, or in patients with longstanding uncontrolled diabetes mellitus ("diabetic cystopathy"), who generally have additional clinical evidence of autonomic neuropathy.

REFERENCES

Jacobsen, S. J., Jacobson, D. J., Girman, C. J. *et al.* (1997). Natural history of prostatism: risk factors for acute urinary retention. *Journal of Urology*, **158**, 481–7.

Orr, P. H., Nicolle, L. E., Duckworth, H. *et al.* (1996). Febrile urinary infections in the institutionalized elderly. *American Journal of Medicine*, **100**, 71–7.

BIBLIOGRAPHY

Loeb, M., Bentley, D. W., Bradley, S. *et al.* (2001). Development of minimum criteria for the initiation of antibiotics in residents of long-term care facilities: results of a consensus conference. *Infection Control and Hospital Epidemiology*, **22**, 120–4.

Medina, J. J., Parra, R. O., and Moore, R. G. (1999). Benign prostatic hypertrophy (the aging patient). *Medical Clinics of North America*, **83**, 1213–29.

Meigs, J. B., Barry, M. J., Giovannucci E. *et al.* (1999). Incidence rates and risk factors for acute urinary retention: the Health Professionals Follow-up Study. *Journal of Urology*, **162**, 376–82.

Nicolle, L. E. (2003). Asymptomatic bacteriuria: when to screen and when to treat. *Infectious Disease Clinics of North America*, **17**, 367–94.

Prather, C. M. and Ortiz-Camacho, C. P. (1998). Evaluation and treatment of constipation and fecal impaction in adults. *Mayo Clinic Proceedings*, **73**, 881–7.

Price, H., McNeal, J. E., and Stamey, T. A. (1990). Evolving patterns of tissue composition in benign prostatic hyperplasia as a function of specimen size. *Human Pathology*, **21**, 578–85.

Saint, S. (2000). Clinical and economic consequences of nosocomial catheter-related bacteriuria. *American Journal of Infection Control*, **28**, 68–75.

Saint, S. and Lipsky, B. (1999). Preventing catheter-related bacteremia: should we? Can we? How? *Archives of Internal Medicine*, **159**, 800–8.

Tambyah, P. A. and Maki, D. G. (2000). Catheter-associated urinary tract infection is rarely symptomatic. *Archives of Internal Medicine*, **160**, 678–82.

Case 35

▶▶ Erectile dysfunction

Mr. J is a 74-year-old man with a history of hypertension and hyperlipidemia. He comes in at the suggestion of a nurse at a community center where he recently underwent screening for prostate cancer. He was told that his prostate-specific antigen (PSA) level was 4 ng/ml and that he ought to discuss this with his physician.

The patient's physical examination is significant for mild muscle atrophy, blood pressure of 140/85, mild gynecomastia, and decreased dorsalis pedis pulses. Prostate gland is diffusely enlarged but there are no palpable nodules. Genitalia are normal, although testicles are mildly atrophic.

The patient used to smoke heavily but quit 1 year ago at your recommendation. He is currently taking hydrochlorothiazide, aspirin, sertraline, and enalapril.

You discuss the PSA level and establish a plan for follow up, reassuring him that the level is likely to be elevated for reasons other than prostate cancer. While the patient is dressing, his wife takes you aside and tells you that her husband has been totally uninterested in any kind of sexual activity and that he is unable to initiate an erection. This problem has been making him progressively more depressed. She wonders if you could prescribe sildenafil (Viagra) for him.

Questions

1. What factors could be contributing to his erectile dysfunction (ED)?
2. What investigations should be performed?
3. Mr. J's testosterone level is 180 ng/dl ($n = 200–800$). Does he suffer from male "andropause?"
4. What effects would be expected from testosterone replacement? From sildenafil? From enhanced sexual activity?

Case Studies in Geriatric Medicine, Judith C. Ahronheim *et al.* Published by Cambridge University Press.
© J. C. Ahronheim, Z.-B. Huang, V. Yen, C. M. Davitt, and D. Barile

Answers

1. ED – the inability to attain and maintain an erection of sufficient rigidity for sexual intercourse during 50% or more of attempts – increases in incidence with age and affects up to 67% of men aged 70 and 75% of those aged 80. However, ED correlates with the medical conditions that cause ED rather than with age alone. Mr. J has several risk factors for ED, including hypertension, a history of cigarette smoking, a history of depression, and use of antihypertensive and antidepressant medication. Antihypertensive medications have often been implicated in ED and, although this may be true for some (e.g. diuretics), it has not been shown for others (e.g. angiotensin-converting enzyme inhibitors). In trials of hypertension treatment, subjects on placebo may have the same overall incidence of ED as subjects on active treatment. Many medications have been implicated, but it is not always possible to know whether the medication is at fault because the cause of ED is often multifactorial, with other etiologies including neurologic, hormonal, and psychogenic factors.

   Multiple factors could well exist in this patient. In addition to medications, physical findings suggest peripheral vascular disease and hypogonadism. Atherosclerosis and atherogenic risk factors (such as hyperlipidemia, diabetes, and smoking) may lead to impaired vascular flow to the corpus cavernosum. The patient's muscle and testicular atrophy, as well as his gynecomastia, suggest "hypogonadism," which is very common in late life (see below) and which is associated with loss of libido as well as ED. If his prior sexual function was normal, this hypogonadism is likely to have been acquired late in life.

2. Although a number of investigations could be performed, and a thorough physical examination is essential, the history may often be the most useful part of the evaluation, especially in older men. It would be important to inquire about the nature, onset, and duration of the patient's problem – whether it began or worsened when chlorthalodone or sertraline was begun, whether it was associated with any specific life event, or whether there has been a progressive worsening of his symptoms over a longer period of time. Other important information might be occurrence of ED around times of stress, presence of morning erections, and retained ability to masturbate, all of which suggest a psychogenic cause. Likewise, it would be important to ascertain whether the problem is loss of libido as opposed to ED, or both.

   A thorough vascular examination should evaluate all lower extremity pulses and the groin should be examined for bruits. Neurologic examination should include assessment of visual fields (abnormal in the presence of a pituitary mass) and also of sensory systems to rule out peripheral and autonomic neuropathy. Unfortunately, many findings are nonspecific in elderly individuals – for example, visual fields may be compressed in glaucoma, and loss of body hair as well as sarcopenia may be normal variants of aging, rather than resulting from hypogonadism.

3. Controversy exists as to whether "andropause" – an age-related decrease in sex steroids in males analogous to menopause – is a definable condition and whether it has clinical significance. The concept of the andropause is derived from epidemiologic data showing an increasing prevalence with age of hypogonadism, as defined by a total serum testosterone level less than approximately 300–325 ng/dl. Importantly, epidemiologic data are limited by methodologic issues – for example, whether data were cross-sectional or longitudinal, degree of reliability of stored specimens in longitudinal studies, or whether total or free (bioavailable) testosterone was assayed, and how the assay was performed. With age, sex hormone-binding globulin increases, so total serum testosterone may appear normal while free levels are low. A large longitudinal study demonstrated that, by age 80 years, 50% of men have low total testosterone levels, but 91% have low free testosterone as determined by the free testosterone index (total testosterone/SHBG; see Harman *et al.*, 2001). However, the normal range of testosterone for the elderly is not really clear, because there is no clinical parameter that can be used to validate a particular level in serum. Likewise, endocrinologic parameters are not helpful because luteinizing hormone does not always increase and upper levels of normal are also unclear. Finally, assays of free testosterone are not always reliable.

In contrast to menopause, which may be associated with dramatic symptoms, age-associated hypogonadism appears to be more gradual in onset. Moreover, it may be quite incorrect to apply to the older man what is known about hypogonadism in younger men – namely, it is not at all certain whether symptoms associated with hypogonadism in younger men, such as loss of energy and vigor, decreased libido, and osteoporosis, are due to hormonal changes in older men or whether those symptoms are due to other factors associated with aging.

Finally, comorbidities, including poor nutritional status, and medications, such as glucocorticoids and alcohol, can lower serum testosterone levels.

4. Given the multiple factors that could be causing this patient's ED, it is unlikely that testosterone replacement would improve his sexual function. Even in patients whose only finding is a low testosterone level, testosterone can improve libido but may fail to improve ED.

In contrast to menopause, which is associated with identifiable symptoms that respond to estrogen, age-associated hypogonadism in men is not associated with well-defined symptoms known to respond to hormones. Symptoms commonly associated with the aging process are similar to those seen in younger patients with low testosterone levels, including decreased libido, ED, low energy, diminished strength, mood, and vigor, and even falling asleep after dinner. Among younger men with gonadal failure – such as Kleinfelter's syndrome – low testosterone-related syndromes such as osteoporosis and decreased lean body mass have been clearly shown to respond to hormone replacement. However, in the elderly, the data are not at all clear. Limited data suggest that testosterone replacement therapy in hypo-gonadal elderly may improve body composition, physical function, bone mineral density (no fracture data available), sexual function, well being, and some aspects of cognitive function, but it is doubtful that testosterone replacement can reverse a state of overall frailty, whether hypogonadism is present or not, because "frailty" in late life may indicate a confluence of more than one age-related physiologic change or pathologic state rather than a low testosterone level. Indeed, these conditions are more likely to be the cause of low testosterone levels.

The safety of long-term testosterone replacement has not been determined. It does not appear to cause prostate cancer de novo, although whether it stimulates occult cancers, increases prostate volume, and exacerbates urinary symptoms has not been fully resolved. The patient's mild elevation in PSA is consistent with enhanced prostate volume seen in benign prostatic hyperplasia, and, at his age, is not a cause for immediate alarm, but, if testosterone were given, close follow up would be needed because of the high prevalence of occult prostate cancer in older men and because of the theoretical risk that the hormone could stimulate an occult cancer.

Risks of testosterone replacement are reviewed in the references (see Rhoden and Morgentaler, 2004; Snyder, 2004). At this point, it would seem more useful to re-evaluate the need for finding alternatives for potentially problematic medications, such as the thiazide diuretic and sertraline, rather than to add testosterone, which might increase libido without enhancing performance.

Sildenafil (Viagra) has been increasingly used for the management of ED. It is an oral phosphodiesterase (PDE5) inhibitor which potentiates the nitric oxide–cyclic GMP response of corpus cavernosum smooth muscle to sexual arousal. It has been shown to increase the duration and number of erections in a randomized, placebo-controlled trial of men aged 20–87 years (average, 57; see Goldstein *et al.*, 1998), and may be equally effective in "elderly" men (average age, 69 years; see Wagner *et al.*, 2001). This drug, furthermore, may be effective in patients with diverse etiologies, including cardiovascular disease, diabetes, prostate surgery, spinal cord injury, medication, and psychogenic and mixed causes.

Adverse reactions of sildenafil include headache, dizziness, flushing, dyspepsia, and nasal congestion. Sildenafil can also produce transient abnormal color/light perception vision through inhibitory activity against PDE6, which is involved in phototransduction. Priapism has been rarely reported. Overall, sildenafil seems to be quite safe; however, it potentiates the hypotensive effects of nitrate prepa-rations, and fatal drops in blood pressure have been reported in patients using both medications. The drug is metabolized in the liver by CYP3A4 to an inactive metabolite, and, although there is a theoretical risk of drug–drug interactions, clinically important interactions are unusual with ordinary use of sildenafil, probably because of its short half-life (approximately 4 hours). Additional agents (vardenafil and tadalafil) are now available. Little data currently exist regarding their use in older men, but caution is called for, especially with tadalafil, which has a 36-hour half-life in nonelderly men.

The efficacy and relative safety of sildenafil has markedly reduced the use of treatments for ED, such as corpus cavernosum injections of prostaglandin or other vasodilators, intraurethral suppositories of prostaglandin, and vacuum pump/occlusion procedures, which are invasive, uncomfortable, or cumbersome. Another drug, yohimbine, a selective alpha-2 adrenergic blocking agent, should theoretically *produce* ED through its release of norepinephrine at nerve terminals (including the penis), by causing vasoconstriction. Yohimbine (derived from the bark of *Corynanthe yohimbe*, once believed to be an aphrodisiac) has been available for a number of years, but clinical trials have not demonstrated great efficacy and the drug is not widely used.

An additional concern for older patients is the increased metabolic demands accompanying suddenly increased sexual activity in patients who may have underlying atherosclerotic heart disease. The average metabolic expenditure for male-on-top coitus is 3.3 METs (1 MET is the energy expenditure at rest, equivalent to approximately 3.5 ml of O_2/min/kg body weight, compared with an adequate exercise tolerance test, which is generally greater than 5 METs).

Limited study of this question includes a double-blind, placebo-controlled, crossover study of sildenafil in older men (mean age 65) with ED and known coronary artery disease (Arruda-Olson *et al.*, 2002). Subjects, who received sildenafil or placebo 1 hour before undergoing supine bicycle echocardiography, demonstrated no differences in ischemic events or measured echocardiographic outcomes, except for lower resting systolic blood pressure with sildenafil. Given the modest energy expenditure of sexual activity, it is unlikely that increased sexual activity alone would be harmful in an older man, even one with coronary artery disease, assuming sildenafil were not given with nitrates.

Caveat

Prostate cancer screening using PSA is not generally recommended in men over the age of 70 or 75 years. There is a very high prevalence of occult prostate cancer in elderly men, but this disease generally has a long natural history and the risks of investigation and treatment generally (though not always) outweigh the benefits. Despite this, older men (like Mr. J) are frequently screened. Unfortunately, the resultant treatment, such as radical prostatectomy, radiation, or hormones, commonly produce ED, sometimes permanently.

REFERENCES

Arruda-Olson, A. M., Mahoney, D. W., Nehra, A. *et al.* (2002). Cardiovascular effects of sildenafil during exercise in men with known or probable coronary artery disease: a randomized crossover trial. *Journal of the American Medical Association*, **287**, 719–25.

Goldstein, I., Lue, T. F., Padma-Nathan, H. *et al.* (1998). Oral sildenafil in the treatment of erectile dysfunction. *New England Journal of Medicine*, **338**, 1397–404.

Harman, S. M., Metter, E. J., Tobin, J. D. *et al.* (2001). Longitudinal effects of aging on serum total and free testosterone levels in healthy men: Baltimore Longitudinal Study of Aging. *Journal of Clinical Endocrinology and Metabolism*, **86**, 724–31.

Rhoden, E. L. and Morgentaler, A. (2004). Risks of testosterone-replacement therapy and recommendations for monitoring. *New England Journal of Medicine*, **350**, 482–92.

Snyder, P. J. (2004). Hypogonadism in elderly men – what to do until the evidence comes. *New England Journal of Medicine*, **350**, 440–2.

Wagner, G., Montorsi, F., Auerbach, S. *et al.* (2001). Sildenafil citrate (Viagra) improves erectile function in elderly patients with erectile dysfunction. *Journals of Gerontology Series A: Biological Sciences and Medical Sciences*, **56**, M113–19.

BIBLIOGRAPHY

Behre, H. M., Bohmeyer, J., and Nieschlag, E. (1994). Prostate volume in testosterone-treated and untreated hypogonadal men in comparison to age-matched normal controls. *Clinical Endocrinology (Oxf)*, **40**, 341–9.

Bross, R., Javanbakht, M., and Bhasin, S. (1999). Anabolic interventions for aging-associated sarcopenia. *Journal of Clinical Endocrinology and Metabolism*, **84**, 3420–30.

Bunting, P. S. (2002). Screening for prostate cancer with prostate-specific antigen: beware the biases. *Clinica Chemica Acta*, **315**, 71–97.

Cheitlin, M. D., Hutter, A. M., Brindis, R. G. *et al.* (1999). ACC/AHA expert consensus document: use of sildenafil (Viagra) in patients with cardiovascular disease. *Journal of the American College of Cardiology*, **33**, 273–82.

Coley, C. M., Barry, M. J., and Fleming, C. (1997). Clinical guidelines. Part II: Early detection of prostate cancer. Part II: Estimating the risks, benefits, and costs. *Annals of Internal Medicine*, **126**, 468–79.

De Berardis, G., Franciosi, M., Belfiglio, M. *et al.*, for the Quality of Care and Outcomes in Type 2 Diabetes (QuED) Study Group (2002). Erectile dysfunction and quality of life in type 2 diabetic patients: a serious problem too often overlooked. *Diabetes Care*, **25**, 284–91.

Feldman, H. A., Goldstein, I., Hatzichristou, D. G. *et al.* (1994). Impotence and its medical and psychosocial corrrelates: results of the Massachusetts Male Aging Study. *Journal of Urology*, **151**, 54–61.

Grimm, R. H., Grandits, G. A., Prineas, R. J. *et al.*, for the TOMHS Research Group (1997). Long term effects on sexual function of 5 antihypertensive drugs and nutritional hygienic treatment in hypertensive men and women – Treatment of Mild Hypertension Study (TOMHS). *Hypertension*, **29**, 8–14.

Johannes, C. B., Araujo, A. B., Feldman, H. A. *et al.* (2000). Incidence of ED in men 40–69 years old: longitudinal results from the Massachusetts Male Aging Study. *Journal of Urology*, **163**, 460–3.

Kenny, A. M., Prestwood, K. M., Gruman, C. A. *et al.* (2002). Effects of transdermal testosterone on lipids and vascular reactivity in older men with low bioavailable testosterone levels. *Journals of Gerontology Series A: Biological Sciences and Medical Sciences*, **57**, M460–5.

Kim, Y. C. (1999). Testosterone supplementation in the aging male. *International Journal of Impotence Research*, **11**, 343–52.

Matsumoto, A. M., Sandblom, R. E., Schoene, R. B. *et al.* (1985). Testosterone replacement in hypogonadal men: effects on obstructive sleep apnea, respiratory drives, and sleep. *Clinical Endocrinology (Oxf)*, **22**, 713–21.

Morley, J. E., Charlton, E., Patrick, P. *et al.* (2000). Validation of a screening questionnaire for androgen deficiency in aging males. *Metabolism*, **49**, 1239–42.

Sih, R., Morley, J. E., Kaiser, F. E. *et al.* (1997). Testosterone replacement in older hypogonadal men: a 12-month randomized controlled trial. *Journal of Clinical Endocrinology and Metabolism*, **82**, 1661–7.

Snyder, P. J., Peachey, H., Hannoush, P. *et al.* (2001). Effect of testosterone treatment on body composition and muscle strength in men over 65 years of age. *Journal of Clinical Endocrinology and Metabolism*, **84**, 2647–53.

▶▶ Vaginal bleeding

An 88-year-old woman with advanced Alzheimer's disease has been residing in a nursing home for 2 years. She does not speak, is incontinent, and cannot feed herself. She receives no medication except for a "bowel regimen" that consists of a stool softener, milk of magnesia, and occasional tap water enemas. She has otherwise been remarkably healthy.

One day, the nurse notices blood on the patient's incontinence pants (adult diapers) and reports to the physician that the patient has vaginal bleeding. Her son cannot remember if she had ever taken estrogen but states that she rarely went to doctors and did not like to take medications.

Questions

1. What is the best way to confirm the presence of vaginal bleeding?
2. What are the common causes of postmenopausal bleeding?
3. What is the next step in this patient?
4. How can her problem be handled?

Answers

1. Since bloodstains can indicate bleeding from the gastrointestinal or urinary tract, a bimanual examination of the vagina should be performed. Insertion of a tampon into the patient's vagina can also confirm whether the suspected site is, indeed, vaginal.
2. The most common cause of postmenopausal uterine bleeding in the elderly is endometrial polyps, which may be benign, hyperplastic, or malignant. Endometrial

Case Studies in Geriatric Medicine, Judith C. Ahronheim *et al.* Published by Cambridge University Press.
© J. C. Ahronheim, Z.-B. Huang, V. Yen, C. M. Davitt, and D. Barile

hyperplasia is a more common cause in women who have taken postmenopausal estrogens, but occasionally is due to endogenous estrogen production by an ovarian tumor. Atypical endometrial hyperplasia is a precursor of endometrial carcinoma, an important malignancy that increases in incidence with age. Invasive cervical cancer (unlike carcinoma in situ) also increases in incidence with age, and can present with bleeding. Vulvar and vaginal cancer, though relatively uncommon, affect the elderly more commonly than the young. Uterine myomas are estrogen sensitive and tend to regress after the menopause, but these occasionally transform into sarcoma, a rare tumor that generally presents later in life.

A "benign" form of postmenopausal bleeding is atrophic vaginitis. This condition is characterized by atrophy, friability, and erosions, is due to an estrogen-depleted state, and is more likely to produce bleeding when there is trauma to the mucosa. This "trauma" in an older woman can be a speculum examination or sexual intercourse. Excoriations of the vulva can also cause bleeding; patients at risk are those with vulvar lichen sclerosus et atrophicus, an inflammatory condition that is more common in late life and is associated with atrophic epithelium (sometimes of "cigarette paper" appearance). Bleeding from excoriations may be particularly problematic in patients with dementia, especially if ordinary nail care is neglected.

Even if "benign" conditions, such as atrophic vaginitis or vulvar excoriations, are present, other causes of bleeding must be considered.

3. The next step is to examine the patient, first by digital examination and then with a speculum. The vulva should also be closely inspected for evidence of neoplasia, excoriations, or friable skin due to lichen sclerosus. Bleeding from the vaginal wall due to atrophic vaginitis is typically minimal if no trauma occurs. Atrophic epithelium appears pale, smooth, and shiny, and is often the result of longstanding estrogen deficiency. Atrophic vaginitis may be associated with introital stenosis and decreased vaginal depth, both predisposing to trauma during speculum examination.

This patient was found to have an incarcerated vaginal pessary (see Figure 15), which had been inserted prior to her admission to the nursing home. Thus, the device has been in place for 2 years at the very least. Vaginal pessaries are sometimes used in women who have limited activity or who refuse or are not candidates for surgery. Indications for a pessary may include stress incontinence, vaginal vault prolapse, cystocele, enterocele, rectocele, uterine prolapse, and as a temporizing measure prior to surgery.

4. Often, an incarcerated pessary can be removed manually without complications, but, if it does not come out readily, topical estrogen treatment for a few days may facilitate removal. Surgical intervention is usually not required.

The pessary can be inserted by a health professional or by the patient herself if able. Vaginal estrogen cream may improve the elderly patient's tolerance of the

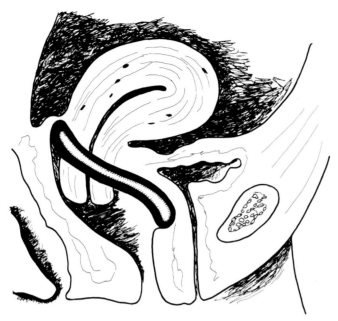

Figure 15   Pessary positioned in the vagina supports the uterus and surrounding structures.

pessary. However, most pessaries need to be removed, cleaned, and reinserted on a regular basis. An ignored pessary can become a nidus for infection, can become incarcerated, ulcerate, and even erode into adjacent organs. The healthcare provider who inserts a pessary must provide or arrange follow up care for the patient. As this case points out, pessaries should not be used in patients with poor cognitive function unless close follow up care is assured. Likewise, it highlights the need for routine vaginal examination of women upon admission to a long-term care facility.

The approach to vaginal bleeding in patients with dementia should be handled on an individual basis. Digital examination is usually warranted but further workup should be guided by weighing the burdens of investigations (such as transvaginal ultrasound or endometrial biopsy) and resulting treatments against any expected benefits.

Caveat

In postmenopausal women on hormone replacement therapy (HRT), abnormal bleeding is defined by what is expected to occur according to her specific HRT regimen. Sequential dosing delivers continuous estrogen during the cycle with progestin added for only 10–14 days. This method induces a monthly menstrual-like bleeding in most women. Continuous combined therapy includes a fixed dose of progestin daily in combination with estrogen. This results in atrophy of the endometrium and subsequent amenorrhea, so, except for minimal spotting in the first few months of treatment, bleeding requires evaluation.

BIBLIOGRAPHY

Gull, B., Carlsson, S. A., Karlsson, B. *et al.* (2000). Transvaginal ultrasound of the endometrium in women with postmenopausal bleeding: is it always necessary to perform an endometrial biopsy? *American Journal of Obstetrics and Gynecology*, **182**, 509–15.

Karlsson, B., Granberg, S., Wilkland, M. *et al.* (1995). Transvaginal ultrasonography of the endometrium in women with postmenopausal bleeding – a Nordic multicenter study. *American Journal of Obstetrics and Gynecology*, **172**, 1488–92.

Paley, P. J. (2001). Screening for major malignancies affecting women: current guidelines. *American Journal of Obstetrics and Gynecology*, **184**, 1021–30.

Rubin, S. C. (1987). Postmenopausal bleeding: etiology, evaluation, and management. *Medical Clinics of North America*, **71**, 59–69.

Viera, A. J. and Larkins-Pettigrew M. (2000). Practical use of the pessary. *American Family Physician*, **61**, 2719–29.

Case 37

▶▶ "Mother is not herself"

A 78-year-old woman with a history of left hip fracture develops intermittent pain in her right buttock, attributed to sciatica. Her fracture had been repaired with a hemiarthroplasty but she developed acetabular erosion and degenerative arthritis of the left hip. She has been treated with acetaminophen and ibuprofen for her pains and ambulates with difficulty, using a cane. She is now brought to the office by her daughter, who says her mother is "not herself." She is depressed, not eating, and complains all the time of "one thing or another . . . aches, pains, you name it." The patient concurs, and says, "I feel like an old woman." She has been feeling weak, has "pains all over," and can hardly get out of bed in the morning.

On physical examination, the patient is of average build and has a depressed affect. She has slight kyphosis and there is decreased range of motion of her left hip. There is tenderness of the right buttock in the distribution of the sciatic nerve but this pain is difficult to localize, as the patient winces often during the rheumatologic examination. Muscle strength seems to be diminished, but the patient does not appear to be making a true effort on testing. Wrist and knee joints are not red or swollen. She has Heberden's and Bouchard's nodes in the joints of both hands.

Blood tests are ordered and the patient is instructed to return in 2 weeks. Celocoxib is increased to 200 mg bid and nortriptyline 25 mg daily is added in an effort to treat the depressive symptoms and to "augment pain control."

Question

What is the differential diagnosis?

Case Studies in Geriatric Medicine, Judith C. Ahronheim *et al.* Published by Cambridge University Press.
© J. C. Ahronheim, Z.-B. Huang, V. Yen, C. M. Davitt, and D. Barile

Answer

The patient has a complex of symptoms which could be attributed to individual pathology, including degenerative arthritis of the left hip, sciatica, and a number of rheumatologic disorders, including osteoarthritis, rheumatoid arthritis, fibromyalgia, and polymyositis. However, her aches and pains, weakness, muscle tenderness, headaches, and depression are all strongly suggestive of polymyalgia rheumatica (PMR). This syndrome has many nonspecific features, and symptoms are commonly misdiagnosed as osteoarthritis or other rheumatologic disorders, are attributed to depression or "old age," or are overlooked if the symptoms are mingled with other rheumatologic signs and symptoms, as they are in this patient.

The clinical syndrome of PMR consists of pain and stiffness in the neck, shoulder, and pelvic girdles, sometimes accompanied by weight loss and fever. Morning stiffness is common, may be severe, and is similar to that seen in rheumatoid arthritis and some other collagen vascular diseases. Further questioning revealed that this patient had recently and rather abruptly developed a new set of symptoms – namely, proximal muscle weakness and morning stiffness. A focused examination revealed that most of the pain she experienced during the examination was due to muscle tenderness.

A week later, the patient's daughter calls to report that her mother has noticed "bumps on her head" and, on two occasions, complained of blurred vision in her right eye.

Questions

1. What is going on now?
2. How can the diagnosis be confirmed?
3. What treatment should be given?
4. How should the patient be followed for this condition?

Answers

1. Blurred vision raises the possibility that the patient has temporal arteritis (TA). PMR is sometimes accompanied by visual disturbances and other symptoms of TA, including headache and jaw claudication. PMR and TA are inflammatory conditions; in TA, inflammatory changes in medium- and large-sized arteries can occur anywhere in the body, so symptoms can be very varied. The onset of blurred vision

in a patient with symptoms of PMR is alarming because these could be premonitory signs of TA involving branches of the ophthalmic artery. Occlusion of the posterior ciliary artery, which nourishes the optic nerve head, can produce ischemic optic neuropathy and unilateral visual loss. This patient's two episodes of blurred vision suggest transient ischemia, which can also occur in TA, so immediate attention is required.

Involvement of other arteries can produce symptoms such as ear pain, hoarseness, respiratory disorders, and even stroke. There should always be a high index of suspicion of TA if an elderly person develops peculiar symptoms that are not explained by other pathology. On physical examination, this patient had scalp tenderness over the distribution of inflamed temporal arteries bilaterally, which she had noted as "bumps" on her head.

2. Although this patient has hip and buttock pain, her presentation is very typical for TA. A careful history and focused physical examination enable this diagnosis to be made clinically, but the workup should include an erythrocyte sedimentation rate (ESR) and, in suspected TA, a confirmatory temporal artery biopsy. Biopsy reveals granulomatous arteritis with giant cells, smooth muscle necrosis, destruction of internal elastic membrane, intimal fibrosis, and nonspecific inflammation. Other nonspecific laboratory abnormalities may occur, including anemia and elevated alkaline phosphatase. Inflammatory markers, such as interleukin-6, may be more sensitive than ESR (see Weyand *et al.*, 2000), but are generally not available in the primary care setting.

If the presentation includes tender, swollen temporal artery, greatly elevated ESR, and dramatic response to corticosteroids, many argue that a biopsy would not change the treatment and needs not be done. Others would argue that potentially dangerous treatment demands as much diagnostic certainty as possible; also, if there is any doubt about the diagnosis (e.g. a normal ESR or sudden visual loss without systemic symptoms), a biopsy should be done. However, biopsy may be negative, since pathology in the affected artery has "skip areas." Negative biopsy should not deter treatment if clinical suspicion is strong. Likewise, if TA is suspected, there is some risk of permanent visual loss, and corticosteroids should be started prior to obtaining the biopsy, which involves some delay.

3. Because of the likelihood that the patient has TA involving branches of the ophthalmic artery, high-dose corticosteroid treatment should be given, and biopsy can be scheduled. Prednisone 60 mg per day is a generally accepted initial treatment. In cases of actual visual loss, and because of the danger of damage to the other eye, high-dose intravenous corticosteroids are recommended – e.g. 250 mg of methylprednisolone administered slowly every 6 hours for 3–5 days, followed by oral corticosteroid therapy. Although not rigorously studied, a high-dose intravenous regimen may prevent additional visual loss in some patients (see Liu, 1994).

However, there is little evidence that this is more likely to reverse visual loss than oral corticosteroids.

Corticosteroid treatment is likely to reduce or eliminate systemic symptoms such as pains, weakness, and depression, within a day or two. This relief is quite dramatic, and persistence of symptoms should put the diagnosis in doubt. In elderly people, it is not uncommon for some symptoms to persist if they are due to unrelated pathology. In this case, the patient continued to have left hip pain from sequelae of her fracture. Her right buttock pain, which was due to radiculopathy, diminished somewhat. In total unilateral loss of vision, there is rarely a complete return of vision, although this patient's visual symptoms were consistent with transient ischemia rather than full-blown ischemic neuropathy. Her other symptoms resolved rapidly on oral corticosteroids and blurred vision did not recur. Nortriptyline was discontinued.

For patients with suspected TA but no visual disturbances, oral prednisone therapy 40–60 mg per day is recommended. Once clinical symptoms resolve and the ESR returns to normal (usually 2–4 weeks), steroid therapy is tapered slowly, with a dose reduction not to exceed 10% of the total daily dose every 2 weeks. During the taper, the patient must be closely monitored (see below).

In PMR without temporal arteritis, symptoms quickly resolve on small doses of oral corticosteroids – approximately 15–20 mg of prednisone per day. Typically, the response is dramatic, with symptoms improving within 48–72 hours after the initiation of therapy. Once symptoms are controlled, the dose is tapered slowly over several weeks.

4. Despite resolution of symptoms, many patients develop recurrent symptoms during taper or after discontinuation of corticosteroids. Once asymptomatic, patients should have close clinical monitoring with periodic determination of ESR, and should be treated if ESR starts to rise or – since ESR may not rise during relapse – if symptoms recur. Relapses are most likely to occur during the first 18 months of therapy and during the first year after cessation of therapy, but some patients experience relapse after many years.

Because of the tendency for corticosteroids to produce osteoporosis, patients who are expected to be taking corticosteroids for prolonged periods, regardless of age, should receive osteoporosis prophylaxis. This issue is discussed further in Case 25.

Caveats

1. Because of the "skipping" nature of TA, biopsy segments are obtained serially along the temporal artery unless there are localizing signs of inflammation. If the biopsy

results are negative but TA is still strongly suspected, biopsy of the opposite side is recommended. Biopsies may remain positive for approximately 7 days into the course of steroid therapy, and sometimes longer.

2. ESR is not always elevated in PMR or TA. In one small study of biopsy-proven TA, 24% of patients had a normal ESR at the time of diagnosis (Weyand *et al.*, 2000). Additional patients may have a normal ESR that later rises or may fail to show an increase in ESR during a clinical relapse. Explanations for low or normal ESR in PMR and TA include technical reasons, such as low temperature or delay in processing blood, and hypofibrinogenemia, which may decrease the ESR by decreasing rouleaux formation and sedimentation. Additionally, prior glucocorticoid use may lower the ESR at presentation.

REFERENCES

Liu, G. T. (1994). Visual morbidity in giant cell arteritis. Clinical characteristics and prognosis for vision. *Ophthalmology*, **101**, 1779–85.

Weyand, C. M., Fulbright, J. W., Hunder, G. G. *et al.* (2000). Treatment of giant cell arteritis: interleukin-6 as a biologic marker of disease activity. *Arthritis and Rheumatism*, **43**, 1041–8.

BIBLIOGRAPHY

Gonzalez-Gay, M. A., Blanco, R., Rodriguez-Valverde, V. *et al.* (1988). Permanent visual loss and cerebrovascular accidents in giant cell arteritis: predictors and response to treatment. *Arthritis and Rheumatism*, **41**, 1497–504.

Hazleman, B. (2000). Laboratory investigations useful in the evaluation of polymyalgia rheumatica and giant cell arteritis. *Clinical and Experimental Rheumatology*, **18**, S29–31.

Salvarani, C. and Hunder, G. G. (2001). Giant cell arteritis with low erythrocyte sedimentation rate: frequency of occurrence in a population-based study. *Arthritis Care and Research*, **45**, 140–5.

Salvarani, C., Cantini, F., Boiardi, L. *et al.* (2002). Polymyalgia rheumatica and giant-cell arteritis. *New England Journal of Medicine*, **347**, 261–71.

Weyand, C. M. and Goronzy, J. J. (2003). Giant-cell arteritis and polymyalgia rheumatica. *Annals of Internal Medicine*, **139**, 505–15.

Case 38

▸▸ "Failure to thrive"

An 89-year-old man comes to your office complaining of "fuzziness." The symptoms began soon after taking his morning medications, and, although he gradually felt better throughout the day, he has noted sweating, chills, and back pain. He took his temperature, which was normal.

The patient has a history of prostate cancer, which was diagnosed 8 years ago on the basis of a markedly elevated prostate-specific antigen (PSA) of 50 ng/ml. He was treated with radiation of the prostate, and he also receives an injection of leuprolide every 6 weeks, which cause him "annoying sweats." He has had episodes of dizziness in the past, but his current symptoms are dissimilar. He has a history of coronary artery disease, and a permanent pacemaker was implanted 5 years ago for syncope related to atrial flutter. He also has a history of recurrent low back pain, which has been attributed to degenerative disc disease, and a recent workup has shown no evidence of metastatic disease to the spine or elsewhere. He also has a history of fecal impaction; stool guaiacs have been normal and colonoscopy has been scheduled.

In addition to leuprolide, the patient takes diltiazem 180 mg, amiodarone 200 mg, warfarin 4 mg, isosorbide mononitrate 20 mg, and pravachol 20 mg daily, plus laxatives as needed.

On physical examination, the patient is alert and interactive. He weighs 150 pounds, which is unchanged from his previous examination a few weeks ago. Blood pressure is 160/60 supine and sitting. Pulse is 60 and regular. Lungs are clear. There is a short systolic murmur at the left sternal border with a musical quality; the murmur has been present on previous examinations. Electrocardiogram shows sinus rhythm with some paced beats, and is unchanged. Blood tests are done and the patient is reassured and sent home. White blood count is normal; hemoglobin is unchanged at 11.8 gm/dl ($n = 11.4-16.7$), and international normalized rate (INR) is 2.4.

Case Studies in Geriatric Medicine, Judith C. Ahronheim *et al.* Published by Cambridge University Press.
© J. C. Ahronheim, Z.-B. Huang, V. Yen, C. M. Davitt, and D. Barile

On follow up 1 month later, the patient reports he had a slight cough, sore throat, a temperature of 100 °F, and myalgias earlier in the week. The cough and sore throat have cleared up, but he feels weak and complains of pain in his neck and lower back. On examination, he looks a bit tired but perks up when engaged in conversation and jokes readily. Blood pressure is 140/60 supine, 130/58 sitting, and pulse is 64 and regular. Oral temperature is 98 °F. His weight is 146 pounds. Throat looks normal and lungs are clear on auscultation. There is pain in the right side of the neck on palpation and on lateral movement. There is no muscle weakness or tenderness, and the physician's impression is that the patient is recovering from a viral syndrome and has deconditioning superimposed on his "usual enhanced sensitivity to illness." He encourages the patient to eat and drink and call if there are more problems. He prescribes acetaminophen and orders stool for occult blood, X-rays of the cervical spine and chest, and blood tests. Repeat complete blood count shows a normal white blood cell count with "no toxic appearing lymphocytes." Hemoglobin is 10.4 g/dl, hematocrit 30.3% ($n = 33.5–49.0$), and mean corpuscular volume (MCV), platelet count, and creatine kinase are normal. Additional blood tests are ordered.

The patient returns 2 weeks later, accompanied by his wife. He continues to feel weak and complains of cold intolerance and his wife states he has "not been well" for several weeks and doesn't have a good appetite. The patient says his temperature at home has been 98–99 °F, but his wife says it was "almost 101° yesterday." Now the oral temperature is 98.3 °F, blood pressure is 146/80, pulse is 60 and regular. His weight is 144 pounds. He appears pale but there is no icterus. Heart and lung examination are unchanged. There is minimal tenderness over the lumbar spine and paraspinal muscles. There is no leg edema. Cervical spine X-rays which were done 1 week before show arthritic changes and reversal of the normal lordotic curve, but no fracture or osteolytic or osteoblastic lesions. Chest X-ray shows cardiomegaly and prominent pulmonary vasculature but no infiltrates or nodules. Three stool guaiacs are negative. Serum iron and total iron-binding capacity (TIBC) are low, ferritin is 45 μg/l ($n = 20–380$), and B12 is 586 ng/l ($n = 200–1100$). Serum protein electrophoresis shows polyclonal gammopathy and albumin of 2.9 gm/dl ($n = 3.5–5.0$). Erythrocyte sedimentation rate (ESR) is 40 mm/h ($n = 0–20$), and serum creatinine is 1.4 mg/dl. Urinalysis shows 1+ protein but no other abnormalities.

The physician is troubled by the patient's nonspecific symptoms and weight loss, and admits him to the hospital with the diagnosis of "failure to thrive."

Questions

1. What could be causing the patient's "failure to thrive?"
2. What aspects of the physical examination are particularly important in this patient?
3. What is the significance of the patient's anemia?

Answers

1. "Failure to thrive" is a term commonly applied to elderly patients who have weight loss, weakness, or other symptoms of inanition that do not point to a specific organ system. However, such presentations require close attention, as remediable problems are often at their source. Common causes of nonspecific presentations in the elderly include cancer, depression, hyperthyroidism, and tuberculosis, and all need to be considered in this patient. Progression of cancer would be important to consider, given his past history, and his history of fecal impaction should direct investigation to a possible bowel malignancy. Thyroid disease should be considered, especially given his treatment with amiodarone, and tuberculosis should always be considered in an elderly person with weight loss or recurrent fever. These conditions, as well as atypical presentations, are discussed elsewhere in this volume (see Cases 15, 30, and 40).

   On admission, chest X-ray showed increased pulmonary vascular congestion suggesting congestive heart failure, which raised the possibility of a cardiac cause of his problem and blood cultures were ordered. Blood cultures grew gram-positive streptococci in pairs and chains in six out of six bottles, and intravenous antibiotics were begun. Transesophageal echocardiogram (TEE) confirmed endocarditis of the mitral valve.

   Bacterial endocarditis in the elderly may present with altered mental status, weight loss, anorexia, myalgias, uremia, and fever of unknown origin, but, as in this patient, fever may be attenuated (see Case 41). Septic cerebral emboli are sometimes misdiagnosed as strokes of atherosclerotic origin. Although these presentations may occur in younger adults, nonspecific symptoms may result in misdiagnosis in the elderly because of their subtlety as well as their resemblance to other common diseases of late life.

   Intravenous antibiotics were begun. Three days later, while reading the newspaper, the patient noticed a partial cut in his left field of vision. He had no other neurologic signs or symptoms and INR remained in the therapeutic range. The deficit was attributed to septic embolization.

2. A careful search should be made for the source of the infection. Sites of infection in the elderly that are commonly overlooked include the mouth, toes, skin, abdomen, and pelvis. Skin ulcers, cellulitis, osteomyelitis, smouldering gallbladder disease, and other genitourinary and gastrointestinal disease may all lead to bacteremia and endocarditis. This patient had a cardiac pacemaker, but there was no redness, swelling, or tenderness of the chest wall and no evidence of pacemaker wire involvement on TEE. Pacemaker endocarditis is uncommon but should be considered, even years after pacemaker insertion (see Laguno *et al.*, 1998). Dental caries in the elderly may be far advanced before pain occurs, and often form on the root surface, which is probably related to gingival recession; however, dental source of infection tends to be a less common source of endocarditis in elderly patients compared with younger adults (see Tomas-Carmona *et al.*, 2003). This patient had no recent dental work, although he did have gingival recession and a partial denture; the denture was removed for the examination, but no disease was obvious to the internist.

The patient's organism was identified as *Streptococcus bovis*, which is more commonly seen in elderly than younger adult patients with endocarditis. It is often associated with colonic cancer and other gastrointestinal neoplasms, but has been associated with other possible portals of entry. This patient's colonoscopy revealed hemorrhoids, severe diverticulosis of the sigmoid and descending colon, and four sessile polyps, which were excised endoscopically. Biopsy showed tubulovillous adenoma of one polyp in the cecum. An occasional complication of *S. bovis* bacteremia pertinent to this patient is spondylitis, which again is more common in the elderly. Despite his musculoskeletal symptoms, he had no evidence of vertebral or disc infection.

3. Normal values for hemoglobin and hematocrit do not change with age. The patient's mild normochromic normocytic anemia was consistent with anemia of chronic disease, as would be expected in subacute bacterial endocarditis. However, iron deficiency, a hypochromic microcytic anemia, cannot be ruled out in elderly patients with normal red blood cell (RBC) indices and would have been an important consideration in this patient despite his negative stool guaiacs. Measures of iron status are unreliable in patients with acute or chronic illness and are particularly unreliable in the elderly. TIBC is often low in elderly patients with iron deficiency anemia. TIBC is a measure of binding sites in circulating transferrin, and depends on adequate protein status (see Case 7). Moreover, iron is required for protein synthesis, which may be impaired in elderly patients, particularly in the setting of disease. Serum ferritin rises with age, since iron stores tend to increase with age. In addition, ferritin exists in many tissues and can be released rapidly into

the serum when there is tissue disruption, such as inflammation, and a "low–normal" serum ferritin might actually indicate critically low iron stores. This patient's polyclonal gammopathy and elevated ESR reflected inflammation of his infection. Serum iron is always low when marrow stores are absent, but can be low when stores are abundant because it is not released by the bone marrow in chronic disease.

B12 deficiency, which is associated with macrocytic anemia, cannot be ruled out on the basis of a normal MCV. Mixed microcytic and macrocytic anemias are common in the elderly, and, at any age, anemia is often associated with anisocytosis (mixed populations of large and small red cells), with MCV reflecting the average RBC diameter. Serum B12 levels are often low in older patients, despite the absence of anemia or other abnormalities. This patient's serum B12 level was well within the normal range.

Caveats

1. Elderly patients with unexplained anemia, with or without associated symptoms, sometimes are found to have myelodysplastic syndrome. This condition increases in incidence with age and is the most common hematologic malignancy among the elderly. Patients whose disease is discovered incidentally do not necessarily need treatment as elderly patients with specific "low-risk" bone marrow findings are likely to die of unrelated causes. However, because myelodysplasia can lead to significant anemia or acute myeloid leukemia, patients with unexplained anemia should be followed closely and bone marrow performed, if appropriate.

2. The standard Schilling test, which measures absorption of free cobalamin, may fail to detect food cobalamin malabsorption in the elderly. Full-blown autoimmune atrophic gastritis is not usually the cause of this subtle malabsorption, which is due to age-related atrophic gastritis and its associated hypochlorhydria. Since acid is required for the release of cobalamin from food, many elderly patients cannot extract vitamin B12 from dietary sources, although they would be able to absorb free cobalamin given in the Schilling test. A "food Schilling test" has been devised in order to overcome this problem, but neither this nor the standard Schilling test is often used today because they are cumbersome and the diagnosis is generally made with serum measurements of homocysteine and methylmalonic acid. Unfortunately, in elderly patients, there is uncertainty over whether elevations in these tests imply vitamin deficiency or represent false-positive results.

3. The incidence of root (cervical) caries increases markedly with age. Root caries are distinguished from coronal caries by their location, and often go unnoticed unless a specific examination is made of this location. Gingival recession exposes

the root surface of teeth to the oral environment, making the surface suscept-ible to destructive lesions. Dental care in the United States has improved to the extent that increasing numbers of older adults retain their teeth. Along with this dental longevity has come an increase in the prevalence of gingival recession. Age and gingival recession are the major risk factors in the development of root caries.

REFERENCES

Laguno, M., Miro, O., and Font, C. (1998). Pacemaker-related endocarditis. Report of 7 cases and review of the literature. *Cardiology*, **90**, 244–8.

Tomas Carmona, I., Limeres Posse, J., Diz Dios, P. *et al.* (2003). Bacterial endocarditis of oral etiology in an elderly population. *Archives of Gerontology and Geriatrics*, **36**, 49–55.

BIBLIOGRAPHY

Anaf, V., Noel, J. C., Thys, J. P. *et al.* (2001). A first case of *Streptococcus bovis* bacteremia and peritonitis from endometrial cancer origin. *Acta Chirurgica Belgica*, **1011**, 38–9.

Carmel, R., Sinow, R. M., Siegel, M. E. *et al.* (1988). Food cobalamin malabsorption occurs frequently in patients with unexplained low serum cobalamin levels. *Archives of Internal Medicine*, **148**, 1715–19.

Dhawan, V. K. (2002). Infective endocarditis in elderly patients. *Clinical Infectious Diseases*, **34**, 806–12.

Green R. (1996). Screening for vitamin B12 deficiency: caveat emptor. *Annals of Internal Medicine*, **125**, 509–11.

Guyatt, G. H., Patterson, C., Ali, M. *et al.* (1990). Diagnosis of iron-deficiency anemia in the elderly. *American Journal of Medicine*, **88**, 205–9.

Heiro, M., Nikoskelainen, J., Engblom, E. *et al.* (2000). Neurologic manifestations of infective endocarditis: a 17-year experience in a teaching hospital in Finland. *Archives of Internal Medicine*, **160**, 2781–7.

Loh, K. C. (2000). Amiodarone induced thyroid disorders: a clinical review. *Postgraduate Medical Journal*, **76**, 133–40.

Moreillon, P. and Que, Y. A. (2004). Infective endocarditis. *Lancet*, **363**, 139–49.

Pergola, V., Di Salvo, G., Habib, G. *et al.* (2001). Comparison of clinical and echocar-diographic characteristics of *Streptococcus bovis* endocarditis with that caused by other pathogens. *American Journal of Cardiology*, **88**, 871–5.

Rimon, E., Levy, S., Sapir, A. *et al.* (2002). Diagnosis of iron deficiency anemia in the elderly by transferrin receptor-ferritin index. *Archives of Internal Medicine*, **162**, 445–9.

Sarkisian, C. A. and Lachs, M. S. (1996). Failure to thrive in older adults. *Annals of Internal Medicine*, **124**, 1072–8.

Seichter, U. (1987). Root surface caries: a critical literature review. *Journal of the American Dental Association*, **115**, 305–10.

Sharma, J. C. and Ray, S. N. (1984). Value of serum ferritin as an index of iron deficiency in elderly anemia patients. *Age and Ageing*, **13**, 248–50.

Songy, W. B., Ruoff, K. L., Facklam, R. R. *et al.* (2002). Identification of *Streptococcus bovis* biotype I strains among *S. bovis* clinical isolates by PCR. *Journal of Clinical Microbiology*, **40**, 2913–18.

Thomson, W. B. (2004). Dental caries experience in older people over time: what can the large cohort studies tell us? *British Dental Journal*, **196**, 89–92.

Williamson, P. J., Kruger, A. R., Reynolds, P. J. *et al.* (1994). Establishing the incidence of myelodysplastic syndrome. *British Journal of Haematology*, **87**, 743–5.

Case 39

▶▶ Three hospitalized patients with agitation

Mrs. T

Mrs. T, an 89-year-old woman with dementia, was admitted to the hospital for control of agitation. Eight months prior to admission, she sustained a hip fracture, underwent surgical repair, and was able to return home, although she required the care of a live-in attendant. Three months later, she was noted to be agitated and was treated with lorazepam. Agitation continued and the dose was gradually increased to 0.5 mg qid. Trazodone 50 mg per day was added with no effect.

On admission, Mrs. T was said to be "crying, yelling, and babbling." She was thin, frail appearing, and reportedly did not cooperate during an attempt at a physical examination because she became agitated and thrashed about when approached. She was able to walk about with assistance, but screamed intermittently.

Trazodone and lorazepam were continued. Haloperidol 0.5 mg was given without effect and the dose was increased to 1 mg.

Questions

1. What could account for the lack of efficacy of Mrs. T's medications?
2. What factors might have led to the misdiagnosis?

Answers

1. Although sedating medications may reduce agitation and aggressiveness in patients with dementia, they are not always effective. Lorazepam and other benzodiazepines produce disinhibition and can, paradoxically, increase agitation in patients with

Case Studies in Geriatric Medicine, Judith C. Ahronheim *et al.* Published by Cambridge University Press.
© J. C. Ahronheim, Z.-B. Huang, V. Yen, C. M. Davitt, and D. Barile

dementia. Trazodone is an antidepressant medication with sedating properties and, although sometimes useful, would not be expected to reduce agitation in severe cases. Haloperidol and other neuroleptics may reduce agitation that is produced by frightening hallucinations or delusions, but, if agitation has a different cause, doses high enough to produce deep sedation might be needed to reduce agitation.

Mrs. T was not adequately evaluated to determine an underlying cause of agitation. Loud screams are not typical in agitation due to impaired cognition or psychiatric disturbances in dementia, and a painful condition should be strongly considered in this patient. Although she did not cooperate fully for a full examination, a cursory examination revealed a large, rock-hard mass in her left breast, and a large mass in the left axilla of similar consistency. Her agitation was markedly exacerbated when her left arm was moved and evaluation of her admission chest X-ray revealed a lytic lesion in the left proximal humerus suggesting metastatic cancer.

Opioid analgesics were given and her agitation improved markedly.

2. This case illustrates the common failure of clinicians to interpret nonverbal expressions of pain in patients with dementia and other neurologic impairments. Such patients may not be able to express specific symptoms in the same way as a normal adult, and agitated behaviors may be the manifestation of a number of diseases. The inability to articulate the cause of pain or discomfort often leads to underdiagnosis and undertreatment of pain, and, in dementia, agitation is mistakenly assumed to be related to dementia alone. A poorly tested assumption exists that aging and dementia are associated with diminished pain perception.

Mr. U

Mr. U is an 80-year-old man with progressive supranuclear palsy (PSP) who is admitted to the hospital for treatment of urosepsis. After a stormy course, which included several days in the intensive care unit, he improves. He is able to eat and drink when fed, although he requires frequent, small feeds throughout the day.

Prior to his acute illness, Mr. U was wheelchair bound, and had difficulty communicating because of very severe dysarthria and slow, virtually unintelligible verbal responses. At this point, in consultation with his family, a decision is made to avoid further invasive treatments, a "comfort care plan" is instituted, and discharge to a nursing home is planned.

After several days, he begins to appear uncomfortable and is seen rubbing his abdomen. Abdominal examination is unrevealing. Fentanyl transdermal patch is instituted. The patient's discomfort persists and he begins to appear agitated. "Rescue" doses of oxycodone are given to supplement the transdermal opioid, and sedation is considered.

Question

What could be causing Mr. U's agitation?

Answer

The prior decision to institute "comfort care" may have encouraged Mr. U's physicians (unlike Mrs. T's physicians) to consider pain management, but again there was a failure to diagnose the cause of the problem. The evaluation of a patient who has difficulty communicating must include a complete, directed physical examination, with particular attention to often neglected aspects, such as evidence of injury, skin inflammation or disruption, contractures that could cause pain, evidence of bladder distention, and any pathology in the feet, heels, and mouth. Sometimes weak or immobile patients are extremely uncomfortable when they cannot change their position in a bed or chair and exhibit significant relief when others assist them in changing their position.

Review of nursing notes revealed that Mr. U had not moved his bowels in more than 1 week, and the patient confirmed this by nodding when he was asked. His immobility elevated his risk for constipation and he developed a fecal impaction, which was worsened by opioids. Manual disimpaction and enemas relieved his discomfort and analgesics were not needed.

Miss. V

Miss. V, an 85-year-old woman with Alzheimer's disease, is hospitalized for cellulitis and is treated with intravenous antibiotics. She is instructed not to get out of bed without assistance, but at night she begins to climb out of bed and a vest restraint is applied. "I have to go to the bathroom," the patient says, and the nurse explains that she has an indwelling catheter and does not need to use the toilet.

Half an hour later, the nurse sees that Miss. V has become tangled in her restraint in an apparent effort to get out of bed and she appears to be pulling out her intravenous line. Wrist restraints are applied and haloperidol 0.5 mg is given but her agitation continues.

Questions

1. Why is Miss. V agitated?
2. What alternatives to her management exist?

Answers

1. Although it is tempting to conclude that this patient is agitated because she has dementia, her agitation results from specific responses that dementia creates. She is unfamiliar with the hospital environment and at home is used to getting out of bed to go to the bathroom at night; she cannot remember the instructions to stay in bed; she is annoyed by the unfamiliar device in her arm; the indwelling catheter produces urethral irritation which she interprets as the need to urinate; she is tied by a restraint and has the natural reaction to try to get rid of it; and she is further restrained at the wrist which likely frightens her and worsens her agitation. This common scenario occurs frequently in the hospital setting and often leads to serious morbidity.

2. Any unnecessary or painful device should be removed. This would include the mechanical restraints, which will merely worsen Miss. V's agitation and could cause injury, and the bladder catheter, for which there does not appear to be an indication (see Cases 33 and 34). If Miss. V has urinary frequency from detrusor instability, timed voiding with assistance from staff will reduce her need to get out of bed. The intravenous line can be covered with a secure bandage, which acts as a camouflage. Oral antibiotics should be substituted if possible.

   Interpersonal methods should be used whenever possible. A family member or volunteer should be enlisted to engage and distract the patient, and to remind her that she is in the hospital being treated for an infection. If this is not possible, it is helpful to seat the patient in a reclining chair near the nurse's station where available staff can observe and interact with her.

   Sedatives should be strictly avoided in these situations. Neuroleptics themselves may produce akathisia, a state of restlessness and constant change in position. Akathisia is often misinterpreted as agitation, leading to increase rather than decrease in the neuroleptic dose, with consequent worsening of restlessness. Benzodiazepines, even in small doses, can produce severe sedation, leading to falls, aspiration, or deconditioning.

BIBLIOGRAPHY

Ferrell, B. A., Ferrell, B. R., and Rivera, L. (1995). Pain in cognitively impaired nursing home patients. *Journal of Pain and Symptom Management*, **10**, 591–5.

Frampton, M. (2003). Experience assessment and management of pain in people with dementia. *Age and Aging*, **32**, 248–51.

Huffman, J. C. and Kunik, M. E. (2000). Assessment and understanding of pain in patients with dementia. *Gerontologist*, **40**, 574–81.

Jonsson, C. O., Malhammar, G., and Waldton, S. (1977). Reflex elicitation thresholds in senile dementia. *Acta Psychiatrica Scandinavica*, **55**, 81–96.

Krulewitch, H., London, M. R., Skakel, V. J. *et al.* (2000). Assessment of pain in cognitively impaired older adults: a comparison of pain assessment tools and their use by nonprofessional caregivers. *Journal of the American Geriatrics Society*, **48**, 1607–11.

Manfredi, P. L., Breuer, B., Meier, D. E. *et al.* (2003). Pain assessment in elderly patients with severe dementia. *Journal of Pain and Symptom Management*, **225**, 48–52.

McCormick, W. C., Kukill, W. A., Belle, G. *et al.* (1994). Symptom patterns and comorbidity in the early stages of Alzheimer's disease. *Journal of the American Geriatrics Society*, **42**, 517–21.

Parmelee, P. A., Smith, B., and Katz, I. R. (1993). Pain complaints and cognitive status among elderly institution residents. *Journal of the American Geriatrics Society*, **41**, 517–22.

Teri, L., Logsdon, R. G., and McCurry, S. M. (2002). Nonpharmacological treatment of behavioral disturbance in dementia. *Medical Clinics of North America*, **86**, 641–56.

Teri, L., Logsdon, R. G., Peskind, E. *et al.* (2000). Treatment of agitation in Alzheimer's disease: a randomized, placebo-controlled trial. *Neurology*, **55**, 1271–8.

Case 40

►► Weight loss

An 80-year-old man visits his doctor complaining that he has been constipated for 1 week. When he moved his bowels, there was blood on the toilet tissue but he had no other gastrointestinal symptoms or prior history of severe constipation. He admits to anorexia for several weeks, has been unable to sleep, and thinks he has lost "a lot of weight." The patient has a history of systolic heart murmur and colonic polyps, and was recently diagnosed as having systolic hypertension for which hydrochlorothiazide was prescribed.

He has no history of surgery, psychiatric illness, blood transfusions, or drug or alcohol abuse. He denies fevers, palpitations, and cough, but has recently had two episodes of substernal pain radiating to the left arm, which he feels were brought on by anxiety. Electrocardiogram (EKG) during these episodes revealed left ventricular hypertrophy by voltage criteria, and was unchanged from previous EKGs.

On physical examination, the patient has kyphosis and appears extremely underweight. Blood pressure is 120/80. Pulse is 88 and regular. His thyroid gland is not palpable. There is no proptosis. Lungs are clear. There is a grade II/VI systolic ejection murmur heard at the base, without radiation. Abdomen is scaphoid; no masses are felt. Rectal examination is normal, and stool is guaiac negative. The patient weighs 120 pounds, 14 pounds less than 3 months before.

Chest X-ray revealed no infiltrates. Blood tests are sent and a colonoscopy is scheduled.

Case Studies in Geriatric Medicine, Judith C. Ahronheim *et al.* Published by Cambridge University Press.
© J. C. Ahronheim, Z.-B. Huang, V. Yen, C. M. Davitt, and D. Barile

Questions

1. What is the differential diagnosis?
2. What accounts for the patient's constipation? Kyphosis? Heart murmur? Overall presentation?
3. How should this condition be managed?

Answers

1. Weight loss in older adults of any age can be due to a number of conditions, including malignancy (often in the gastrointestinal tract), other gastrointestinal illness, endocrinologic disease, such as diabetes mellitus and hyperthyroidism, and psychologic factors. Tuberculosis may present with weight loss and failure to thrive, but is unlikely in the absence of fever, cough, or an abnormal chest X-ray. In the setting of constipation and rectal bleeding, colorectal cancer should be strongly considered in this patient.

   This patient underwent colonoscopy which revealed internal hemorrhoids and no masses. His laboratory studies were consistent with hyperthyroidism: free T_4 of 2.4 ng/dl ($n = 0.7$–1.8) and thyroid-stimulating hormone (TSH) of <0.03 mU/l ($n = 0.40$–5.50). Hyperthyroidism is an important cause of weight loss and, when it presents in late life, the classic signs of hyperthyroidism, such as goiter and exophthalmos as seen in Graves's disease, are uncommon. The patient's radioactive iodine uptake was "low–normal," but the scan revealed two demarcated areas in the left lobe intensely concentrating the radiopharmaceutical and suppressing the right lobe, and was considered to be diagnostic of hyperfunctioning nodules. The thyroid scan in Graves's disease would show diffuse and homogeneous uptake, usually elevated at 24 hours.

2. Although diuretic therapy might have been a contributing factor, the constipation was due to hyperthyroidism, and it resolved when the hyperthyroidism was treated. More than 20% of elderly hyperthyroid patients present with constipation, rather than classic symptoms of diarrhea or hyperdefecation. The mechanism is not known, but may be related to the increased number of beta-adrenergic receptors that accompany hyperthyroidism. The increased beta sensitivity of gut smooth muscle would result in relaxation and inhibition of motility and, perhaps, constipation if the gut were predisposed. The tendency for healthy elderly to develop constipation may partly explain this phenomenon.

Kyphosis due to osteoporosis is less common in elderly men than in women. However, hyperthyroidism can accelerate bone loss and could have been a contributing factor in this patient, depending on the duration. Causes of secondary osteoporosis in men are discussed in detail in Case 25.

Hyperthyroidism can produce a flow murmur or accentuate an existing murmur, but this patient's heart murmur antedated the onset of hyperthyroidism by years. Approximately 80% of 80-year-olds have systolic murmurs (see Case 2).

Absence of goiter may be related to age-related decrease in size of the thyroid, and difficulty palpating a gland which is situated below the clavicle owing to thoracic deformity, such as kyphosis. Furthermore, Graves's disease accounts for a smaller proportion of hyperthyroidism cases in the elderly, whereas multinodular goiter or a solitary nodule are more common. However, among older patients with Graves's disease, a goiter is not palpable in the majority (see Diez, 2003).

Atypical presentations of hyperthyroidism in the elderly may be due to the presence of subclinical disease in at least one organ system, with the most vulnerable organ "hit" first. For example, the most apparent presenting symptom in a patient with cardiovascular disease might be atrial fibrillation or congestive heart failure, while confusion or apathy might be prominent in a patient with central nervous system disease.

Tachycardia, weight loss, and apathy are the most common signs of hyperthyroidism in the elderly. Approximately 15% of hyperthyroid patients over the age of 60 present with the triad of weight loss, anorexia, and constipation, the "gastrointestinal" presentation described in this case. Compared with younger adults with hyperthyroidism, older patients more frequently have anorexia and atrial fibrillation, and less frequently have hyperactive reflexes, tremor, heat intolerance, sweating, increased appetite, and nervousness.

A large proportion of hyperthyroid patients over 75 do not have tachycardia. This may be because of underlying conduction system disease or concurrent use of negative chronotropic medications.

3. Antithyroid agents such as the thionamides propylthiouracil (PTU) and methimazole are often given prior to radioactive iodine, since radiation-induced thyroiditis with a transient rise in thyroid hormone levels may occur shortly after radioactive iodine treatment and could be harmful to someone with underlying cardiac disease. Thionamides act by blocking iodine uptake and organification, so they must be discontinued several days before radioiodine administration, at which time a significant rise in thyroid hormone levels may occur. The clinical significance of this is probably minimal, but beta-blockers are also generally given to relieve or prevent symptoms of sympathetic discharge such as tremor, anxiety, and palpitations, until the patient is euthyroid. Although beta-blockers can inhibit

deiodinase activity and reduce conversion of T4 to T3, this effect may be also clinically negligible. Interestingly, this patient's constipation was relieved shortly after propranolol was instituted.

Methimazole is generally preferred over PTU in the elderly because it can be administered once daily and appears to have a lower incidence of agranulocytosis. However, long-term use of these antithyroid medications is associated with a higher rate of agranulocytosis (0.3%) than in younger adults, so radioactive iodine (RAI) is the preferred treatment, especially in toxic nodular disease, which does not remit after thionamide therapy. RAI is also more cost effective. The disadvantage of definitive treatment with RAI is that, if the patient is lost to follow up, secondary hypothyroidism may go undetected until serious problems develop.

Caveats

1. The antiarrhythmic agent amiodarone, widely used for both ventricular and atrial arrhythmias, contains 37% iodine and causes overt thyroid dysfunction in 14–18% of patients, both hyper- and hypothyroidism. The hyperthyroidism can be caused by the iodine load itself, usually in a gland with pre-existing abnormalities, or by a destructive thyroiditis accompanied by very high serum interleukin-6 levels.
2. The presence of a tremor in an elderly person is a nonspecific sign, and any kind of tremor can be accentuated by hyperthyroidism. The careful observer can note, however, that uncomplicated "senile" essential tremor has a lower frequency and greater amplitude than hyperthyroid tremor. Parkinsonian tremor is, likewise, different in quality and occurs in conjunction with other physical signs.
3. "Subclinical" hyperthyroidism – a suppressed TSH but normal T4 and T3 levels – is technically an asymptomatic condition, but research has shown it is associated with a 3-fold increase in atrial fibrillation risk over 10 years, accelerated bone loss, and, possibly, greater overall mortality. Further research is needed to determine if treatment of the chemical abnormalities alone reduces morbidity and mortality.

REFERENCE

Diez, J. J. (2003). Hyperthyroidism in patients older than 55 years: an analysis of the etiology and management. *Gerontology*, **49**, 316–23.

BIBLIOGRAPHY

Attia, J., Margetts, P., and Guyatt, G. (1999). Diagnosis of thyroid disease in hospitalized patients. *Archives of Internal Medicine*, **159**, 658–65.

Bauer, D. C., Ettinger, B., and Browner, W. S. (1998). Thyroid function and serum lipids in older women. A population based study. *American Journal of Medicine*, **104**, 546–51.

Bilezikian, J. P. and Loeb, J. N. (1983). The influence of hyperthyroidism and hypothyroidism on alpha- and beta-adrenergic receptor systems and adrenergic responsiveness. *Endocrine Reviews*, **4**, 378–88.

Cooper, D. S. (1998). Subclinical thyroid disease: a clinician's perspective. *Annals of Internal Medicine*, **129**, 135–8.

Greenspan, S. L. and Greenspan, F. S. (1999). Effect of thyroid hormone on skeletal integrity. *Annals of Internal Medicine*, **130**, 750–8.

Hak, A. E., Pols, H. A., van Hemert, A. M. *et al.* (2000). Subclinical hypothyroidism is an independent risk factor for atherosclerosis and myocardial infarction in elderly women: the Rotterdam study. *Annals of Internal Medicine*, **132**, 270–8.

Helfand, M. and Redfern, C. C. (1998). Clinical Guideline, Part 2. Screening for thyroid disease: an update – American College of Physicians. *Annals of Internal Medicine*, **129**, 144–58.

Jaeschke, R., Guyatt, G., Gerstein, H. *et al.* (1996). Does treatment with L-thyroxine influence health status in middle aged and older adults with subclinical hypothyroidism? *Journal of General Internal Medicine*, **11**, 744–9.

Klein, I. and Ojamaa, K. (2001). Thyroid hormone and the cardiovascular system. *New England Journal of Medicine*, **344**, 501–9.

Lankisch, P. G., Gerzmann, M., Gerzmann, J. F. *et al.* (2001). Unintentional weight loss: diagnosis and prognosis. The first prospective follow-up study from a secondary referral center. *Journal of Internal Medicine*, **249**, 41–6.

Martino, E., Bartalena, L., Bogazzi, F. *et al.* (2001). The effects of amiodarone on the thyroid. *Endocrine Reviews*, **22**, 240–54.

Mokshagundam, S. and Barzel, U. S. (1993). Thyroid disease in the elderly. *Journal of the American Geriatrics Society*, **41**, 1361–9.

Sawin, C. T., Geller, A., Wolf, P. A. *et al.* (1994). Low serum thyrotropin concentration as a risk factor for atrial fibrillation in older persons. *New England Journal of Medicine*, **331**, 1249–52.

Toft, A. D. (2001). Subclinical hyperthyroidism. *New England Journal of Medicine*, **345**, 512–16.

Trivalle, C., Doucet, J., Chassagne, P. *et al.* (1996). Differences in the signs and symptoms of hyperthyroidism in older and younger patients. *Journal of the American Geriatrics Society*, **44**, 50–3.

Woeber, K. A. (2000). Update on the management of hyperthyroidism and hypothyroidism. *Archives of Internal Medicine*, **160**, 1067–71.

▸▸ Hypothermia

An 80-year-old woman was brought to the hospital after being found unresponsive in her home. It was a cold January day, and her apartment reportedly "seemed cold," but the heat in her apartment appeared to be functioning. No medical history is available, but a long-time neighbor mentions that she last saw her 1 week ago, and she appeared confused at the time.

On examination, the patient is moderately obese and does not respond to deep painful stimuli. Her rectal temperature is 90 °F, blood pressure 120/98, pulse 50 and regular, and respiratory rate 8 per minute. Her skin has an orange tint. Neck examination reveals bilateral carotid bruits but the thyroid gland is not palpable and there are no masses. Her heart sounds are distant, rales are heard on lung examination at the left base, and bowel sounds are absent. The relaxation phase of the biceps reflex is delayed. There is bilateral peripheral edema.

In the emergency room, abnormal laboratory findings included serum sodium 128 mg/dl, hematocrit 29.4%, with normochromic, normocytic indices, and creatine kinase 480 U/l ($n = 50$–250). On arterial blood gas determination, pH is 7.30, pCO_2 55 mm Hg, and pO_2 80 mm Hg.

Electrocardiogram reveals sinus bradycardia at a rate of 48 beats per minute, with low voltage. Chest X-ray shows cardiomegaly and haziness at the left base, suggesting infiltrate or effusion. Abdominal X-ray shows a bowel gas pattern consistent with ileus.

Questions

1. What is the differential diagnosis?
2. What could have led to this patient's severe condition?

Case Studies in Geriatric Medicine, Judith C. Ahronheim *et al*. Published by Cambridge University Press.
© J. C. Ahronheim, Z.-B. Huang, V. Yen, C. M. Davitt, and D. Barile

3. How are the other abnormalities explained?
4. How should she be treated?
5. What age-related factors predispose the elderly to hypothermia?

Answers

1. Hypothermia – defined as core body temperature less than 35 °C – can be due to decreased heat production, increased heat loss, or impaired neuroregulation of body temperature. Important causes of decreased heat production in the elderly include abnormal metabolic states, especially hypothyroidism, hypoadrenalism, hypoglycemia, and malnutrition. Increased heat loss can occur as a result of exposure to a cold environment ("accidental hypothermia") or in burns. Impaired neuroregulation of body temperature can be seen in Parkinson's disease, stroke, autonomic neuropathy, brain neoplasm, and certain other neurologic impairments, especially if the thermal centers of the anterior preoptic as well as posterior hypothalmus are involved. These can impair autonomic and endocrine mechanisms of heat conservation, as well as behavioral responses, such as seeking a warmer environment. Hypothermia can also occur in sepsis, uremia, and pancreatitis.

   In the winter time, the most common cause of hypothermia in a home-bound elderly person would be exposure to a cold environment, but there is evidence from this patient's examination of another etiology. The necklace scar, as seen in Figure 16, suggests a history of thyroid surgery, and other findings on the examination suggest hypothyroidism, including absent bowel sounds, abnormal reflexes, and abnormal skin complexion. Other findings, such as bradycardia and edema, although nonspecific in an 80-year-old, are consistent with this diagnosis. Her low core body temperature, respiratory depression, and coma could be explained by hypothyroidism alone – notably, myxedema coma, a state of extreme, decompensated hypothyroidism, induced by a precipitating event. Bradycardia in the setting of hypothyroidism also supports the diagnosis of hypothyroidism. Tachycardia in this setting would raise the suspicion of hypoglycemia, hypovolemia, or a medication known to interfere with central thermoregulation.

   The patient was treated for myxedema coma. Subsequently, laboratory results revealed thyroid-stimulating hormone (TSH) of 69 mU/l ($n = 0.4$–5.50) with a free thyroxine level of 0.2 ng/dl ($n = 0.7$–1.8).

2. Thyroxine maintains metabolic rate by increasing the activity of sodium–potassium ATPase. In hypothyroidism, basal metabolic rate (BMR) can be reduced by 50%, increasing the risk of hypothermia. Myxedema coma may occur if a serious stressor

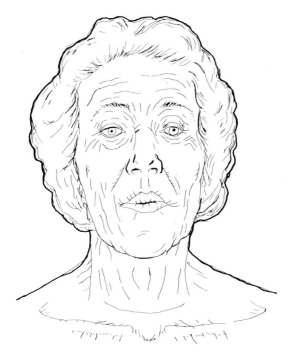

Figure 16   The patient had a transverse ("necklace") scar on her neck indicating prior thyroid surgery.

is superimposed on inadequately treated hypothyroidism. Important precipitants of myxedema coma include stroke, pulmonary embolism, myocardial infarction, or, as in this case, exposure to a cold environment. Medications, including sedatives, hypoglycemic agents, clonidine, digoxin, phenothiazines, opioids, and alcohol, can predispose to hypothermia, by interfering with central thermoregulation. It would be important for someone to look carefully in the patient's apartment for medications.

Another factor in this patient might have been failure to recognize symptoms of hypothyroidism earlier in its clinical course. Hypothyroidism increases in incidence with age, but "typical" signs and symptoms, such as constipation, brittle hair, and dry skin, are nonspecific, and bradycardia, fatigue, and other symptoms may be attributed to nonthyroid illness common in late life.

3. This patient has a number of physical and laboratory abnormalities that exist in severe hypothyroidism and that are reversible with treatment. The orange tint reflects decreased metabolism of carotene, with deposition in the skin. Her necklace scar suggests that her hypothyroidism may be the result of thyroidectomy (rather than Hashimoto's autoimmune thyroiditis, which is the most common cause in the elderly). The surgery could have been performed for cancer or nodular disease of the gland, or possibly for hyperthyroidism.

The distant heart sounds, as well as the low voltage on electrocardiogram, may reflect pericardial effusion, which is seen in 25% of myxedematous patients. Hyponatremia reflects the requirement of thyroid hormone for adequate delivery of solute to the distal nephron (diluting segments) in the process of free water generation and clearance. The patient's respiratory acidosis and low respiratory rate reflect central hypoventilation, although, in her case, pneumonia may be a cofactor. A pleural effusion (with or without pneumonia) would not be surprising; like pericardial effusion, pleural effusion can occur due to membrane permeability.

4. The diagnosis must be made on clinical grounds and treatment initiated without delay. Initially, thyroxine 200–300 μg is given intravenously, to fill thyroid-binding globulin sites, and thereafter 50–100 μg of thyroxine is given daily intravenously until the patient is able to take hormone by mouth. The use of the active form of thyroid hormone, triiodothyronine (T3), has not been shown to have clear-cut benefit over thyroxine (T4) in myxedema coma.

In addition to thyroid hormone, 100 mg hydrocortisone should be given initially for possible adrenal insufficiency, which may occur in some patients with hypothalamic or pituitary hypothyroidism. Although hypothermia in this case could be fully explained by decompensated primary hypothyroidism, it could also be explained by hypopituitarism. Adrenal insufficiency also sometimes occurs in patients with primary hypothyroidism, which sometimes coexists with other autoimmune diseases such as Addison's disease; in such cases, borderline hypoadrenalism can be unmasked when the enhanced metabolic state induced by thyroid hormone administration increases the clearance of cortisol.

Supportive treatment includes mechanical ventilation if necessary, passive rewarming with blankets, or active rewarming by direct application of heat externally via a heating blanket, or, internally, via warmed enteral fluids or heated intravenous fluids. Active external rewarming techniques should be applied with extreme caution in geriatric patients, who are at risk of cardiovascular collapse if vasodilation is extreme. In addition, comorbidities, such as infection, should be treated. Hyponatremia generally should be corrected at the rate that it developed, but if this is unclear, generally no more than a 1 mEq/h correction should be undertaken, because of a risk of central pontine demyelination syndromes sometimes seen after a too rapid, uncontrolled correction.

In less urgent situations, replacement of thyroxine in elderly patients at risk for cardiac disease is generally initiated at a low dose and titrated upward at 6–8-week intervals, because of concern that thyroid hormone could exacerbate angina or cause myocardial infarction by increasing chronotropy and inotropy. In fact, such events are rare and angina generally improves, presumably because thyroid hormone improves the efficiency of myocardial oxygen consumption and decreases systemic vascular resistance. T3 is known to have a direct vasodilatory effect on vascular smooth muscle cells – it binds to nuclear receptors in the cardiac myocyte and initiates transcription of structural and regulatory proteins in the heart. Finally, although hyperthyroidism predisposes to atrial arrhythmias, hypothyroidism predisposes to ventricular arrhythmia, related to prolonged Q-T interval.

5. Normally, body temperature is precisely regulated via interactions between peripheral cold receptors in the skin (which greatly outnumber heat receptors), the thermoregulatory centers in the hypothalmus, various neuroendocrine and metabolic reactions, and, ultimately, the effector organs in the cardiovascular, neuromuscular, and respiratory systems. Elderly patients often have functional alterations and loss of reserve and adaptability in most of these areas; as such, body temperature can be easily affected by ambient temperature and patients are more susceptible to increases and decreases in temperature. The risk is further elevated if the patient also has a decreased sensation of cold and lowered ability or perceived need to perform adaptive behavior – such as seek a warmer environment. Finally, heat generation may be impaired. Physical activity and shivering can increase heat production 5-fold, but basal and activity-generated thermogenesis is significantly lower with aging. Basal metabolic rate (BMR) declines from approximately 37 kcal/m^2/h at age 30 years to 33 kcal/m^2/h by age 80, and there is also a decrease in muscle mass with aging, and a decreased BMR response to sympathomimetic amines. In addition, levels of growth hormone and insulin-like growth factor-1 appear to decline with age; these substances are associated with decreased muscle mass and alterations in counterregulatory glucose production, both of which can contribute to hypothermia.

Caveats

1. Thyroid function tests performed on patients with acute nonthyroidal illness are often abnormal. This "euthyroid sick" syndrome is confirmed when thyroid function tests normalize after the patient has recovered. This subject is reviewed in the references (see Chopra, 1997).

2. Because of the nonspecific presentation of thyroid disease in the elderly, all elderly persons should be screened for "asymptomatic" disease using the sensitive TSH test with confirmatory free thyroxine if the TSH is abnormal. Although clinical benefits of treating such patients are uncertain, and parameters for treatment are controversial, patients like the present one might have avoided serious illness if screening and careful follow up had been performed.

REFERENCE

Chopra, I. J. (1997). Euthyroid sick syndrome: is it a misnomer? *Journal of Clinical Endocrinology and Metabolism*, **82**, 329–34.

BIBLIOGRAPHY

Attia, J., Margetts, P., and Guyatt, G. (1999). Diagnosis of thyroid disease in hospitalized patients: a systematic review. *Archives of Internal Medicine*, **159**, 658–65.

Diekman, T, Lansberg, P. J., Kastelein, J. J. *et al.* (1995). Prevalence and correction of hypothyroidism in a large cohort of patients referred for dyslipidemia. *Archives of Internal Medicine*, **155**, 1490–5.

Hak, A. E., Pols, H. A., Visser, T. J. *et al.* (2000). Subclinical hypothyroidism is an independent risk factor for atherosclerosis and myocardial infarction in elderly women: the Rotterdam study. *Annals of Internal Medicine*, **132**, 270–8.

Harchelroad, F. (1993). Acute thermoregulatory disorders. *Clinics in Geriatric Medicine*, **9**, 621–39.

Helfand, M., Redfern, C. C., Sox, H. C., and the Clinical Efficacy Assessment Subcommittee, American College of Physicians (1998). Position paper: screening for Thyroid Disease. *Annals of Internal Medicine*, **129**, 141–3.

Hollowell, J. G., Staehling, N. W., Flanders, W. D. *et al.* (2002). Serum TSH, T(4), and thyroid antibodies in the United States population (1988 to 1994): National Health and Nutrition Examination Survey (NHANES III). *Journal of Clinical Endocrinology and Metabolism*, **87**, 489–99.

Jaeschke, R., Guyatt, G., Gerstein, H. *et al.* (1996). Does treatment with L-thyroxine influence health status in middle aged and older adults with subclinical hypothyroidism? *Journal of General Internal Medicine*, **11**, 744–9.

Klein, I. and Ojamaa, K. (2001). Thyroid hormone and the cardiovascular system. *New England Journal of Medicine*, **344**, 501–9.

Larson, E. B., Reifler, B. V., Sumi, S. M. *et al.* (1986). Diagnostic tests in the evaluation of dementia: a prospective study of 200 elderly outpatients. *Archives of Internal Medicine*, **146**, 1917–22.

Mokshagundam, S. P. and Barzel, U. S. (1993). Thyroid disease in the elderly. *Journal of the American Geriatrics Society*, **41**, 1361–9.

Sawin, C. T., Geller, A., Hershman, J. M. *et al.* (1989). The aging thyroid. The use of thyroid hormones in older persons. *Journal of the American Medical Association*, **261**, 2653–5.

Umpierrez, G. E. (2002). Euthyroid sick syndrome. *Southern Medical Journal*, **95**, 506–13.

U.S. Preventive Services Task Force (2004). Clinical Guidelines: screening for thyroid disease. Recommendation statement. *Annals of Internal Medicine*, **140**, 125–7.

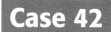

Case 42

▸▸ Hyperthermia

The daughter of an 83-year-old female patient calls you one July afternoon stating that she has not heard from her mother in 3 days and that she is not answering phone calls. She is concerned because there is a heat wave in town and she knows her mother does not have air conditioning. The patient has congestive heart failure and Parkinson's disease with moderate dementia and hallucinations. She is being treated with furosemide, levodopa/carbidopa, and enalapril. A small dose of olanzapine was recently started.

Emergency medical personnel and the building superintendent enter the apartment and find the patient in her bed, unresponsive. Her rectal temperature is 105 °F. Her pulse is 100, respiratory rate is 28, and blood pressure is 80/50. She has a very dry mouth and axillae. She has mild cogwheel rigidity. Her skin is hot and dry. Laboratory results reveal white blood cell count 30 000/mm^3, blood urea nutroten 70 mg/dl, and serum creatinine 6.9 mg/dl. Liver function tests, including prothrombin time and partial thromboplastin time, are elevated. Creatine kinase (CK) measures 8000 U/l ($n = 50-250$). Thyroid function test results are pending.

Questions

1. What could be causing her elevated temperature?
2. What age-related changes affect thermoregulation and predispose the elderly to heat stroke and its consequences?
3. How should she be treated?
4. How can heat stroke be prevented in the elderly?

Case Studies in Geriatric Medicine, Judith C. Ahronheim *et al.* Published by Cambridge University Press.
© J. C. Ahronheim, Z.-B. Huang, V. Yen, C. M. Davitt, and D. Barile

Answers

1. The differential diagnosis of fever is broad, and includes infection, drug reactions, hyperthyroidism, malignancy, and others. However, extreme elevation of temperature often indicates some state of thermal dysregulation, with imbalance between heat production and heat loss. Hyperthermia has generally been defined as temperature greater than 40 °C (104 °F), although patients can develop heat-related syndromes – including malignant hyperthermia – at lower temperatures.

    This patient had "heat stroke," a clinical syndrome consisting of central nervous system (CNS) symptoms, such as delirium, seizures, or coma, accompanying an acute failure to maintain normal body temperature. "Classic" heat stroke occurs in the setting of exposure to high environmental temperatures, and generally affects the very young or the very old, or those with underlying conditions that impair thermoregulation, such as cardiovascular, psychiatric, neurologic, or metabolic disease, or those using anticholinergic, diuretic, or certain other drugs. In contrast, exertional heat stroke is related to strenuous exercise during periods of high ambient temperature and humidity, and thus generally occurs in younger adults, such as army recruits or athletes. Although encephalopathy is a defining feature, heat stroke is actually a syndrome of multiorgan failure in which CNS symptoms predominate. The syndrome, with a mortality as high as 50%, has been attributed to a systemic inflammatory response to heat involving the endothelial cells, inflammatory mediators of the immune system such as IL (interleukin)-1, TNF (tumor necrosis factor)-alpha, IFN (interferon)-gamma, and the coagulation system in a cascade of interactions that is similar to exposure to endotoxin, as in septic states. The mechanism is reviewed in detail in the references (see Bouchama and Knochel, 2002).

    In milder forms of heat illness – such as heat exhaustion – thermoregulation is maintained, the systemic inflammatory response does not occur, and CNS and other organ functions are maintained. As such, these milder varieties improve upon lowering of the core temperature.

    Although elevated ambient temperature is a likely precipitant in this patient, other conditions, such as sepsis or thyroid storm, should be considered, as these can present with fever, tachycardia, and mental status changes. Diaphoresis is typically present in the hyperthyroid state and in fevers related to infection, but elderly hyperthyroid patients typically have far fewer clinical findings of hyperthyroidism than younger patients (see Case 40), and thyroid storm is rare at any age. In her case, thyroid-stimulating hormone (TSH) was 0.4 mU/l ($n = 0.4–5.50$) and free T4 was 0.6 ng/dl ($n = 0.7–1.8$). TSH in the low range, with a slightly low free T4, was consistent with "euthyroid sick syndrome" (see Case 41).

The recent addition of the "atypical" neuroleptic olanzapine to the patient's drug regimen raises the possibility of "neuroleptic malignant syndrome" (NMS), or "drug-induced central hyperthermic" syndrome, an idiosyncratic reaction to certain medications characterized by muscle rigidity, hyperthermia, autonomic instability, and altered mental status. The hyperthermia mainly arises from heat generated by excess muscular activity, which presents as rigidity, and CK levels are often highly elevated. NMS is not related to drug dosage or duration, although the majority of cases occur within the first 30 days (usually the first 3–9 days) of using the drug, and intramuscular injection of higher potency neuroleptics seems to impose a higher risk.

Virtually any drug that blocks dopamine receptors or inhibits dopamine release has been implicated, including neuroleptics, lithium, metoclopramide, and others, although it is difficult to delineate the precise contribution of pharmacologic and other contributing factors in individual cases that comprise the literature (e.g. see Assion *et al.*, 1998). Acute alterations and reduction in central dopaminergic (primarily D2) activity – including sudden withdrawal of Parkinson's medications or rapid increases in neuroleptic medication – may cause the syndrome. While epidemiologic data seem to imply an increased incidence of NMS in the setting of high ambient temperatures, this hypothesis has not been substantiated. However, this elderly patient's use of dopaminergic medications, with their effects on autonomic function, could have predisposed her to ambient heat-associated hyperthermia (see below).

2. The elderly are more prone to heat stroke because of impaired homeostatic mechanisms directed toward heat dissipation. Approximately one-third of deaths related to heat exposure are among people over 75 years old. People who are poor or socially isolated are also at elevated risk, possibly in part because of a lack of access to air conditioning.

Normally, four main mechanisms are employed to dissipate body heat when the core temperature rises: vasodilatation, sweating, decreased heat production, and adaptive behavior. The physiologic processes are integrated by the thermoregulatory center in the preoptic nucleus of the anterior hypothalmus, where the neuroendocrine and metabolic responses to temperature input from skin receptors, abdominal viscera, great vessels, and spinal cord are orchestrated. As such, CNS pathology, especially involving these areas, could predispose to disruptions in thermal stability. Normally, radiative heat loss from peripheral vasodilatation and evaporative heat loss from sweating account for most of the heat loss in normal thermoregulation. Vasodilatation occurs via inhibition of the sympathetic centers in the hypothalmus that cause vasoconstriction. Large increases in cardiac output are required to bring about the blood flow needed to shunt blood from the central circulation (the intestines and kidneys) to the periphery (the muscles and skin) in order to facilitate heat dissipation. Skin blood flow has been estimated to increase by up to 300%. In the elderly, shunting of blood to the periphery may lead to relative hypoperfusion of the mesentery and, if splanchnic blood flow is already compromised, intestinal hyperpermeability and ischemia may occur, resulting in the release of endothelial cell cytokines and vasoactive factors, which serve as the source of the systemic inflammatory response in heat stroke. When ambient temperature exceeds body temperature, sweating remains the principal heat-dissipating mechanism. Sweating itself removes heat from the body, with an estimated 1 kcal of heat removed per 1.7 ml sweat, but the maximum sweat rate in the elderly is reduced by an estimated 50%. In addition, the thresholds of temperature or environmental conditions at which sweating is initiated seem to be higher in later life, under experimental and pharmacologic conditions (see Brody, 1994).

Perception of temperature and thirst are also altered in late life, and elderly individuals often fail, or are unable, to perform adaptive behaviors in response to heat, such as wearing appropriate clothing, going out of doors, seeking air conditioning, or obtaining cold fluids. Medications may exacerbate these problems: anticholinergics or neuroleptics may lead to further hypohidrosis, diuretics to hypovolemia, and beta-blockers to a fixed cardiac output.

3. Treatment is generally directed toward reducing core temperature and supporting organ systems. Unfortunately, normalization of body temperature may not be enough to prevent the inflammatory response and progression to multiorgan failure in heat stroke.

Placing the patient in an air-conditioned environment, spraying cold water or applying ice to the skin, and fanning should act to transfer heat from the core to the environment. However, such direct methods of lowering skin temperature produce vasoconstriction and shivering, which would tend to counteract cooling efforts somewhat. Thus, it is theoretically preferable to use tepid water rather than ice water for external cooling, but no controlled studies have compared different temperatures or methods of cooling, such as gastric or peritoneal lavage with cool water. Likewise, the role of antipyretics has not been adequately evaluated in heat stroke.

Supportive treatment often requires mechanical ventilation and the management of other derangements that result from hyperthermic stress, such as cardiac decompensation, seizures, and hepatic and renal failure.

Public health measures and education should be used to prevent heat-related death in the elderly – e.g. encouraging the use of air-conditioned public places such as shopping malls, senior centers, or libraries during times of severe heat.

Caveats

1. Although NMS has been reported in elderly patients, it has most often been reported in patients younger than age 65, and mostly in males. However, the prevalence and epidemiology depend greatly on the diagnostic criteria used, and it may well be under-recognized in the elderly.
2. NMS should not be confused with the serotonin syndrome, a toxic reaction to medications that stimulate serotonin receptors, such as selective serotonin reuptake inhibitors, meperidine, monoamine oxidase inhibitors, and others. The serotonin syndrome is characterized by agitation, diarrhea, myoclonus, and, unlike NMS, usually has an abrupt onset following ingestion of the responsible medications. Hyperthermia, rigidity, and marked elevations of CK levels are unusual.

REFERENCES

Assion, H. J., Heinemann, F., and Laux, G. (1998). Neuroleptic malignant syndrome under treatment with antidepressants? A critical review. *European Archives of Psychiatry and Clinical Neuroscience*, **348**, 231–9.

Bouchama, A. and Knochel, J. P. (2002). Heat stroke. *New England Journal of Medicine*, **346**, 1978–88.

Brody, G. M. (1994). Hyperthermia and hypothermia in the elderly. *Clinics in Geriatric Medicine*, **10**, 213–29.

BIBLIOGRAPHY

Addonizio, G. (1987). Neuroleptic malignant syndrome in elderly patients. *Journal of the American Geriatrics Society*, **35**, 1011–12.

Adityanjee, Aderibigbe, Y. A., and Mathews, T. (1999). Epidemiology of neuroleptic malignant syndrome. *Clinical Neuropharmacology*, **22**, 151–8.

Birmes, P., Coppin, D., Schmitt, L. *et al.* (2003). Serotonin syndrome: a brief review. *Canadian Medical Association Journal*, **168**, 1439–42.

Centers for Disease Control and Prevention (2002). Heat related deaths – four states, July–August 2001, and United States, 1979–1999. *Morbidity and Mortality Weekly Report*, **51**, 567–70.

Harchelroad, F. (1993). Acute thermoregulatory disorders. *Clinics in Geriatric Medicine*, **9**, 621–37.

Wongsurawat, N., Davis, B. B., and Morley, J. E. (1990). Thermoregulatory failure in the elderly. *Journal of the American Geriatrics Society*, **38**, 899–906.

▸▸ A centenarian

A 102-year-old African American woman comes to the emergency room of a large teaching hospital because of weakness. She is found to have atrial fibrillation with a ventricular rate of 38 beats per minute. She admits to mild lightheadedness but no loss of consciousness or falls.

On physical examination, she is alert, oriented, and in no acute distress. Blood pressure is 158/70. In the left breast, there is a movable, rock-hard mass measuring 5 × 5 cm in diameter. There is no ulceration or erythema. She has no hepatomegaly or jaundice, and there are no palpable lymph nodes on examination. Neurologic examination is normal.

Her clinic chart is retrieved and reviewed. At age 93, she developed a mass in her right breast but was thought to be too old for surgery. Two years later, her presumed breast cancer was treated with hormones and radiation therapy. At age 97, she developed a lump in her left breast. Aspiration biopsy revealed "carcinoma, small cell type," but she and her physicians felt that she was too old for treatment. She did well and continued to visit the clinic, where she was treated for chronic atrial fibrillation with digoxin. Digoxin had recently been discontinued because of occasional pulse rates under 60.

She thinks it is quite remarkable that she has lived so long, she says, smiling slightly and sighing. The patient is a widow, who lives alone and cares for herself. She is active in her church and has a lot of friends. Her picture was recently in the newspaper on the occasion of her 102nd birthday.

Cardiology consult is called. The consultant is reluctant to insert a pacemaker "because of the patient's age and advanced cancer." She is admitted to the hospital's intermediate care unit for observation.

Case Studies in Geriatric Medicine, Judith C. Ahronheim *et al.* Published by Cambridge University Press.
© J. C. Ahronheim, Z.-B. Huang, V. Yen, C. M. Davitt, and D. Barile

Questions

1. Is this patient too old for pacemaker placement?
2. How should decisions about invasive treatments be made very late in life?
3. Are breast cancers in older women less aggressive than in younger women?
4. How does the life expectancy of an African American woman differ from her white counterpart?

Answers

1. Symptomatic bradycardia with atrial fibrillation is clearly an indication for pacemaker placement, and is consistent with American College of Cardiology/American Heart Association practice guidelines (see Gregoratos, 2002). If a patient meets criteria for pacemaker placement, age alone should not be an obstacle to obtaining this treatment. In general, if the patient's life expectancy is considered "reasonable" by doctor and patient standards, then pacemaker insertion may be appropriate at any age. The average life expectancy for a 100-year-old black female is 2.7 years (no data exist for 102-year-olds). Given this women's comorbid conditions, her life expectancy may be considerably less.

   Whether to insert a pacemaker in a 102-year-old patient depends not on outcomes data, which are lacking for that age group, but on other factors, such as projected life span and expected impact on quality of life. One randomized controlled comparison of ventricular pacing and dual chamber pacing in subjects 65 years of age and older showed that quality of life improved significantly after pacemaker insertion (see Lamas *et al.*, 1998). However, the average age of study subjects was 76 (range 65–96), almost 30 years younger than the patient in question, making it difficult to extrapolate such findings to this unusual situation. Since her anticipated life expectancy without cancer is short, attention should be focused on her interests regarding goals of care.

2. As in the case of the pacemaker decision discussed above, all treatment decisions for very old individuals should be based on the anticipated life expectancy and the patient's goals of care, whether the treatment is uncomplicated medical therapy or major surgery. Because of the paucity of data available on very old patients, treatment decisions need to be carefully individualized.

Limited data available on centenarians appear to support the principle that age alone is a poor predictor of outcome. As discussed in Case 12, very elderly surgical patients may have a similar survival rate and outcome as their peers not undergoing surgery. These and other positive outcomes may be related, not surprisingly, to the observation that centenarians represent an elite group of individuals who have lived healthy lives and undergo a relatively "rapid terminal decline" (see Hitt *et al.*, 1999).

3. The biologic nature of this patient's breast cancer seems to be quite indolent, and, despite the local tumor growth, it has not interfered with her function or quality of life. Like many elderly cancer patients, she has developed cardiac disease which is more likely than the cancer to threaten her life and her quality of life. Although breast cancer after menopause tends to be less aggressive than in young women, the biologic nature of a particular cancer cannot be predicted at the time of diagnosis, with some very old women having aggressive cancers. There has been an overall increase in the incidence in cancer in recent years, even among the oldest old. However, autopsy studies continue to show an increased incidence, with age, of malignant tumors undetected during life. These tumors tend to be nonmetastatic and are infrequently the cause of death. It is not certain if this is due to indolent tumor growth, or because of the greater likelihood of death from other causes very late in life.

It is important to recognize that data about cancers in the elderly may be difficult to interpret. Whereas autopsy data suggest an increased incidence of indolent tumors, survival data show overall higher cancer mortality rates in late life. Older patients with metastatic cancer may have been diagnosed late, and this may reflect obstacles to diagnosis or treatment rather than tumor biology. Such obstacles include patient or physician biases about screening or treating older individuals, or failure to report or note symptoms. Observed decreased survival time could be related to a direct impact of comorbid illnesses, or to the impact of comorbidity on host vulnerability, rather than the biologic nature of the cancer itself. For example, expression of genes that promote resistance to chemotherapeutic agents is much more common in older adults with acute myelocytic anemia, although subgroups of older patients respond well, and comorbidity also plays a role in poor prognosis.

Biologic explanations for indolent tumors include intrinsic factors of the tumor itself, T-cell immunosenescence, and decreased response to angiogenic stimuli and other tumor growth factors. Tumor growth requires immunologic help, and tumor-enhancing mechanisms involving T lymphocytes are less active with age. Indolent breast cancer in late life has been explained by both of these mechanisms, with the important caveat that some women have breast cancers with a very aggressive course (see Balducci and Extermann, 2000). In general, immunosenescence theoretically should favor the growth of highly immunogenic tumors, and this has been demonstrated in some animal studies.

Table 1 Life expectancy (years) in United States, 2001.

	At birth	At age 75	At age 85	At age 100
All Americans	*77.2*	*11.5*	*6.5*	*2.7*
White men	75.0	10.2	5.6	2.3
Black men	68.6	9.3	5.7	2.9
White women	80.2	12.3	6.7	2.5
Black women	75.5	11.7	7.0	3.0

Data from National Center for Health Statistics (2004).

Some tumors tend to be more aggressive in late life. Late-life thyroid carcinoma is usually of the aggressive anaplastic type. Acute leukemia may be more aggressive in late life and nodular melanoma is aggressive at any age. The complex aspects of biology of cancer and aging is reviewed in detail in the references (see Ershler and Longo, 1997; Balducci and Extermann, 2000).

4. As of 2001, life expectancy at birth of a black American female was 75.5 years as compared with 80.2 years for a white American female (figures for males are 68.6 and 75.0 years, respectively). The racial gap narrows progressively, so, by age 81, a black woman's life expectancy is equal to a white woman's (8.7 years for both), and, by age 84, black and white men have the same life expectancy (6.0 years). The average life expectancy at age 100 is approximately 2.7 years for Americans overall, but, at this age, African Americans have a slight edge (see Table 1). Data on life expectancy among other races and ethnic groups in the United States are limited.

Life expectancy varies widely among the world's nations (see Central Intelligence Agency, 2003).

Caveats

1. Although many people claim to be centenarians, there is not always written verification of their claims. Pockets of very old people have been described in various places in the world, including Ecuador, Soviet Georgia, and west Pakistan, where long-lived individuals have made all sorts of claims as to the reasons for their longevity. However, when documentation was sought, it was not forthcoming or did not exist. It has been concluded that many claims of extreme old age are due to various incentives – old-age pension, veneration, and regional publicity. Because of this, and because of questions regarding validity of centenarian age in the U.S. census, recent population-based studies of centenarians have sought to validate self- or

family report of a centenarian's actual age, and, in at least one study, these methods were generally reliable (see Perls *et al.*, 1999).

2. When interpreting figures of life expectancy, it is important to know whether those figures are for birth, midlife, or late life. Although average life expectancy for American males and females at birth leapt 32 years – from 47 years in 1900 to 77 in 2000 – there was an unimpressive 4-year increase in life expectancy at age 75 during that same time. Thus, Americans making it to age 75 in the year 1900 lived, on average, to age 82, while the average 75-year-old person in 2000 would live until age 86. There does not appear to have been any increase in maximal attainable life span, which is approximately 110 years.

REFERENCES

Balducci, L. and Extermann, M. (2000). Cancer and aging: an evolving panorama. *Hematology/Oncology Clinics of North America*, **14**, 1–16.

Central Intelligence Agency (2003). CIA – The World Factbook. http://www.odci.gov/cia/publications/factbook/rankorder/2102rank.html; accessed February 28, 2005.

Ershler, W. B. and Longo, D. L. (1997). Aging and cancer: issues of basic and clinical science. *Journal of the National Cancer Institute*, **89**, 1489–97.

Gregoratos, G. (2002). ACC/AHA/NASPE 2002 guideline update for implantation of cardiac pacemakers and antiarrhymia devices: summary article. A report of the American College of Cardiology/American Heart Association Task Force on Practice Guidelines. *Circulation*, **106**, 2145–61.

Hitt, R., Young-Xu, Y., Silver, M. *et al.* (1999). Centenarians: the older you get, the healthier you have been. *Lancet*, **354**, 652.

Lamas, G. A., Orav, J. E., and Stambler, B. S. (1998). Quality of life and clinical outcomes in elderly patients treated with ventricular pacing as compared with dual-chamber pacing. *New England Journal of Medicine*, **338**, 1097–104.

National Center for Health Statistics (2004). United States Life Tables, 2001. *National Vital Statistics Reports*, **52**, 7–26. http://www.cdc.gov/nchs/data/nvsr/nvsr52/nvsr52_14.pdf; accessed February 19, 2004.

Perls, T. T., Bochen, K., Freeman, M. *et al.* (1999). Validity of reported age and centenarian prevalence in New England. *Age and Ageing*, **28**, 193–7.

BIBLIOGRAPHY

Adami, H., Malker, B., Holmberg, L. *et al.* (1986). The relation between survival and age at diagnosis in breast cancer. *New England Journal of Medicine*, **315**, 559–63.

Berlin, N. I. (1995). The conquest of cancer. *Cancer Investigations*, **13**, 540–50.

Gregoratos, G. (1999). Permanent pacemakers in older persons. *Journal of the American Geriatric Society*, **47**, 1125–35.

Nybo, H., Petersen, H. C., Gaist, D. *et al.* (2003). Predictors of mortality in 2,249 nonagenarians – the Danish 1905-Cohort Study. *Journal of the American Geriatrics Society*, **51**, 1365–73.

Olshansky, S. J., Carnes, B. A., and Desesquelles, A. (2001). Prospects for human longevity. *Science*, **291**, 1491–2.

Rose, J. H., O'Toole, E. E., and Dawson, N. V. (2000). Age differences in care practices and outcomes for hospitalized patients with cancer. *Journal of the American Geriatric Society*, **48** (5 Suppl), S25–32.

Saltzein, S. L., Behling, C. A., and Baergen, R. N. (1998). Features of cancer in nonagenarians and centenarians. *Journal of the American Geriatric Society*, **46**, 994–8.

Stanta, G., Campagner, L., Cavallieri, F. *et al.* (1997). Cancer of the oldest old. What we have learned from autopsy studies. *Clinics in Geriatric Medicine*, **13**, 55–68.

Stone, R. M. (2002). The difficult problem of acute myeloid leukemia in the older adult. *CA Cancer Journal for Clinicians*, **52**, 363–71.

Suen, K. C., Lau, L. L., and Yermakov, V. (1974). Cancer and old age. An autopsy study of 3535 patients over 65 years old. *Cancer*, **33**, 1164–8.

Warner, M. A., Saletel, R. A., and Schroeder, M. S. (1998). Outcomes of anesthesia and surgery in people 100 years of age and older. *Journal of the American Geriatric Society*, **46**, 988–93.

Wilson, T. M., Crawford, K. L., and Shabot, M. M. (2000). Intensive care unit outcomes of surgical centenarians: the "oldest old" of the new millennium. *American Surgeon*, **66**, 870–3.

Index